Harrison's PRINCIPLES OF INTERNAL MEDICINE

PreTest® Self-Assessment and Review

For use with the 11th edition of
HARRISON'S PRINCIPLES OF INTERNAL MEDICINE

Editors

EUGENE BRAUNWALD, A.B., M.D., M.A. (Hon.), M.D. (Hon.) Hersey Professor of the Theory and Practice of Physic and Herrman Ludwig Blumgart Professor of Medicine, Harvard Medical School; Chairman, Department of Medicine, Brigham and Women's and Beth Israel Hospitals, Boston

KURT J. ISSELBACHER, A.B., M.D. Mallinckrodt Professor of Medicine, Harvard Medical School; Physician and Chief, Gastrointestinal Unit, Massachusetts General Hospital, Boston

ROBERT G. PETERSDORF, A.B., M.D., M.A. (Hon.), D.Sc. (Hon.), M.D. (Hon.), L.H.D. (Hon.) Professor of Medicine, Dean and Vice Chancellor, Health Sciences, University of California School of Medicine, San Diego, La Jolla

JEAN D. WILSON, M.D. Professor of Internal Medicine, The University of Texas Southwestern Medical School, Dallas

JOSEPH B. MARTIN, M.D., Ph.D., F.R.C.P.(C), M.A. (Hon.) Julieanne Dorn Professor of Neurology, Harvard Medical School; Chief, Neurology Service, Massachusetts General Hospital, Boston

ANTHONY S. FAUCI, M.D. Chief, Laboratory of Immunoregulation and Director, National Institute of Allergy and Infectious Diseases, National Institutes of Health, Bethesda

McGRAW-HILL BOOK COMPANY
Health Professions Division
PreTest Series

New York St. Louis San Francisco Auckland Bogotá
Hamburg London Madrid Mexico Milan
Montreal New Delhi Panama Paris San Juan
São Paulo Singapore Sydney Tokyo Toronto

NOTICE

Medicine is an ever-changing science. As new research and clinical experience broaden our knowledge, changes in treatment and drug therapy are required. The editors and the publisher of this work have made every effort to ensure that the drug dosage schedules herein are accurate and in accord with the standards accepted at the time of publication. Readers are advised, however, to check the product information sheet included in the package of each drug they plan to administer to be certain that changes have not been made in the recommended dose or in the contraindications for administration. This recommendation is of particular importance in regard to new or infrequently used drugs.

Harrison's
**PRINCIPLES OF INTERNAL MEDICINE
PreTest® Self-Assessment and Review**

Copyright © 1987 by McGraw-Hill, Inc. All rights reserved. Printed in the United States of America. Except as permitted under the United States Copyright Act of 1976, no part of this publication may be reproduced or distributed in any form or by any means, or stored in a data base or retrieval system, without the prior written permission of the publisher.

23456789   SEMSEM   8943210987

ISBN 0-07-051947-1

This book was set in Times Roman by Monotype Composition Company; the editors were J. Dereck Jeffers and Eileen J. Scott; the consulting editor was Muriel Stangler; the production supervisor was Avé McCracken.

Semline, Inc., was printer and binder.

Library of Congress Cataloging-in-Publication Data

Harrison's principles of internal medicine : PreTest
  self-assessment and review.

  "For use with the 11th edition of Harrison's
principles of internal medicine."
    Bibliography: p.
    1. Internal medicine—Examinations, questions, etc.
I. Harrison, Tinsley Randolph, Date.
II. Braunwald, Eugene, Date. III. Principles
of internal medicine. [DNLM: 1. Internal Medicine—
examination questions. WB 18 H322]
RC58.H37   1987   616.0076   86-21380
ISBN 0-07-051947-1

CONTENTS

List of Contributors — v

Introduction — vii

Infectious Diseases
    Questions 1–127 — 1
    Answers, Explanations, and References — 17

Disorders of the Heart and Vascular System
    Questions 128–226 — 35
    Answers, Explanations, and References — 50

Disorders of the Respiratory System
    Questions 227–268 — 63
    Answers, Explanations, and References — 70

Disorders of the Kidney and Urinary Tract
    Questions 269–312 — 79
    Answers, Explanations, and References — 89

Disorders of the Alimentary Tract and Hepatobiliary System
    Questions 313–408 — 97
    Answers, Explanations, and References — 116

Immunologic, Allergic, and Rheumatic Disorders
    Questions 409–482 — 131
    Answers, Explanations, and References — 141

Disorders of the Hematopoietic System
    Questions 483–526 — 155
    Answers, Explanations, and References — 162

Neoplasia
    Questions 527–570 — 171
    Answers, Explanations, and References — 179

Endocrine, Metabolic, and Genetic Disorders
    Questions 571–696 — 187
    Answers, Explanations, and References — 206

Dermatologic Disorders
    Questions 697–719 — 231
    Answers, Explanations, and References — 237

Disorders of the Nervous System and Muscles
    Questions 720–835 — 243
    Answers, Explanations, and References — 255

Bibliography — 267

Appendix
    Laboratory Values of Clinical Importance — A-1

Color Plates

LIST OF CONTRIBUTORS

Kenneth Bauer, M.D.
Assistant Professor of Medicine
Harvard Medical School
Associate Physician
Beth Israel Hospital
Boston, Massachusetts

Barbara Clark, M.D.
Clinical and Research Fellow in Medicine
Harvard Medical School
Beth Israel Hospital
Boston, Massachusetts

Placido B. Grino, M.D.
Postdoctoral Research Fellow
Department of Internal Medicine
University of Texas Health Science Center
Dallas, Texas

Walter Koroshetz, M.D.
Research Fellow in Neurology
Massachusetts General Hospital
Boston, Massachusetts

Leonard S. Lilly, M.D.
Assistant Professor of Medicine
Harvard Medical School
Associate Physician
Brigham and Women's Hospital
Boston, Massachusetts

Norman Nishioka, M.D.
Research Fellow in Medicine
Harvard Medical School
Clinical and Research Fellow in Medicine
Massachusetts General Hospital
Boston, Massachusetts

Sharon Reed, M.D.
Assistant Professor
Division of Infectious Diseases
University of California, San Diego
La Jolla, California

Allan Ropper, M.D.
Associate Professor of Neurology
Harvard Medical School
Director, Neurological/Neurosurgical Intensive Care Unit
Massachusetts General Hospital
Boston, Massachusetts

Marc Schieber, M.D.
Assistant Professor
Department of Anatomy and Neurobiology
Washington University School of Medicine
St. Louis, Missouri

Arthur J. Sober, M.D.
Associate Professor of Dermatology
Harvard Medical School
Head, Pigmented Lesion Clinic
Massachusetts General Hospital
Boston, Massachusetts

J. Woodrow Weiss, M.D.
Assistant Professor of Medicine
Harvard Medical School
Associate Physician
Beth Israel Hospital
Boston, Massachusetts

K. Randall Young, M.D.
National Institutes of Health
Bethesda, Maryland

INTRODUCTION

Harrison's Principles of Internal Medicine: PreTest Self-Assessment and Review has been designed to provide physicians with a comprehensive, relevant, and convenient instrument for self-evaluation and review within the broad area of internal medicine. Although it should be particularly helpful for residents preparing for the American Board of Internal Medicine (ABIM) certification examination and for board-certified internists preparing for recertification, it should also be useful for internists, family practitioners, and other practicing physicians who are simply interested in maintaining a high level of competence in internal medicine. Study of this self-assessment and review book should help to (1) identify areas of relative weakness; (2) confirm areas of expertise; (3) assess knowledge of the sciences fundamental to internal medicine; (4) assess clinical judgment and problem-solving skills; and (5) introduce recent developments in general internal medicine.

This book consists of more than 800 multiple-choice questions that (1) are representative of the major areas covered in *Harrison's Principles of Internal Medicine,* ed. 11, and (2) parallel the format and degree of difficulty of the questions on the examination of the American Board of Internal Medicine. Each question is accompanied by an answer, a paragraph-length explanation, and a reference to a specific chapter in *Harrison's,* as well as in some cases references to more specialized textbooks and current journal articles. A list of normal values used in the laboratory studies in this book can be found in the Appendix, following a Bibliography listing all the sources used for the questions. All color plates referred to in the text are found in the back of the book. All this material was prepared by physicians representing the major subspecialities in internal medicine under the supervision of *Harrison's* editors—Eugene Braunwald, M.D., Kurt J. Isselbacher, M.D., Robert G. Petersdorf, M.D., Joseph B. Martin, M.D., Jean D. Wilson, M.D., and Anthony S. Fauci, M.D.

We have assumed that the time available to the reader is limited; as a result, this book can be used profitably a chapter at a time. By allowing no more than two and a half minutes to answer each question, you can simulate the time constraints of the actual board exams. When you finish answering all the questions in a chapter, spend as much time as necessary verifying answers and carefully reading the accompanying explanations. If after reading the explanations for a given chapter, you feel a need for a more extensive and definitive discussion, consult the chapter in *Harrison's* or any of the other references listed.

Based on our testing experience, on most medical examinations, examinees who answer half the questions correctly would score around the 50th or 60th percentile. A score of 65 percent would place the examinee above the 80th percentile, whereas a score of 30 percent would rank him or her below the 15th percentile. In other words, if you answer fewer than 30 percent of the questions in a chapter correctly, you are relatively weak in that area. A score of 50 percent would be approximately average, and 70 percent or higher would probably be honors.

We have used three basic question types in accordance with the format of the ABIM certification and recertification exams. Considerable editorial time has been spent trying to ensure that each question is clearly stated and discriminates between those physicians who are well prepared in the subject and those who are less knowledgeable.

This book is a teaching device that provides readers with the opportunity to evaluate and update their clinical expertise, their ability to interpret data, and their ability to diagnose and solve clinical problems.

INFECTIOUS DISEASES

DIRECTIONS: Each question below contains five suggested answers. Choose the **one best** response to each question.

1. Which of the following organisms would be LEAST likely to be recovered from a bone marrow culture?

(A) *Salmonella*
(B) *Mycobacterium*
(C) *Histoplasma*
(D) *Streptococcus*
(E) *Staphylococcus*

2. Which of the following organisms would be LEAST likely to cause infection in a patient with acquired immunodeficiency syndrome (AIDS)?

(A) Cytomegalovirus
(B) *Cryptococcus neoformans*
(C) *Pneumocystis carinii*
(D) *Pseudomonas aeruginosa*
(E) *Mycobacterium avium intracellulare*

3. A patient is examined for presumed septic arthritis. Joint fluid is aspirated, but the sample inadvertently is left at the bedside for several hours. Culturing which of the following organisms would be most affected by the delay in delivery of the specimen to the laboratory?

(A) *Neisseria gonorrhoeae*
(B) *Staphylococcus aureus*
(C) *Streptococcus pyogenes*
(D) *Haemophilus influenzae*
(E) *Salmonella choleraesuis*

4. A 23-year-old graduate student complains of burning on urination and a vaginal discharge. On physical examination, a bilateral groin rash, generalized vaginal erythema, and a whitish vaginal discharge are observed; the remainder of the physical examination is negative. The laboratory test most likely to detect a specific host-defense defect causing this clinical problem would be

(A) blood glucose concentration
(B) blood urea nitrogen concentration
(C) serum immunoglobulin A concentration
(D) serum immunoglobulin E concentration
(E) serum complement concentration

5. The most common source for bacterial infection of intravenous cannulas is

(A) contamination of fluids during the manufacturing process
(B) contamination of fluids during cannula insertion
(C) contamination at the site of entry through the skin
(D) contamination during injection of medications
(E) seeding from remote sites due to intermittent bacteremia

6. A 73-year-old previously healthy man is hospitalized because of the acute onset of dysuria, urinary frequency, fever, and shaking chills. His temperature is 39.5°C (103.1°F), blood pressure is 100/60 mmHg, pulse is 140/min, and respiratory rate is 30/min. Which of the following interventions would be the most important in the treatment of this acute illness?

(A) Catheterization of the urinary bladder
(B) Initiation of antibiotic therapy
(C) Infusion of Ringer's lactate solution
(D) Infusion of dopamine hydrochloride
(E) Intravenous injection of methylprednisolone

7. Infection with *Pseudomonas* organisms is frequently associated with each of the following EXCEPT

(A) osteomyelitis developing after a nail puncture wound of the foot
(B) ecthyma gangrenosum
(C) both a mild and an invasive form of otitis externa
(D) meningitis in neonatal infants
(E) endocarditis in drug addicts

8. A 17-year-old pregnant girl is hospitalized 2 days after she inserted a metal rod into her uterus during an abortion attempt. She has a temperature of 40.5°C (104.9°F), shaking chills, and a purulent vaginal discharge; blood pressure is normal. Which of the following laboratory results would be LEAST consistent with a diagnosis of septic abortion?

(A) White blood cell count: 30,000/mm³ with occasional metamyelocytes, many band neutrophils, and toxic granulation
(B) Prothrombin time: 16 s (control 12 s)
(C) Arterial blood gases: pH 7.30; P_{O_2} 90 mmHg; P_{CO_2} 30 mmHg
(D) Urinalysis: pH 5.0; glucose negative; protein 2+; RBC 3+; many RBC casts
(E) Serum chemistries: Na⁺ 138 meq/L; K⁺ 4.0 meq/L; Cl⁻ 100 meq/L; HCO₃⁻ 20 meq/L; creatinine 1.0 mg/dL

9. Tomorrow, a 68-year-old man is to undergo a transurethral resection for benign prostatic hypertrophy that has caused lower urinary tract obstruction and repeated urinary tract infections. He has a history of congestive heart failure. His urine cultures have grown *Escherichia coli*, *Klebsiella*, and enterococci on several separate occasions. His most recent quantitative urine culture grew only 5000 organisms; the laboratory did not identify them. The best therapeutic plan for this man would be to give

(A) gentamicin before and after surgery
(B) carbenicillin before and after surgery
(C) ampicillin and gentamicin before and after surgery
(D) gentamicin before surgery and gentamicin and carbenicillin after surgery
(E) no antibiotics before surgery but ampicillin after surgery

10. The most common cause of "traveler's diarrhea" ("turista") in Americans traveling abroad is

(A) *Staphylococcus aureus*
(B) *Clostridium perfringens*
(C) *Escherichia coli*
(D) *Bacillus cereus*
(E) rotavirus

11. Vaginitis due to *Gardnerella vaginalis* (formerly called *Haemophilus vaginalis*) is treated most effectively with

(A) sulfonamides
(B) tetracycline
(C) ampicillin
(D) nystatin
(E) metronidazole

12. Antibiotic prophylaxis would most likely be of benefit for persons undergoing

(A) vaginal hysterectomy
(B) splenectomy
(C) coronary artery bypass surgery
(D) ligation of fallopian tubes
(E) open biopsy of the kidney

13. Pneumococcal vaccination would be LEAST beneficial for which of the following individuals?

(A) A 20-year-old woman with sickle-cell anemia
(B) A 24-year-old man with nephrotic syndrome
(C) A 28-year-old man who recently had a splenectomy following a car accident
(D) A 42-year-old woman with multiple myeloma
(E) A 70-year-old woman in good health

14. All the following factors are thought to contribute to the pathogenicity of staphylococci EXCEPT

(A) penicillinase production
(B) coagulase production
(C) enterotoxin production
(D) exotoxin production
(E) leukocidin production

15. Which of the following organisms is most likely to cause infection of a shunt implanted for treatment of hydrocephalus?

(A) *Staphylococcus epidermidis*
(B) *Staphylococcus aureus*
(C) *Corynebacterium diphtheriae*
(D) *Escherichia coli*
(E) *Bacteroides fragilis*

16. A 14-year-old girl has fever, headache, pain on swallowing, and loss of voice. Her cervical lymph nodes are tender to palpation. Of these signs and symptoms, which is LEAST suggestive of a diagnosis of streptococcal pharyngitis?

(A) Fever
(B) Headache
(C) Pain on swallowing
(D) Loss of voice
(E) Tender cervical lymph nodes

17. Meningococcal meningitis can be prevented by the administration of all the following preparations EXCEPT

(A) group A vaccine
(B) group B vaccine
(C) group C vaccine
(D) sulfonamides
(E) rifampin

18. A 27-year-old heterosexual man has a urethral discharge. Intracellular gram-negative diplococci are seen in the exudate, and treatment with a single oral dose of amoxicillin (3 g) plus oral probenicid (1 g) is recommended. One week later the man returns, again complaining of urethral discharge. Which of the following statements is the LEAST likely explanation for this clinical situation?

(A) The man did not take the prescribed medications
(B) The organism was resistant to amoxicillin
(C) The man had a chlamydial infection as well as a gonococcal infection
(D) The man has become infected again
(E) Single-dose therapy for gonorrhea is outmoded

19. A 60-year-old insulin-dependent man with diabetes mellitus has had purulent drainage from his left ear for one week. Suddenly, fever, increased pain, and vertigo develop. The most likely causative agent is

(A) *Aspergillus*
(B) *Mucor*
(C) *Pseudomonas*
(D) *Staphylococcus aureus*
(E) *Haemophilus influenzae*

20. Typhoid fever can be characterized by all the following statements EXCEPT

(A) the illness usually is acquired from ingestion of contaminated food, water, or milk
(B) leukopenia is more common than leukocytosis in acutely ill individuals
(C) rose spots are usually present at the time the fever begins
(D) chloramphenicol is not effective in preventing relapse
(E) adults are more likely to become chronic carriers than are children

21. *Haemophilus influenzae* infections occur with increased frequency in association with all the following conditions EXCEPT

(A) alcoholism
(B) sickle cell disease
(C) splenectomy
(D) agammaglobulinemia
(E) chronic granulomatous disease

22. To determine whether a child with paroxysmal coughing and gasping has whooping cough, a physician would do best to order

(A) white blood cell count and differential
(B) Gram stain of the sputum
(C) blood cultures
(D) chest x-ray
(E) lateral x-ray of the neck

23. Of the following infections, which is most frequently associated with hypersensitivity reactions, such as erythema nodosum, erythema multiforme, arthritis, and arthralgias?

(A) Histoplasmosis
(B) Cryptococcosis
(C) Aspergillosis
(D) Blastomycosis
(E) Coccidioidomycosis

24. A 9-month-old boy is hospitalized because of high fever and vomiting. Lumbar puncture reveals many polymorphonuclear leukocytes, a low glucose, high protein, and pleomorphic gram-negative bacilli. The best initial choice for antibiotic therapy would be

(A) carbenicillin
(B) chloramphenicol
(C) ampicillin
(D) chloramphenicol and carbenicillin
(E) chloramphenicol and ampicillin

25. All the following are characteristic clinical features of chancroid EXCEPT

(A) initial presentation as a tender papule
(B) development of painful genital ulcers
(C) tender, enlarged inguinal lymph nodes
(D) *Haemophilus ducreyi* isolated from bacteriologic cultures
(E) response to ampicillin therapy

26. A 62-year-old gardener who has chronic lymphocytic leukemia develops lymphangitis and a painless, nodular lesion on his wrist. Subsequently, he becomes severely ill with cavitary right-upper-lobe pneumonia; *Sporothrix schenckii* is isolated. He should be treated with

(A) chloramphenicol
(B) potassium iodide
(C) penicillin
(D) amphotericin B
(E) flucytosine

27. Four days after he and his friends were killing muskrats along a rural creek, a boy becomes ill with headache, fever, and a macular rash. On examination, axillary adenopathy is noted, but otherwise the examination is normal. Which of the following tests would be most helpful in proving that this boy has tularemia?

(A) Blood culture
(B) Aspiration of an axillary lymph node
(C) Determination of serum agglutinins for *Francisella tularensis*
(D) Bone-marrow culture
(E) Examination of his friends

28. A 10-year-old boy is seen in a rural Arizona clinic because of prostration, fever of 40°C (104°F), and severe headache. Examination is negative for rash, stiff neck, joint tenderness, and chest and abdominal abnormalities. However, several tender, enlarged lymph nodes are palpated in the left axilla, which is very edematous. The test most likely to be of greatest help in the immediate management of this boy would be

(A) blood culture
(B) examination of a blood smear
(C) biopsy of an axillary lymph node
(D) aspiration of an axillary lymph node
(E) surgical excision of an axillary node

29. Which of the following organisms often causes diarrhea, confusion, and delirium in conjunction with pneumonia?

(A) *Legionella pneumophila*
(B) *Francisella tularensis*
(C) *Mycoplasma pneumoniae*
(D) *Haemophilus pneumoniae*
(E) *Klebsiella pneumoniae*

30. *Listeria monocytogenes* most frequently causes which of the following infections?

(A) Endocarditis
(B) Peritonitis
(C) Hepatitis
(D) Meningitis
(E) Conjunctivitis

31. Which of the following signs and symptoms is LEAST characteristic of diphtherial infections of the upper respiratory tract?

(A) Gray-white pharyngeal membrane
(B) Temperature greater than 38.9°C (102°F)
(C) Sore throat
(D) Pain on swallowing
(E) Hoarseness

32. Which of the following findings would NOT be consistent with a diagnosis of cutaneous anthrax?

(A) A history of handling animal hides
(B) A vesicular skin lesion that develops into a painless ulcer
(C) Regional lymphadenopathy
(D) A Gram stain showing gram-negative bacilli
(E) Low-grade fever and malaise

33. Which of the following infectious disorders frequently develops in persons who have bartonellosis?

(A) Pneumococcal bacteremia
(B) *Salmonella* bacteremia
(C) *Haemophilus influenzae* pneumonia
(D) *Pneumocystis carinii* pneumonia
(E) Herpes zoster eruption

34. Which of the following pleural-fluid profiles is most suggestive of tuberculous pleuritis?

Fluid sample	Color	pH	Protein, g/dL	Glucose, mg/dL	LDH, units/mL	WBC Total (per mm³)	% Lymphocytes
A	Clear yellow	7.15	3.5	20	600	2000	95
B	Thick green	7.00	4.0	20	600	10,000	50
C	Clear yellow	7.30	1.5	80	150	200	50
D	Pink-tinged	7.40	3.0	80	600	3000	50
E	Clear yellow	7.30	3.5	60	150	2000	95

(LDH, lactate dehydrogenase; WBC, white blood cell count)

(A) Sample A
(B) Sample B
(C) Sample C
(D) Sample D
(E) Sample E

35. A 27-year-old woman returned from a camping trip in New England. Two weeks later a small red papule developed which expanded into a large annular lesion. She also had headache, fever, chills, malaise, and fatigue. Which of the following studies would be most useful to confirm the diagnosis of Lyme disease?

(A) Skin biopsy
(B) Giemsa or Wright stain of a blood smear
(C) Culture of skin or blood in Kelly's modified medium
(D) Acute and convalescent serologic studies after several weeks of symptoms
(E) Examination of cerebrospinal fluid

36. A 10-year-old child has malaise, a low-grade fever, and cervical lymphadenopathy. Biopsy of a cervical lymph node reveals granulomatous inflammation; the culture grows *Mycobacterium scrofulaceum*. The best treatment for this child would be

(A) excision of the infected nodes
(B) isoniazid and ethambutol
(C) streptomycin, isoniazid, and ethambutol
(D) rifampin, isoniazid, and ethambutol
(E) observation until the results of sensitivity studies are available

37. A 40-year-old Canadian who operates a tropical fish store sees his physician because of a nonhealing ulcer on his left arm. He is afebrile and gives no history of night sweats, weight loss, or other constitutional symptoms. Biopsy of the lesion shows granulomatous inflammation and rare acid-fast organisms. A tuberculin test is negative. This man most likely has an infection caused by

(A) *Mycobacterium tuberculosis*
(B) *Mycobacterium ulcerans*
(C) *Mycobacterium kansasii*
(D) *Mycobacterium marinum*
(E) *Mycobacterium fortuitum*

38. Legionnaire's disease is characterized by all the following statements EXCEPT

(A) the disease is not spread from person to person
(B) diarrhea, nausea, and vomiting often are prominent early symptoms
(C) chest x-ray usually shows few abnormalities, while chest examination usually is markedly abnormal
(D) fever is usually prolonged
(E) therapy with erythromycin is recommended

39. Which of the following tests is LEAST useful for recognizing infections caused by the "newly discovered" *Legionella* species (e.g., the Pittsburgh pneumonia agent)?

(A) Direct fluorescent antibody staining
(B) Indirect fluorescent antibody staining
(C) Paired serologic testing
(D) Culture of sputum
(E) Culture of a lung aspirate

40. Which of the following serologic tests would be most helpful in determining if a newborn infant of a mother with syphilis had acquired the infection in utero?

(A) Quantitative Venereal Disease Research Laboratories (VDRL) test
(B) Fluorescent *Treponema pallidum* antibody-absorption (FTA-ABS) test using IgG antibody
(C) *T. pallidum* immobilization (TPI) test
(D) *T. pallidum* hemagglutination (TPHA) test
(E) None of the above

41. The diagnosis of relapsing fever (*Borrelia* infection) usually is made by

(A) serologic testing
(B) blood culture
(C) examination of blood smears
(D) lymph-node aspiration
(E) lumbar puncture

42. The characteristic "sulfur granules" of actinomycosis are composed chiefly of

(A) organisms
(B) neutrophils and monocytes
(C) monocytes and lymphocytes
(D) eosinophils
(E) calcified cellular debris

43. Antigen testing of blood and cerebrospinal fluid is most useful in the diagnosis of

(A) histoplasmosis
(B) blastomycosis
(C) cryptococcosis
(D) coccidioidomycosis
(E) sporotrichosis

44. In which of the following infections are the pulmonary lesions most often calcified?

(A) Histoplasmosis
(B) Cryptococcosis
(C) Aspergillosis
(D) Blastomycosis
(E) Coccidioidomycosis

45. Impaired immune competence is the predisposing factor in about half of all individuals who develop

(A) histoplasmosis
(B) coccidioidomycosis
(C) blastomycosis
(D) cryptococcosis
(E) sporotrichosis

46. A 50-year old woman presents with fever, abdominal cramps, and watery diarrhea one week after finishing an oral course of ampicillin for cystitis. The best way to document pseudomembranous colitis caused by *Clostridium difficile* is

(A) stool culture
(B) a rise in serologic titers to *C. difficile*
(C) the presence of characteristic pseudomembranes on endoscopy
(D) cytopathic effect of stool filtrate on tissue culture monolayers
(E) Gram stain of the stool showing sheets of neutrophils and gram-positive rods

47. Recommended therapy for persons who have dermatophytosis, otherwise known as ringworm, includes all the following agents EXCEPT

(A) clotrimazole
(B) griseofulvin
(C) undecylenic acid
(D) amphotericin
(E) ketoconazole

48. Factors contributing to blindness in persons who have trachoma include all the following EXCEPT

(A) superficial corneal vascularization
(B) corneal abrasion by eyelashes
(C) bacterial superinfection
(D) inflammatory destruction of the lacrimal glands
(E) glaucoma due to limbic obstruction

49. A 28-year-old woman who works in a poultry processing factory develops an acute febrile illness. Which of the following signs and symptoms is LEAST suggestive of the diagnosis of psittacosis?

(A) Shaking chills with fever to 40.6°C (105°F)
(B) Severe headache
(C) Nonproductive cough
(D) Stiff back and neck
(E) Diarrhea

50. Which of the following characteristics would be most useful in distinguishing between mumps and acute bacterial parotitis?

(A) Age of the individual
(B) Presence or absence of fever
(C) Presence or absence of warmth and tenderness over the parotid glands
(D) Gram stain of parotid secretions
(E) Serum amylase concentration

51. Which of the following is LEAST suggestive of infection with poliovirus?

(A) Low-grade fever and malaise with complete resolution in two to three days
(B) Biphasic illness with several days of fever, then meningeal symptoms and asymmetric flaccid paralysis 5 to 10 days later
(C) Descending motor paralysis with preservation of muscle reflexes and sensation
(D) Failure to isolate a virus from the cerebrospinal fluid in the presence of marked meningismus
(E) Recovery of function up to six months after initial paralysis

52. A 58-year-old schoolteacher is hospitalized after 10 days of a respiratory illness. For 2 days he has had a dramatically worsening cough and shortness of breath. He also has had severe malaise, myalgias, arthralgias, rhinorrhea, and pharyngitis and has lost 2.7 kg (6 lb). No sputum or respiratory secretions can be collected. Chest x-ray shows a diffuse bronchopneumonia.

Which of the following antibiotics would NOT be acceptable for the initial treatment of this man's illness?

(A) Penicillin G
(B) Nafcillin
(C) Vancomycin
(D) Cephalothin
(E) Clindamycin

53. A 26-year-old garage mechanic has been ill for 3 days with fever, malaise, cough, and mild shortness of breath. On physical examination there is no evidence of pharyngitis or lymphadenopathy; only a few scattered pulmonary rhonchi, and no wheezes or rales, are heard on chest auscultation. Chest x-ray, however, shows changes of bronchopneumonia.

Assuming the person has no history of drug allergy, oral antibiotic therapy should begin with

(A) chloramphenicol
(B) erythromycin
(C) tetracycline
(D) penicillin V potassium
(E) cephalexin

54. Acyclovir is NOT indicated for treatment of which of the following?

(A) Herpes encephalitis
(B) Mucocutaneous herpes infection in immunocompromised patients
(C) Prophylactically to prevent herpes infection during periods of immunosuppression
(D) Herpes zoster in elderly patients to prevent dissemination and post-herpetic neuralgia
(E) Chronic suppression of frequently recurring genital herpes

55. Urinary tract infections would be LEAST likely to develop in association with

(A) diabetes mellitus
(B) sickle cell anemia
(C) hyperparathyroidism
(D) gout
(E) Wilson's disease

56. Brain abscess can be best identified by which of the following diagnostic tests?

(A) CT scanning
(B) Radionuclide scanning with technetium 99m
(C) Gallium-labeled neutrophil scanning
(D) Ultrasonography
(E) Arteriography

57. Which of the following agents is the most frequent cause of nonepidemic, sporadic encephalitis in the United States?

(A) Togavirus
(B) Picornavirus
(C) Rubella virus
(D) Epstein-Barr virus
(E) Herpes simplex virus

58. A 29-year-old patient with acquired immunodeficiency syndrome (AIDS) has abdominal cramps and profuse watery diarrhea. The best way to establish the diagnosis of cryptosporidiosis is

(A) stool culture
(B) Gram stain of stool
(C) acute and convalescent serologic studies
(D) wet mount of stool
(E) acid-fast staining of concentrated stool

59. There has been an outbreak of infections caused by methicillin-resistant *Staphylococcus aureus* in the Surgical Intensive Care Unit. The most effective means of limiting the spread is

(A) treatment with cephalosporins to which most strains are sensitive
(B) treatment with nafcillin and gentamicin, which have a synergistic effect
(C) use of high-dose nafcillin alone, and isolation
(D) treatment with vancomycin
(E) minimizing use of any antibiotics in the affected patients because resistance will rapidly develop in other bacteria

60. A 40-year-old Filipino man has hypopigmented macular lesions and a palpably enlarged ulnar nerve. The diagnosis of leprosy can best be established by

(A) positive lepromin skin test
(B) culture of material obtained on skin biopsy
(C) development of erythema and swelling of the lesions after a trial of dapsone therapy
(D) demonstration of acid-fast organisms in skin or nerves
(E) none of the above; leprosy is a clinical diagnosis

61. All of the following groups have an increased risk of infection with *Giardia lamblia* EXCEPT

(A) campers in mountainous areas
(B) patients receiving chemotherapy
(C) toddlers in day-care centers
(D) patients with IgA deficiency
(E) male homosexuals

62. A 35-year-old Samoan presents with recurrent fever, headache, photophobia, and painful lymphangitis in his left leg. The best way to diagnose filariasis caused by *Wucheria bancrofti* is

(A) biopsy of any inflamed lymph nodes to demonstrate the adult worm
(B) serologic studies
(C) intense itching occurring after a single dose of diethylcarbamazine
(D) demonstration of microfilariae after injection of blood into mice
(E) demonstration of microfilariae in blood taken between 9 P.M. and 2 A.M.

INFECTIOUS DISEASES

DIRECTIONS: Each question below contains five suggested answers. For **each** of the five alternatives of **each** item, you are to respond either YES (Y) or NO (N). In a given item all, some, or none of the alternatives may be correct.

63. Which of the following statements concerning fever are true?
 (A) "Fever blisters" occur with approximately the same frequency in most infections in which fever is above 38.3°C (101°F) for at least 2 to 3 days
 (B) Fever is of benefit in bacterial infections, because it accelerates phagocytosis and bacterial killing by polymorphonuclear leukocytes
 (C) The simplest and best method to reduce fever in young adults is to sponge the extremities with alcohol
 (D) Morphine sulfate is often effective in relieving the rigors that accompany rapid defervescence in febrile individuals
 (E) Bacterial abscesses usually cause intermittent fevers

64. Nosocomial infections can be described by which of the following statements?
 (A) R factors can readily transfer antibiotic resistance from one gram-negative bacterium to another
 (B) Even with the best of care, bladder catheters lead to urinary tract infections in more than 50 percent of cases in which the catheter remains in place for at least 5 days
 (C) There is a greater risk of local phlebitis with plastic cannulas than with stainless steel needles
 (D) Intravenous cannulas should not be left in place more than 72 hours
 (E) Health-care workers who are seropositive for hepatitis B surface antigen should not engage in obtaining blood samples

65. Which of the following statements concerning laboratory diagnosis of microbial infections are true?
 (A) Infection with *Borrelia recurrentis* and *Plasmodium vivax* can be recognized by examining Wright's-stained blood smears
 (B) *Nocardia* and *Mycobacterium* are both acid-fast organisms
 (C) *Legionella pneumophila* can be detected in sputum by immunofluorescent staining
 (D) A single negative throat culture for *Streptococcus pyogenes* is typically sufficient to exclude the diagnosis of streptococcal pharyngitis
 (E) In cases of partially treated meningitis, gram-positive organisms tend to take up the blue dye with increased avidity, so that the organism appears darker than normal

66. Which of the following statements concerning infections in immunocompromised individuals are true?
 (A) Pneumococci are the organisms most frequently isolated from splenectomized individuals who develop bacteremic illnesses
 (B) Monthly gamma globulin injections are useful in preventing infection in individuals with multiple myeloma and hypogammaglobulinemia
 (C) The most common cause for enhanced susceptibility to infection in individuals receiving cyclophosphamide is neutropenia
 (D) Deficiencies involving early complement components generally are associated with more severe infectious problems than are deficiencies of late components
 (E) Long-term high-dose glucocorticosteroid therapy is thought to increase the risk of infection in humans

67. Which of the following statements concerning the pathophysiology of septic shock are true?
 (A) Endotoxemia causes thrombocytopenia and granulocytopenia
 (B) Complement levels (total hemolytic complement and C3 levels) are usually reduced
 (C) Activation of complement, with the liberation of C5a, increases granulocyte margination
 (D) Infusion of prostacyclin, a thromboxane A_2 antagonist, improves the outcome in experimental septic shock
 (E) Naloxone, an endorphin antagonist, worsens the outcome in experimental septic shock

68. Cephalosporin antibiotic agents can be described by which of the following statements?
 (A) Cefazolin is better tolerated than cephalothin when given intramuscularly
 (B) Cefoxitin is inactive in vitro against *Bacteroides fragilis*
 (C) Cefamandole is more active than cephalothin against many gram-negative aerobic organisms
 (D) Cephalosporin therapy is acceptable for most cases of bacterial meningitis
 (E) Cephalosporin therapy is an acceptable alternative to penicillin therapy in individuals known to be allergic to penicillin

69. Which of the following statements about penicillin antibiotic agents are true?

(A) Penicillin G, procaine penicillin, and benzathine penicillin all differ in the rate of absorption from a site of injection
(B) Amoxicillin is not as well absorbed as ampicillin
(C) Neither ampicillin nor carbenicillin is effective against *Klebsiella*
(D) Ticarcillin is similar to carbenicillin except for its somewhat greater activity against *Pseudomonas*
(E) Nafcillin is more effective than methicillin for treating staphylococcal endocarditis

70. Which of the following statements concerning genitourinary infections are true?

(A) A man who has dysuria, no urethral discharge, and only 1 or 2 leukocytes per high-power field on microscopic examination of material obtained by a urethral swab probably has chlamydial urethritis
(B) A man who has a urethral discharge containing many leukocytes but only extracellular gram-negative diplococci should be treated with tetracycline, pending the results of cultures
(C) A woman who has a watery, malodorous vaginal discharge that does not contain *Candida* or *Trichomonas* on microscopic examination should be treated with a sulfonamide vaginal cream for presumed *Gardnerella vaginalis* infection
(D) A pregnant woman who has mucopurulent cervicitis without gram-negative diplococci on Gram stain or *Neisseria gonorrhoeae* isolated on culture should be treated with tetracycline for 1 to 3 weeks
(E) In the United States, the most common cause of ulcerative genital lesions is herpes simplex virus

71. Which of the following statements concerning pneumococcal infection are true?

(A) Infections with type 3 pneumococci are associated with a higher mortality rate than infections with any other type of pneumococci
(B) Individuals who have had a splenectomy for any reason should receive pneumococcal vaccine
(C) Pneumococcal pharyngitis is the most common precipitating event of pneumococcal meningitis in adults
(D) The occurrence of the "crisis" in pneumococcal pneumonia generally corresponds to the time of maximum leukocytosis
(E) Hypogammaglobulinemia is an important factor contributing to the unfavorable prognosis for pneumococcal pneumonia in alcoholic individuals

72. Which of the following statements about the pathogenesis of streptococcal infections are true?

(A) Streptococcal strains without M protein in the cell wall are nonpathogenic
(B) Antistreptolysin O (ASLO) titers are nearly always elevated in persons with poststreptococcal glomerulonephritis
(C) ASLO titers are nearly always elevated in persons with streptococcal pyoderma
(D) Scarlet fever can be caused by group A, C, or G streptococci as well as by certain staphylococci
(E) Streptococcal pyoderma does not lead to acute rheumatic fever

73. Which of the following statements about leptospirosis are true?

(A) Fleas are the most important vector for transmission of *Leptospira* to humans
(B) Leptospirosis usually begins with fever, headache, and myalgias
(C) Leptospiral hepatitis often causes marked hyperbilirubinemia with only moderate transaminasemia
(D) A normal glucose concentration and a moderately elevated white blood cell count (100 to 1000 cells/mm³) are characteristic cerebrospinal fluid findings in leptospiral meningitis
(E) The best way to diagnose acute leptospirosis is by dark-field microscopic examination of blood smears

74. *Neisseria gonorrhoeae* infections can be described by which of the following statements?

(A) Gonococci with pili tend to be avirulent
(B) Strains of *N. gonorrhoeae* that produce β-lactamase are resistant to penicillin but usually are sensitive to "third generation" cephalosporins, such as cefotaxime
(C) Gonococcemia frequently occurs during menstruation
(D) The skin lesions of gonococcemia usually appear first on the distal portions of the extremities
(E) Gonococcal arthritis is usually symmetrical in distribution

75. Which of the following statements concerning *Acinetobacter* are true?

(A) This organism often is confused with *Neisseria* on Gram stain
(B) This organism often is mistakenly identified as a diphtheroid on Gram stain
(C) This organism can be easily mislabeled as a member of the Enterobacteriaceae family when first isolated on routine laboratory culture media
(D) This organism usually is sensitive to penicillin and ampicillin
(E) Organisms of the genus *Acinetobacter* are rarely isolated from normal individuals

76. Which of the following statements concerning melioidosis are true?

(A) Infection usually is caused by person-to-person transmission
(B) Patients with pneumonia usually have relatively few organisms in the sputum
(C) Diagnosis usually depends on serologic testing
(D) Calcification of cavitary lung lesions does not occur
(E) Therapy with a combination of two or three antibiotics is recommended for acutely ill patients

77. Brucellosis can be described by which of the following statements?

(A) Cattle are the most important source of human *Brucella* infections in the United States
(B) Brucellosis is an important cause of abortion in cattle and pigs, but not in humans
(C) Brucellosis should be considered in the differential diagnosis of fever of unknown origin in the United States
(D) *Brucella* cannot be grown in usual blood culture media
(E) A combination of tetracycline and streptomycin is the treatment of choice

78. Cholera can be characterized by which of the following statements?

(A) In endemic areas, it is predominantly a disease of children
(B) The most reliable means of diagnosis is by dark-field microscopy
(C) Oral treatment must include replacement fluids containing glucose and sodium bicarbonate
(D) Treatment with oral tetracycline shortens the duration of diarrhea
(E) Vaccination affords good protection from infection

79. Which of the following statements concerning botulism are true?

(A) Botulinus toxins are the most potent toxins yet discovered
(B) Botulinus toxins are absorbed in the stomach and upper small intestine
(C) Botulinus toxins block cholinergic neurotransmission at the presynaptic level
(D) The therapeutic effect of guanidine hydrochloride results from blocking acetylcholine degradation
(E) Edrophonium (Tensilon) is generally less effective in treating botulism than in treating myasthenia gravis

80. Which of the following statements concerning syphilis are true?

(A) Syphilis acquired by a woman during pregnancy is likely to remain subclinical
(B) All newborn infants of mothers with reactive serologic tests will themselves be reactive
(C) If a person with syphilis goes untreated, the VDRL test will remain reactive indefinitely
(D) Symptomatic neurosyphilis is unlikely in persons treated with at least 6 million units of penicillin G
(E) The major cause of death from untreated syphilis is cardiovascular disease

81. Which of the following statements describe accurately the use of amphotericin B in treating fungal infections?

(A) It usually is best to give an initial test dose of 1 mg intravenously
(B) Alternate-day double-dose administration of amphotericin is as efficacious as daily therapy
(C) Alternate-day double-dose amphotericin therapy causes less fever than daily single-dose therapy
(D) Addition of hydrocortisone to the intravenous infusion is recommended
(E) Side effects of intracisternal administration generally are fewer than those associated with lumbar injections

82. Which of the following statements about mucormycosis are true?

(A) The organism is grown easily from most clinical specimens once an adequate tissue sample is obtained
(B) A characteristic feature of *Mucor* is its tendency to invade blood vessels
(C) In individuals with hematologic malignancies the sinuses are the most frequent site of infection
(D) Diagnosis by serologic testing is not yet clinically practical
(E) The treatment of choice is amphotericin B

83. Which of the following statements about Rocky Mountain spotted fever are true?

(A) Fleas are the characteristic vector of disease spread
(B) The disease is caused by the gram-negative, obligate intracellular organism *Rickettsia rickettsii*
(C) Frank arthritis is a common early manifestation of infection
(D) The initial skin lesions usually appear on the extremities
(E) Treatment of choice consists of early administration of chloramphenicol or tetracycline

84. *Mycoplasma* pneumonia has which of the following characteristics?

(A) The causal organism, *Mycoplasma pneumoniae*, is gram-positive
(B) Persons older than 40 years of age rarely are affected
(C) A fourfold rise in the cold-agglutinin titer within 10 days of the onset of symptoms is specific evidence of this disease
(D) Treatment with tetracycline is effective
(E) Treatment with erythromycin is effective

85. Which of the following statements concerning toxic shock syndrome are true?

(A) It is associated with a staphylococcal exotoxin
(B) Blood cultures are positive for *S. aureus* in approximately 50 percent of patients
(C) Approximately 25 to 30 percent of cases are nonmenstrual
(D) Multiorgan system involvement often occurs
(E) Patients with postoperative staphylococcal wound infections usually have an obvious tissue focus presenting at least one week postoperatively

86. Which of the following statements concerning variola (smallpox) are true?

(A) All of the cutaneous vesicles tend to appear within a few hours of each other
(B) Cutaneous lesions remain infectious until they have healed
(C) Electron microscopic examination of vesicle fluid is helpful in distinguishing between variola and varicella-zoster infection
(D) Thiosemicarbazone is useful for prophylaxis against, but not for treatment of, variola infection
(E) In the United States, smallpox vaccination is required only for certain health workers and travelers to certain African countries

87. For their preventive medical care, which of the following individuals should be seriously considered for, if not in fact given, rabies vaccination?

(A) Letter carriers
(B) Cave explorers
(C) Veterinarians
(D) City park-department workers
(E) Children in families owning more than three dogs

88. Which of the following statements concerning infectious mononucleosis are true?

(A) The most common symptom of infectious mononucleosis is sore throat
(B) In young adults, the incubation period for infectious mononucleosis is 30 to 50 days
(C) The atypical lymphocytes associated with infectious mononucleosis are T cells
(D) Heterophil antibody titers usually decline within 3 to 6 months from the onset of symptoms
(E) Antibodies to Epstein-Barr virus generally persist longer in the circulation than do heterophil antibodies

INFECTIOUS DISEASES

89. Cat-scratch disease can be described by which of the following statements?

(A) Only about half of all cases are associated with cat scratches
(B) Lymph node histopathology usually is characteristic
(C) Lymph node swelling usually lasts no more than 2 weeks
(D) Splenomegaly is common
(E) Treatment with tetracycline is usually effective

90. Which of the following statements describing amebiasis are true?

(A) Humans are the principal reservoir
(B) Amebic liver abscess is characterized by prompt response to therapy with metronidazole
(C) In persons who have received metronidazole for liver abscess, the amebic serology usually reverts from positive to negative within 4 to 6 weeks
(D) If the fluid aspirated from a liver cyst identified by liver-spleen scan contains no polymorphonuclear leukocytes or amebas, then amebic abscess is an unlikely diagnosis
(E) The mortality rate for intestinal amebiasis in the United States is less than 5 percent

91. Which of the following statements concerning malaria are true?

(A) Individuals who lack the Duffy blood-group antigens on their red blood cells are resistant to *Plasmodium vivax* infection
(B) Glomerulonephritis in acute falciparum malaria can be attributed to the deposition of immune complexes along the glomerular basement membrane
(C) In most malarial infections, the appearance of strain-specific antibodies occurs coincidentally with a decrease in the degree of parasitemia
(D) In persons with "tropical splenomegaly," chronic antimalarial therapy causes a regression in splenic enlargement
(E) Travelers to regions with chloroquine-sensitive malaria usually can discontinue prophylaxis a week after leaving an endemic area

92. Toxoplasmosis can be described by which of the following statements?

(A) A pregnant woman who has acquired *Toxoplasma* any time before pregnancy is unlikely to deliver an infected infant
(B) A woman who develops acute toxoplasmosis during one pregnancy is more likely than other women to give birth to an infected child from a subsequent pregnancy
(C) A woman who acquires toxoplasmosis during the last trimester of pregnancy is more likely to deliver an infected infant than if she acquired the infection during the first trimester
(D) Toxoplasmosis in an individual with Hodgkin's disease probably is due to reactivation of a latent infection
(E) Antibody response is not a reliable diagnostic indicator of toxoplasmosis in immunocompromised patients

93. Which of the following statements about *Pneumocystis carinii* pneumonia are true?

(A) Fever and marked tachypnea are early signs
(B) Pleural effusions are common
(C) Pulmonary fibrosis is a common development
(D) Systemic dissemination is extremely rare
(E) Trimethoprim-sulfamethoxazole is the treatment of choice

94. An individual who has liver disease caused by *Schistosoma mansoni* would be likely to have

(A) gynecomastia
(B) jaundice
(C) esophageal varices
(D) ascites
(E) spider nevi

95. Which of the following statements regarding *Shigella* and shigellosis are true?

(A) *S. sonnei* is the isolate most frequently found in the United States
(B) Patients who have had gastric surgery or who are taking antacids have an increased susceptibility to infection
(C) There is increased transmission at day-care centers and among male homosexuals
(D) *Shigella* organisms are locally invasive in the bowel, but positive blood cultures are very unusual
(E) Antibiotic therapy should be avoided since it will increase the carrier rate

96. Which of the following statements concerning extrapulmonary tuberculosis are true?

(A) Pleural effusions associated with tuberculosis usually occur in older patients with reactivation disease developing after an insidious onset
(B) Patients with laryngitis or bronchitis caused by tuberculosis are highly infectious
(C) Pott's disease, with extensive bony involvement of the midthoracic spine and paravertebral cold abscesses, will usually respond well to chemotherapy alone
(D) Cranial nerve findings are frequently associated with tuberculous meningitis because of basilar involvement by infection
(E) The stomach is most likely to be involved in patients with gastrointestinal tuberculosis

97. Which of the following statements about Lyme disease are true?

(A) Transmission occurs only in the northeastern United States
(B) A typical skin lesion, erythema chronicum migrans, usually occurs within a month of the infected tick bite
(C) Constitutional symptoms are very rare at the time of skin involvement
(D) Meningitis is the only form of neurologic involvement
(E) In patients with frank meningitis or significant cardiac conduction defects, parenteral therapy with 20 million units per day of penicillin G for 10 days is indicated

98. Which of the following statements about clostridial infections are true?

(A) Early antibiotic therapy is important after the isolation of clostridia from any wound to prevent more serious disease
(B) Alpha toxin, a lecithinase, is one of the major clostridial toxins
(C) *C. perfringens* is one of the most common causes of food poisoning in the United States
(D) The diagnosis of clostridial myonecrosis can be difficult to make because few organisms are present in the skin lesions
(E) Septicemia with *C. septicum* has been associated with gastrointestinal malignancies

99. Anaerobic organisms should be considered as potential etiologic agents in which of the following patients?

(A) A previously healthy 18-year-old boy with sudden fever, cough, and right lower lobe infiltrate
(B) A 50-year-old man with alcoholism who has marked cellulitis, swelling, and pain of his left lower mandible
(C) A 40-year-old woman with a seizure disorder, low-grade fever, malaise, and a right lower lobe infiltrate
(D) A 50-year-old woman with fever, hypoxia, and pulmonary infiltrates four hours after having general anesthesia for a cholecystectomy
(E) A 38-year-old man with a history of rheumatic fever and severe periodontitis in whom a low-grade fever, malaise, and a new heart murmur develop

100. Which of the following statements about varicella-zoster infection are true?

(A) Once dermatomal herpes zoster develops in a patient, repeated recurrences are the rule
(B) Cerebellar ataxia is a serious complication of varicella in children
(C) Chickenpox is very contagious with attack rates estimated at between 70 and 90 percent
(D) Varicella pneumonitis, the most serious complication of chickenpox, occurs more frequently in adults than in children
(E) If available within 72 hours of exposure, varicella-zoster immune globulin should be given to all patients to prevent development of clinical disease

101. Which of the following statements regarding infection with cytomegalic virus (CMV) are true?

(A) Approximately 60 percent of infants who are breast-fed by seropositive mothers become infected, causing the majority of the cases of cytomegalic inclusion disease in newborn infants
(B) Although 1 percent of newborn infants may be infected with CMV in the United States, less than 5 percent have symptomatic disease
(C) CMV mononucleosis is the most common cause of heterophile-negative mononucleosis
(D) CMV pneumonia, a major cause of morbidity and mortality in bone marrow transplant patients, can be diagnosed only by viral cultures of sputum
(E) Cultures of CMV from urine, saliva, or buffy coat specimens confirm the presence of the virus but do not necessarily imply acute infection

INFECTIOUS DISEASES

102. Which of the following statements about viral gastroenteritis caused by rotavirus and Norwalk virus are true?

(A) Both alter cyclic nucleotide levels, causing a secretory diarrhea
(B) Rotaviruses are the most important causes of severe diarrhea in infants
(C) Rotavirus infection can be diagnosed only retrospectively by serologic methods since isolation from stool is very difficult
(D) Norwalk virus has been associated with both food-borne and water-borne epidemics
(E) Both viruses cause a self-limited disease with vomiting and diarrhea

103. Which of the following statements about influenza infection are true?

(A) Pandemics are caused by several simultaneous point mutations
(B) Immunity is established by the development of antibodies to the neuraminidase preventing release of replicated viral particles
(C) Outbreaks with influenza B tend to be smaller than those with influenza A because the virus does not undergo extensive antigenic shift as it does in influenza A
(D) In a minority of patients, prolonged weakness and fatigue develop, associated with persistent viral shedding
(E) Amantadine or rimantadine may be useful in prophylaxis or therapy of influenza A if started within 48 hours of infection

104. Which of the following statements about tetanus are true?

(A) Neonatal tetanus develops after passage through a contaminated birth canal
(B) If given early enough after exposure, human tetanus immune globulin can significantly modify the course of disease
(C) Tetanus does not recur since lasting immunity develops
(D) Trismus is a common manifestation
(E) In a patient who is uncertain about his or her immunization status, both tetanus toxoid and immune globulin should be given for serious wounds

DIRECTIONS: The groups of questions below consist of four or five lettered headings followed by several numbered items. For each numbered item choose the **one** lettered heading with which it is **most** closely associated. Each lettered heading may be used once, more than once, or not at all.

Questions 105–108

Match each defect in host immunity with the type of infection most commonly associated with it.

(A) *Pneumocystis carinii* infection
(B) Recurrent *Neisseria meningitidis* infections
(C) Recurrent staphylococcal skin abscesses
(D) *Streptococcus pneumoniae* bacteremia
(E) Gram-negative bacteremia

105. Deficiencies of late complement components

106. Post-splenectomy state

107. Abnormal T-cell suppressor/helper ratio in patients with the acquired immunodeficiency syndrome (AIDS)

108. Chronic granulomatous disease

Questions 109–113

For each of the following causes of acute diarrhea, select the most appropriate therapy.

(A) Ampicillin
(B) Trimethoprim-sulfamethoxazole
(C) Quinacrine
(D) Erythromycin
(E) Bismuth subsalicylate

109. Enterotoxigenic *Escherichia coli*

110. *Yersinia enterocolitica*

111. *Shigella flexneri*

112. *Giardia lamblia*

113. *Campylobacter jejuni*

Questions 114–118

Several preventive measures for viral infections are now at hand. For each of the following viral infections select the most appropriate method of prevention.

(A) Inactivated virus vaccination
(B) Attenuated virus vaccination
(C) Passive immunization
(D) Prolonged autoclaving of surgical instruments
(E) Chemoprophylaxis

114. Creutzfeldt-Jakob disease

115. Varicella

116. Influenza A

117. Rubella

118. Smallpox

Questions 119–123

Several mechanisms protect hosts from viral infections. For each cell or humoral factor that follows, select the host-defense function with which it is most likely to be associated.

(A) Blocks viral replication intracellularly
(B) Blocks viral attachment to mucosal surfaces
(C) Blocks viral attachment to host cells
(D) Produces interferon
(E) Produces antibody proteins

119. Immunoglobulin A

120. Immunoglobulin G

121. B lymphocyte

122. T lymphocyte

123. Macrophage

Questions 124–127

For each pathogen listed below, select the clinical sign or symptom most likely to be the presenting complaint of an affected individual.

(A) Jaundice
(B) Rectal itching
(C) Weakness and fatigue
(D) Dysuria
(E) Cutaneous nodules

124. *Enterobius vermicularis*

125. *Necator americanus*

126. *Clonorchis sinensis*

127. *Schistosoma haematobium*

Infectious Diseases

Answers

1. The answer is D. *(Braunwald, ed 11, chap 83.)* Bone marrow cultures are not generally helpful except in the diagnosis of a few specific infections. Organisms that can be recovered are those that tend to survive in mononuclear phagocytes. Of the organisms listed in the question, streptococci are the most readily killed and hence would not likely be isolated from marrow specimens. The others, though more likely to be isolated, are not recovered very frequently.

2. The answer is D. *(Braunwald, ed 11, chap 84.)* Acquired immunodeficiency syndrome is characterized by a decreased helper T-cell-to-suppressor T-cell ratio. The commonly associated infections are those requiring a normal T-cell response. Though sepsis can develop in association with marked neutropenia, organisms such as *Pseudomonas aeruginosa* rarely are a problem.

3. The answer is A. *(Braunwald, ed 11, chap 83.)* As a rule, all clinical tissue or fluid specimens should be delivered to the appropriate laboratory as quickly as possible, preferably within an hour. In the situation described in the question, the organism most likely to be lost would be *Neisseria*. Such a delay also would adversely affect recovery of *Shigella* from stool samples; thus, in cases of suspected shigellosis, stool should be cultured as quickly as possible.

4. The answer is A. *(Braunwald, ed 11, chap 146.)* The physical signs and symptoms listed in the question suggest infection with *Candida albicans*. *C. albicans* infections occur in several clinical settings: diabetes in poor control; broad-spectrum antibiotic therapy; chronic mucocutaneous candidiasis syndrome; and others. Although some of these conditions may be associated with elevated serum levels of immunoglobulins A and E, these are nonspecific findings. On the other hand, a significantly elevated blood glucose concentration would make the diagnosis of diabetes almost certain. In complement deficiency or uremia, the defects in host defense are not characteristically manifested by vaginal candidiasis.

5. The answer is C. *(Braunwald, ed 11, chap 85.)* Cannula infections occur most commonly due to contamination during cannula insertion or manipulation. Although the daily application of an antibacterial ointment is recommended by some authorities, the best way to prevent these infections is to change the cannula periodically, no less often than every 2 or 3 days. An exception is the use of cuffed catheters, which are inserted surgically into the subclavian vein and can be used for many weeks. Cannula infections occur much less frequently as a result of the other factors listed in the question.

6. The answer is B. *(Braunwald, ed 11, chap 86.)* In the case presented, the history and physical examination strongly suggest gram-negative sepsis stemming from a urinary-tract infection. In older men, obstruction due to prostatic hypertrophy is usually the cause. Prompt initiation of appropriate antibiotic therapy is most important. The choice of antibiotics can be guided by the history and microscopic examination of a Gram-stained urine specimen. In the absence of definitive laboratory information, initial treatment with broad-spectrum coverage, such as gentamicin or tobramycin plus ampicillin or a cephalosporin, is indicated. Bladder catheterization may be necessary to relieve the obstruction or monitor urine flow. Intravenous infusion of bicarbonate solutions and Ringer's lactate or dextrose-in-saline solutions is needed acutely to correct acidosis, restore vascular volume, and maintain renal perfusion. Corticosteroids may protect against the lethal effects of endotoxin, but their use is controversial.

7. The answer is D. *(Braunwald, ed 11, chap 105.)* Primary *Pseudomonas* osteomyelitis is very unusual except in intravenous drug addicts, but it should be considered in a nail puncture wound that does not respond to local or oral antibiotic therapy. Ecthyma gangrenosum, an indurated black area approximately 1 cm in diameter with an ulcerated center and surrounding erythema, is highly suggestive of *Pseudomonas* bacteremia. *Pseudomonas* is the most common cause of chronic otitis externa which usually responds to local measures. In diabetics, however, a rapidly invasive form may develop requiring aggressive debridement and antibiotic therapy. *Escherichia coli* is the most frequent cause of gram-negative meningitis in neonatal infants. Development of *Pseudomonas* meningitis usually occurs only after introduction by surgery, trauma, or foreign objects such as shunts. *Pseudomonas* endocarditis usually occurs in intravenous drug users or after open-heart surgery.

8. The answer is D. *(Braunwald, ed 11, chap 86.)* Leukocytosis with a marked shift to immature neutrophils in the blood and prolongation of the prothrombin and partial thromboplastin times frequently occur in persons with sepsis. Metabolic acidosis, reflected by reductions in blood pH and carbon dioxide tension and in serum bicarbonate concentration, is also common. Urinalysis usually shows nonspecific changes; the finding of red-cell casts would be very unusual, unless the affected individual has another cause for renal injury.

9. The answer is C. *(Braunwald, ed 11, chaps 86, 88.)* In the clinical situation described in the question, antibiotic therapy would be recommended both before and after surgery to try to prevent bacteremia and septic shock. On the basis of the information available, the best choice of antibiotics would be ampicillin and gentamicin. Combining carbenicillin and gentamicin probably would be satisfactory as well, although a history of congestive failure is a relative contraindication to the use of carbenicillin, at least in high doses. Gentamicin alone is effective against *Klebsiella* but not against enterococci; carbenicillin is not effective against *Klebsiella*.

10. The answer is C. *(Braunwald, ed 11, chap 89.)* Toxigenic *Escherichia coli* is the major cause of diarrhea ("turista") for Americans abroad. *Staphylococcus aureus*, *Clostridium perfringens*, and *Bacillus cereus* cause various types of acute food poisoning due to bacterial proliferation and elaboration of toxins in improperly stored food. Children throughout the developing world can develop acute diarrhea, similar to traveler's diarrhea, due to rotavirus infection. All five of these agents cause watery diarrhea that generally is without blood, mucus, or fecal leukocytes.

11. The answer is E. *(Braunwald, ed 11, chap 90.)* Epidemiologic studies have established that *Gardnerella vaginalis* is an important cause of vaginitis. Cases of vaginitis not attributable to *Trichomonas vaginalis* or *Candida* infection are often due to this organism. Treatment with sulfonamides and tetracycline was recommended in the past but has been shown to be ineffective. Metronidazole is more effective than ampicillin. Nystatin is effective for treating candidiasis but not bacterial infections.

12. The answer is A. *(Braunwald, ed 11, chap 92.)* Antibiotic prophylaxis with a cephalosporin, usually cefazolin, is of value in association with vaginal and abdominal hysterectomies. Antibiotic prophylaxis is unlikely to be of value in persons undergoing the other surgical procedures listed in the question. In these operations, the tissues involved are generally sterile, and contamination of the surgical field can be avoided readily.

INFECTIOUS DISEASES

13. The answer is E. *(Braunwald, ed 11, chaps 92, 93.)* Sickle-cell disease, multiple myeloma, nephrotic syndrome, splenectomy, and increasing age all predispose persons to pneumococcal infection. The indications for vaccination, however, are most clear for persons with diseases affecting splenic function and immunoglobulin synthesis. Aging impairs the immune response only very modestly; hence, pneumococcal vaccination of older persons should largely be limited to individuals with certain chronic diseases, particularly chronic cardiopulmonary diseases.

14. The answer is A. *(Braunwald, ed 11, chap 94.)* The pathogenicity of staphylococci is related to a number of biologic properties, including the production of coagulase, leukocidin, exotoxin, and enterotoxin. Coagulase and leukocidin are thought to protect staphylococci within a host from being destroyed by phagocytes. Some staphylococcal strains produce an exotoxin that can cause intraepidermal cleavage and bullae formation. Other strains elaborate an enterotoxin that produces gastrointestinal disease. The production of penicillinase, though rendering a pathogenic organism harder to destroy pharmacologically, does not contribute to pathogenicity.

15. The answer is A. *(Braunwald, ed 11, chaps 94, 346.)* Probably because of its ubiquity and ability to stick to foreign surfaces, *Staphylococcus epidermidis* is the most frequent cause of infections of central nervous system shunts, as well as an important cause of infection on artificial heart valves and orthopedic prostheses. *Corynebacterium* species (diphtheroids), just like *S. epidermidis*, colonize the skin. When these organisms are isolated from cultures of shunts, it is often difficult to be sure if they are the cause of disease or simply contaminants. Leukocytosis in cerebrospinal fluid, consistent isolation of the same organism, and the character of a patient's symptoms all are helpful in deciding whether treatment for infection is indicated.

16. The answer is D. *(Braunwald, ed 11, chap 95.)* Streptococcal pharyngitis, usually caused by group A streptococci, is an exceedingly common bacterial infection, especially in school-age and adolescent children. Symptoms commonly include sudden sore throat and pain on swallowing, fever, headache, malaise, anorexia, nausea, and abdominal pain; aside from edema, erythema, and lymphoid hyperplasia of the posterior pharynx, physical signs also include tender, enlarged cervical lymph nodes. Because involvement of the larynx does not occur, loss of voice would not be expected.

17. The answer is B. *(Braunwald, ed 11, chap 103.)* Vaccines prepared from high-molecular-weight antigens of *Neisseria meningitidis*, serotypes A and C, have proved effective, but an effective group B vaccine is not available. Although sulfonamide resistance is an important problem in meningococcal epidemics with sulfonamide-sensitive organisms, sulfonamides remain a good choice for prophylaxis. When sulfonamide-resistant strains are isolated but the sensitivity of the organism is not known, rifampin therapy is generally recommended.

18. The answer is E. *(Braunwald, ed 11, chap 104.)* Single-dose therapy with either oral amoxicillin or ampicillin plus probenicid is still the treatment of choice for gonorrhea. In homosexual men, intramuscular penicillin, rather than oral amoxicillin or ampicillin, is recommended because the organisms tend to be somewhat more penicillin-resistant in these individuals. Noncompliance, antibiotic resistance due to penicillinase production, reinfection, and simultaneous infection with *Chlamydia* are all possible causes for a therapeutic failure.

19. The answer is C. *(Braunwald, ed 11, chap 105.)* *Pseudomonas* organisms can cause a rapidly invasive infection resulting in extensive bony erosion in diabetics. Aggressive surgical debridement and parenteral administration of antibiotics are required for treatment. *Aspergillus* organisms can be isolated frequently from external ear swabs but do not cause invasive disease. Mucormycosis must be considered in any seriously ill diabetic patient with sinus or ocular involvement. Infection usually spreads from the nasal cavity and does not involve the ears. Insulin-dependent diabetics are more likely to have their skin colonized by *S. aureus*, but such colonization is not associated with external otitis. *H. influenzae* is a frequent cause of otitis media, especially in children, but not of otitis externa.

20. The answer is C. *(Braunwald, ed 11, chap 107.)* *Salmonella typhi* survives well in food and water and generally causes infection by penetrating the intestinal mucosa and entering the bloodstream. Usually at the time that affected individuals present with fever and other signs of an acute illness, the white blood cell count is depressed. In contrast, rose spots usually do not occur until the second week of illness. Therapy with chloramphenicol does not prevent relapses but does alter the course of the acute illness. A chronic carrier state can develop in large part because of the propensity of *S. typhi* to seed and inhabit the gallbladder, especially in adults with gallstones.

21. The answer is E. *(Braunwald, ed 11, chap 109.)* Individuals who have sickle-cell disease or agammaglobulinemia and individuals who have been splenectomized have defective opsonization and are more likely to develop infections with encapsulated organisms, like *Haemophilus influenzae*. *H. influenzae* infections also are more common in alcoholic individuals, in part because of abnormal cellular defense mechanisms. Individuals who have chronic granulomatous disease have problems combating infection with *Staphylococcus aureus, Salmonella,* and *Serratia,* but not *H. influenzae*.

22. The answer is A. *(Braunwald, ed 11, chap 109.)* Because a marked lymphocytosis characteristically is observed in children who have *Haemophilus pertussis* infection (whooping cough) and is rare in other respiratory illnesses, white blood cell count with differential would be useful in making the diagnosis. Blood cultures would be negative, and Gram stain of the sputum and chest and neck x-rays would show nonspecific changes. The diagnosis of pertussis is confirmed in most cases by nasopharyngeal culture.

23. The answer is E. *(Braunwald, ed 11, chap 146.)* Coccidioidomycosis, caused by the inhalation of *Coccidioides immitis,* may present clinically with manifestations of hypersensitivity reactions. Arthralgias and frank arthritis (so-called desert rheumatism) as well as such skin reactions as erythema nodosum and erythema multiforme are associated far more frequently with coccidioidomycosis than with the other mycoses listed in the question. Delayed hypersensitivity to *C. immitis* antigens tends to be a good prognostic sign.

24. The answer is E. *(Braunwald, ed 11, chaps 109, 346.)* Although ampicillin alone was recommended for the treatment of *Haemophilus influenzae* meningitis until a few years ago, the emergence of ampicillin-resistant strains now necessitates that all systemic infections potentially due to this organism be treated with chloramphenicol until the results of antimicrobial sensitivities are known. The ampicillin resistance is due to the production of a β-lactamase, which confers resistance to carbenicillin as well. Most authorities therefore recommend beginning therapy with both ampicillin and chloramphenicol, then dropping chloramphenicol if the organism is found to be sensitive to ampicillin. To avoid interference between the drugs, ampicillin should be given 30 to 60 minutes before chloramphenicol.

25. The answer is E. *(Braunwald, ed 11, chap 110.)* *Haemophilus ducreyi* causes painful genital ulcers, which begin as small tender papules. In contrast, syphilitic ulcers are usually painless, and the initial lesions of genital herpes simplex infections are usually vesicular. The organism causing chancroid can be isolated from both the ulcers and affected lymph nodes; in fact, culturing the lymph nodes may produce a pure culture of this organism. Unlike infection with other members of the genus *Haemophilus,* therapy with ampicillin is ineffective in treating chancroid. Trimethoprim-sulfamethoxazole and erythromycin are the antibiotic agents of choice.

26. The answer is D. *(Braunwald, ed 11, chap 146.)* Individuals who have localized sporotrichosis can be treated successfully with potassium iodide. However, systemic infections, particularly pneumonia in immunocompromised individuals, should be treated with amphotericin B. Untreated individuals can develop chronic sporotrichosis.

27. The answer is B. *(Braunwald, ed 11, chap 113.)* Aspiration and culture of an enlarged axillary lymph node would be most helpful in yielding a diagnosis of tularemia in the case described. Blood and bone-marrow cultures rarely are positive for *Francisella (Pasteurella) tularensis.* Agglutinin reactions ordinarily are not positive for at least one week after infection. A wide variety of animals and insects can transmit tularemia to humans.

INFECTIOUS DISEASES

28. The answer is D. *(Braunwald, ed 11, chap 114.)* In the case presented, the diagnosis of plague (*Yersinia pestis* infection) must be considered. To make this diagnosis, affected lymph nodes should be aspirated and the contents Gram-stained. In most cases of bubonic plague, lymph-node aspirates teem with pleomorphic gram-negative bacilli, which can be identified immediately by immunofluorescent staining of the specimen. Blood culture, bone-marrow examination, and lymph-node biopsy might be used to diagnose plague, but with undue delay. In this situation, great care should be exercised in handling the infected materials—there is a significant risk of infection for the laboratory workers.

29. The answer is A. *(Braunwald, ed 11, chap 117.)* Legionnaire's disease is caused by *Legionella pneumophila*. It occurs sporadically or in outbreaks and often begins with myalgias, headache, and fever. Diarrhea and delirium also are early features in many cases. Gastrointestinal symptoms should suggest the possibility of this diagnosis, particularly in persons who have severe pneumonia, scant production of sputum, and other extrapulmonary abnormalities. Of the other organisms listed in the question, all can cause pneumonia; *Mycoplasma pneumoniae* infection is most likely to be confused with Legionnaire's disease.

30. The answer is D. *(Braunwald, ed 11, chap 97.)* *Listeria monocytogenes* is a gram-positive motile bacillus that tends to infect infants as well as persons over the age of 55 years. Major illnesses in both groups are meningitis and other forms of central nervous system infection. Many of the older patients are immunosuppressed because of disease (e.g., cancer), immunosuppressive drug therapy, or both. Endocarditis, peritonitis, hepatitis, and conjunctivitis also can be caused by *Listeria* infection.

31. The answer is B. *(Braunwald, ed 11, chap 96.)* Persons with diphtheria characteristically have a sore throat and experience pain on swallowing; examination reveals a gray-white pharyngeal membrane. Hoarseness and stridor occur when the membrane extends to the larynx, an event that can result in upper airway obstruction. High fever generally is not associated with diphtheria, unless a streptococcal infection is superimposed.

32. The answer is D. *(Braunwald, ed 11, chap 98.)* Anthrax is caused by *Bacillus anthracis*, a gram-positive bacillus. This organism is one of a small group of gram-positive bacilli able to be isolated in the clinical laboratory; others in this group include *B. subtilis*, *Corynebacterium*, *Listeria*, and *Lactobacillus*. Characteristically, persons acquire anthrax from handling infected animal hides or carcasses. As in syphilis, but in very few other infections, the typical skin ulcer and affected lymph nodes are not very tender and constitutional symptoms are mild.

33. The answer is B. *(Braunwald, ed 11, chap 116.)* *Salmonella* bacteremia is a particularly frequent complication of bartonellosis, a peculiar infection associated with hemolytic anemia and occurring predominantly in certain valleys in the Andes Mountains of South America. Salmonellosis is also a problem in other hemolytic disorders, such as sickle cell disease. It is thought that this association is due to an acquired abnormality in the reticuloendothelial cell system. Pneumococcal bacteremia occurs frequently in splenectomized individuals, *Haemophilus influenzae* pneumonia in individuals with agammaglobulinemia, *Pneumocystis carinii* pneumonia in individuals with leukemia, and herpes zoster in individuals with various malignancies (e.g., Hodgkin's disease).

34. The answer is A. *(Braunwald, ed 11, chap 119.)* The diagnosis of a tuberculous pleural effusion is suggested by the following set of pleural-fluid findings; color, clear yellow; pH, < 7.20; protein, > 3.0 g/dL; glucose, < 25 mg/dL; lactate dehydrogenase (LDH), > 450 units/mL; and a lymphocytosis. Tubercle bacilli rarely are identified on a smear of infected pleural fluid, and cultures are positive in no more than one-quarter of cases. Antituberculous treatment usually should commence as soon as the diagnosis is suspected.

35. The answer is D. *(Braunwald, ed 11, chap 127.)* In a patient with Lyme disease, biopsy of the typical skin lesion, erythema chronicum migrans, usually shows nondiagnostic perivascular lymphocytic and histiocytic infiltration. Though hematogenous dissemination of the spirochete causing Lyme disease, *Borrelia burgdorferi*, does occur, it is rarely detected on direct examination. The spirochete has been cultured from blood, skin, and cerebrospinal fluid (CSF), but culture of this organism is not a routine procedure. Frank meningitis with CSF pleocytosis rarely occurs until several weeks or months into the illness. Lymphocytosis and an elevated protein level are typically found but are not diagnostic. The most useful study is a serum determination of IgG antibody titers which are almost uniformly elevated after several weeks of illness.

36. The answer is A. *(Braunwald, ed 11, chap 121.)* Two of the lesser-known species of *Mycobacterium*, *M. scrofulaceum* and *M. avium-intracellulare*, cause lymphadenitis in children. Usually affected are the lymph nodes that drain the buccal mucosa. Both *M. scrofulaceum* and *M. avium-intracellulare* respond poorly to chemotherapy. Treatment of choice, therefore, is prompt lymph-node excision, before rupture has occurred.

37. The answer is D. *(Braunwald, ed 11, chap 121.)* *Mycobacterium marinum* is known as the "swimming pool" or "fishtank" bacillus, because ulcerative cutaneous infections can be acquired from contact with contaminated swimming pools and aquariums. *M. ulcerans* also causes ulcerative skin lesions but characteristically is confined to tropical regions. Other "atypical" mycobacteria that cause cutaneous infections in humans include *M. avium-intracellulare*, *M. scrofulaceum*, *M. kansasii*, and *M. fortuitum*.

38. The answer is C. *(Braunwald, ed 11, chap 117.)* Legionnaire's disease is caused by *Legionella pneumophila*. Person-to-person spread of this soil organism has not been documented. Gastrointestinal symptoms preceding pneumonia are sometimes a clue to the diagnosis. In many cases, chest x-ray shows dense infiltrates despite paucity of physical signs, such as rales or rhonchi; in this regard, the disease resembles *Mycoplasma* pneumonia. Although *L. pneumophila* has been found in vitro to be sensitive to several drugs, erythromycin is the treatment of choice.

39. The answer is D. *(Braunwald, ed 11, chap 117.)* Since the recognition of *Legionella pneumophila*, several other species of *Legionella* have been discovered. These organisms can be detected by silver staining, immunofluorescent staining, and culture of infected materials. It is much better to culture lung tissue or pleural fluid than sputum, because sputum contains a mixture of other organisms, which tend to overgrow *Legionella*. Aside from direct methods of diagnosis, serologic tests run on paired serum specimens also are useful.

40. The answer is E. *(Braunwald, ed 11, chap 122.)* Newborn infants of women who had syphilis during pregnancy will have reactive standard serologic tests, such as the VDRL and fluorescent *Treponema pallidum* antibody-absorption (FTA-ABS) tests, even if they are free of infection, because maternal IgG antibody crosses the placenta and enters the fetal bloodstream. Fetal infection, however, stimulates production of IgM antibody, which does not cross the placenta. Therefore, only an IgM-FTA-ABS test is able to indicate if an infant has syphilis or simply has acquired IgG antibody from the mother. This principle also is used in determining whether neonates have acquired other infections, such as toxoplasmosis, rubella, and cytomegalovirus infection.

41. The answer is C. *(Braunwald, ed 11, chap 126.)* Relapsing fever can be diagnosed by finding spirochetal borreliae in a peripheral blood smear. Sometimes it is necessary to examine thick smears or to use phase microscopy to see the organisms. In the western United States, especially in areas in which tick bites are likely to occur, relapsing fever should be suspected in individuals with acute febrile illnesses characterized by headache, photophobia, and muscle pains.

42. The answer is A. *(Braunwald, ed 11, chap 147.)* In the examination of purulent material from persons suspected of having actinomycosis, it is important to search the material for the characteristic "sulfur granules" and then to examine the granules for organisms. Actinomycetes are gram-positive branching organisms. If they are detected in an individual presenting with a suggestive clinical picture, such as a chronic draining sinus in the oropharyngeal area, the gastrointestinal tract, or the pelvic area, then the diagnosis of actinomycosis is ensured.

INFECTIOUS DISEASES

43. The answer is C. *(Braunwald, ed 11, chap 146.)* Initial diagnosis of cryptococcal meningitis usually is based on finding encapsulated yeast on an India ink preparation. This test, however, is positive in only about half of cases in which the diagnosis is eventually made. Testing of serum and cerebrospinal fluid for cryptococcal antigen is a very helpful adjunctive test, because antigen is found in about 90 percent of cases. In pulmonary cryptococcosis, only about one-third of affected persons are antigen-positive.

44. The answer is A. *(Braunwald, ed 11, chap 146.)* All of the infections listed in the question are associated with pneumonitis, which, however, heals in a slightly different pattern for each infection. Calcifications in healed granulomata are frequent in histoplasmosis. Radiographic findings in children who have had primary histoplasmosis can include spotty calcifications in the lung and hilar lymph nodes; in adults, round accumulations of scar tissue sometimes featuring a central area of calcification (histoplasmomas) may be identified.

45. The answer is D. *(Braunwald, ed 11, chap 146.)* Fungal and yeast infections, predominantly candidiasis, aspergillosis, and mucormycosis, occur frequently in severely immunosuppressed patients, particularly those who have received broad-spectrum antibiotics for a prolonged period. A number of other types of fungal infection occur in these patients. About half of all cases of *Cryptococcus neoformans* infection occur in individuals who have lymphoma, are taking glucocorticosteroids, or are otherwise immunocompromised. The association of cryptococcal meningitis and Hodgkin's disease is important clinically.

46. The answer is D. *(Braunwald, ed 11, chap 101.)* *Clostridium difficile* can be isolated on selective agar media, but this method is not dependable for diagnosis. Pseudomembranous colitis (PMC) is caused by the local action of at least two enterotoxins, toxins A and B. Serologic tests are not helpful. The punctate plaques on a hyperemic mucosa are characteristics of PMC, but similar pathologic changes can be seen with ischemic colitis. The best diagnostic test is the demonstration of *C. difficile* cytotoxin, an assay that can be positive in 24 hours. Clostridia are part of normal fecal flora, so a Gram stain of the stool would not be helpful.

47. The answer is D. *(Braunwald, ed 11, chap 146.)* As primary therapy for dermatophytosis (ringworm), topical undecylenic acid, clotrimazole, and tolnaftate usually are recommended. In severe cases, griseofulvin generally is used, with ketoconazole recommended for griseofulvin-resistant cases. Amphotericin is not a recommended treatment of dermatophytosis.

48. The answer is E. *(Braunwald, ed 11, chap 150.)* Trachoma remains the most important cause of preventable blindness in the world. Blindness occurs primarily because of damage to the cornea and eyelids. Corneal abrasion, scarring of the lids, secondary infections, and loss of lacrimal function are the principal problems.

49. The answer is E. *(Braunwald, ed 11, chap 150.)* Fever, chills, headache, cough, and myalgias are the typical presenting signs and symptoms of psittacosis. Gastrointestinal symptoms also may occur but are much less frequent. The diagnosis of psittacosis usually depends on serologic tests or cultures of respiratory secretions. Even a low-titer positive complement fixation antibody test, in conjunction with the clinical setting described, would strongly suggest the diagnosis of psittacosis and warrant the use of tetracycline.

50. The answer is D. *(Braunwald, ed 11, chap 141.)* Both mumps and bacterial parotitis produce fever, and both may be associated with elevated serum amylase levels because of the release of salivary amylase into the blood. In individuals who have mumps, the parotid glands are usually not as warm and tender as in individuals who have bacterial parotitis. Mumps tends to be a disease of children and young adults, whereas bacterial parotitis tends to affect the elderly. The most useful distinguishing feature, however, is probably the nature of the parotid secretions. In bacterial parotitis, significant numbers of leukocytes and bacteria, usually staphylococci, are found in parotid secretions; in mumps, only a small amount of parotid fluid, and no pus, is observed.

51. The answer is C. *(Braunwald, ed 11, chap 139.)* As many as 90 percent of the patients with poliovirus are asymptomatic or have only a self-limited febrile illness. Paralytic polio is characterized by an initial febrile illness that resolves followed by development of aseptic meningitis and asymmetric paralysis. In contrast to polio, the Guillain-Barré syndrome is characterized by symmetric muscle weakness with frequent paresthesias but normal reflexes. Motor neurons are primarily affected by poliovirus infection resulting in the loss of reflexes and flaccid paralysis. Return of neuronal function may be possible for up to six months after infection.

52. The answer is A. *(Braunwald, ed 11, chap 205.)* The man described in the question has symptoms suggesting influenza complicated by bacterial pneumonia. Pneumococci and staphylococci are the leading pathogens causing secondary bacterial infection in this situation, and effective therapy would include drugs that act against penicillinase-producing staphylococci. The agent of choice is nafcillin or another semisynthetic penicillinase-resistant penicillin; penicillin G would be an ill-advised choice. Other drugs acceptable as alternative therapies would include vancomycin, clindamycin, and cephalothin.

53. The answer is B. *(Braunwald, ed 11, chap 149.)* Most authorities recommend using erythromycin in the treatment of persons who have community-acquired bronchopneumonia because the drug is effective therapy for pneumococcal as well as mycoplasmal infections, the leading causes. It also is an effective treatment for Legionnaire's disease. Tetracycline may not always be effective against pneumococci, and penicillin V potassium and cephalexin are not effective against mycoplasma. Chloramphenicol is too toxic for initial therapy of bronchopneumonia.

54. The answer is D. *(Braunwald, ed 11, chap 129.)* Acyclovir is now the drug of choice in the treatment of herpes encephalitis. It has been shown to be more effective than vidarabine and also has fewer side effects. Acyclovir has been shown both to shorten viral shedding in mucocutaneous infections and to prevent outbreaks in immunocompromised patients. Similarly, acyclovir is useful in immunocompromised patients with herpes zoster, but it is not indicated in nonimmunocompromised patients in whom the risk of dissemination is very small. Both the frequency and the duration of recurrent episodes of genital herpes are reduced on long-term suppressive therapy. As soon as the drug is discontinued, however, infection recurs.

55. The answer is E. *(Braunwald, ed 11, chaps 225, 227.)* Precisely how diabetes mellitus and sickle cell disease predispose to urinary tract infection is unclear. In persons with diabetes, glycosuria and neuropathic changes in bladder function are probably contributory. In association with both diabetes and sickle cell disease, avascular areas in the kidney probably provide sites for bacterial multiplication remote from phagocytic cells. In hyperparathyroidism and gout, stone formation leads to obstruction and infection. Although in Wilson's disease copper is deposited in the kidney and tubular dysfunction occurs, urinary infections generally are not a major problem.

56. The answer is A. *(Braunwald, ed 11, chap 346.)* Computerized tomography scanning is the best test to identify a brain abscess and has largely supplanted arteriography in this setting. Radionuclide scanning is also quite reliable, if CT facilities are not available. Generally, a CT or radionuclide scan is sufficient to rule out the diagnosis of brain abscess; rarely are both a scan and an arteriogram needed to rule out this diagnosis.

57. The answer is E. *(Braunwald, ed 11, chaps 136, 347.)* Among the many viruses that can cause acute encephalitis, the most frequent cause in the United States is herpes simplex. A few years ago, this fact would have been of academic interest only, but with the availability of antiviral chemotherapy, establishment of the specific diagnosis can be fruitful. Brain biopsy and CT scanning are the most helpful procedures for establishing this diagnosis.

58. The answer is E. *(Braunwald, ed 11, chap 161.)* Cryptosporidia, a protozoan, cannot be cultured from the stool. They stain with iodine but not Gram's stain. Investigational serologic tests appear promising but are not readily available. Because of their small size (5 μm) and lack of motility, detection of cysts by wet mounts is very difficult. By using acid-fast stains or rhodamine fluoresence, even a few cysts can be detected easily and the diagnosis of cryptosporidiosis made.

INFECTIOUS DISEASES

59. The answer is D. *(Braunwald, ed 11, chap 88.)* Methicillin-resistant *Staphylococcus aureus* is becoming a major source of morbidity and mortality. In vitro sensitivity testing may demonstrate sensitivity to cephalosporins, but these tests are unreliable and all strains are resistant in vivo. These strains have an altered penicillin-binding protein, and are resistant to all penicillinase-resistant penicillins, alone or in combination with an aminoglycoside. Resistance is not plasmid-mediated, and there is no risk of spread to other bacteria. Administration of vancomycin is the most effective treatment.

60. The answer is D. *(Braunwald, ed 11, chap 120.)* A papular reaction usually develops in patients with tuberculoid leprosy one month after injection of killed suspensions of *Mycobacterium leprae*, but it is not diagnostic since positive reactions occur in nearly all adults. Culture of *M. leprae* is exceedingly difficult and can only be accomplished in mice or armadillos. A minimum of six months is usually required before the results are available; therefore cultures are not practical for diagnosis. Erythema of existing skin lesions with dapsone therapy usually occurs in borderline patients and is not diagnostic. Demonstration of the organism on microscopic examination of a biopsy specimen is the only definitive way to make the diagnosis of leprosy.

61. The answer is B. *(Braunwald, ed 11, chap 160.)* The infective cysts of *G. lamblia* can survive for several months in cold water and have been responsible for large epidemics in communities such as Vail, Colorado. Immunity to giardia is not well understood, but there is no increased incidence in granulocytopenic patients. Intestinal IgA may be important, as deficient patients appear to be at increased risk of infection. Transmission is primarily by the fecal-oral route, resulting in higher incidence in male homosexuals, retarded patients in institutions, and children in day-care centers.

62. The answer is E. *(Braunwald, ed 11, chap 163.)* Adult worms do reside in lymph nodes, but biopsy is relatively contraindicated because of the potential to exacerbate problems with lymphatic drainage. Serologic testing is available at specialized centers using indirect hemagglutination, but cross-reactions with other filariae are common. Intense pruritus and a rash developing after administration of diethylcarbamazine (Mazzotti's test) suggest dermal microfilaria; it typically occurs in patients with onchocerciasis. Maintenance of filariae in cultures or animals is extremely difficult. The best animal model is in cats, but this technique plays no role in clinical diagnosis. Diagnosis is best made by demonstrating microfilariae on a Giemsa stain of blood. *W. bancrofti* microfilariae usually maintain a nocturnal periodicity and are found in the bloodstream in greatest number at night. The exact reason for the periodicity is not known, but it may be related to oxygen tension in the pulmonary vessels.

63. The answer is A-N, B-N, C-N, D-Y, E-Y. *(Braunwald, ed 11, chap 9.)* Fever does little measurably to influence host defense mechanisms and does not influence phagocytosis or the bactericidal action of neutrophils. Fever blisters occur in certain infections, such as pneumococcal pneumonia, malaria, and meningococcemia, but they are rare in other infections, such as tuberculosis and mycoplasma infections. The basis for these associations is not known. Bacterial abscesses infrequently cause relapsing or sustained fever; usually the fever is intermittent. A cool bath or a cooling blanket is much better than an alcohol rub for reducing fever. Morphine, meperidine, and other parenteral opiates can relieve rigors associated with rapid defervescence, blood-product administration, and amphotericin therapy.

64. The answer is A-Y, B-N, C-Y, D-Y, E-N. *(Braunwald, ed 11, chap 85.)* Nosocomial infections often are caused by antibiotic-resistant organisms, which acquire their resistance through R-factor transfer. Preventive measures are key. For example, if catheter care is good, it should be possible to maintain a sterile urinary tract for at least 5 to 7 days in most patients. Intravenous lines of all types tend to become infected after about 3 days; the danger is somewhat less with needles than with plastic cannulas. There is no good evidence to suggest that individuals having hepatitis surface antigen in their blood should be prevented from drawing blood or working directly with patients.

65. The answer is A-Y, B-Y, C-Y, D-Y, E-N. *(Braunwald, ed 11, chap 83.)* Each microbial illness is best diagnosed by a specific set of laboratory procedures. For example, although it is difficult to isolate bacteria from the blood in most bacterial infections, the spirochetes causing relapsing fever can be seen in routine blood smears. In malaria, routine Wright's staining also is sufficient to recognize the parasites in many cases, although thick smears may be necessary. Both *Nocardia* and *Mycobacterium* are acid-fast organisms, a key to their identification in the laboratory. The early diagnosis of *Legionella* has been facilitated by the development of immunofluorescent staining, but it can only be done reliably in reference laboratories having highly skilled technologists. Because a single throat swab can detect about 90 percent of patients with streptococcal pharyngitis, a negative result is very helpful in excluding this diagnosis. In persons with partially treated meningitis, gram-positive organisms may fail to stain well and often appear gram-negative.

66. The answer is A-Y, B-N, C-Y, D-N, E-Y. *(Braunwald, ed 11, chap 84.)* Impaired immune competence increases the risk of infection. Splenectomized individuals, for example, have an increased frequency of bacteremic infections, with pneumococci accounting for about two-thirds of these infections. Gamma globulin therapy is of proven benefit only for individuals with agammaglobulinemia and for prophylaxis for or treatment of certain specific infections; in most individuals with hypogammaglobulinemia, it is of no benefit. Neutropenia is the most common host-defense abnormality associated with cyclophosphamide treatment. Infection is more of a problem for individuals deficient in the late complement components than in complement components C1, C2, and C4, because C3 can be activated by either the classic or the alternate pathway. Long-term high-dose glucocorticosteroid therapy is thought to increase the risk of infection in humans, but this relationship has yet to be proven.

67. The answer is A-Y, B-N, C-Y, D-Y, E-N. *(Braunwald, ed 11, chap 86.)* Granulocytopenia and thrombocytopenia are seen in persons with severe septic shock; they are thought to occur because of direct effects of endotoxin on these cells as well as because of changes in the vascular endothelium. In addition, complement activation, with the generation of C5a, appears to increase granulocyte margination and lead to a further reduction in the blood granulocyte count. Although sepsis leads to complement activation and increased turnover of complement components in the blood, usually the total serum complement and C3 levels remain in the normal range. Both prostacyclin and naloxone are beneficial in the treatment of experimental septic shock; both agents improve tissue blood flow and prevent the severe sequelae of hypotension.

68. The answer is A-Y, B-N, C-Y, D-N, E-Y. *(Braunwald, ed 11, chap 88.)* Cephalosporin antibiotics are an acceptable alternative to penicillin therapy in individuals known to be allergic to penicillin. However, because cephalosporins do not penetrate well into the cerebrospinal fluid, their use is not recommended in individuals with proven or suspected meningitis. Cefazolin is much less painful than cephalothin when given intramuscularly and can be administered less frequently because of a longer blood half-life. Cefoxitin is active against *Bacteroides fragilis*. Cefamandole is more active against many gram-negative aerobes, but most stains of *Klebsiella* resistant to cephalothin are also resistant to cefamandole.

69. The answer is A-Y, B-N, C-Y, D-Y, E-N. *(Braunwald, ed 11, chap 88.)* Procaine and benzathine penicillins are less painful to administer intramuscularly than is penicillin G (benzyl penicillin) and are more apt to sustain low blood levels of antibiotic because of their slower absorption. Amoxicillin is much better absorbed than ampicillin. Neither ampicillin nor carbenicillin is effective against *Klebsiella*; this organism usually is sensitive to cephalosporin and aminoglycoside antibiotics, such as cephalothin and gentamicin, respectively. Ticarcillin is a semisynthetic penicillin that is two to four times as effective against *Pseudomonas* as is carbenicillin. Clinical evidence has not shown therapeutic superiority for nafcillin and oxacillin over methicillin; nafcillin is used frequently because some data suggest that interstitial nephritis is a more common consequence of methicillin therapy.

INFECTIOUS DISEASES

70. The answer is A-N, B-Y, C-N, D-N, E-Y. *(Braunwald, ed 11, chap 90.)* A man who has dysuria but no urethral exudate or leukocytes in a urethral swab specimen probably does not have a chlamydial infection. On the other hand, if he has an exudate in which intracellular gram-negative diplococci are not seen, he should be considered to have chlamydial urethritis and treated presumptively with tetracycline, an antibiotic also effective against gonococci. A pregnant woman with presumed chlamydial cervicitis should be treated with erythromycin, because tetracycline can produce fetal complications. Sulfa creams are ineffective in the treatment of *Gardnerella vaginalis* infections; metronidazole or ampicillin is the preferred form of therapy. Genital ulcers in U.S. residents are due most frequently to herpes simplex virus; elsewhere in the world, syphilis and chancroid are more common.

71. The answer is A-Y, B-Y, C-N, D-N, E-N. *(Braunwald, ed 11, chap 93.)* Type 3 pneumococci cause the most severe of all pneumococcal infections; the reason is not known. All splenectomized individuals, even those without underlying disease, should receive pneumococcal vaccine. The "crisis" in pneumococcal pneumonia ordinarily corresponds to the appearance of type-specific antibodies, not maximum leukocytosis. Alcoholic individuals who develop pneumococcal pneumonia have a poor prognosis for several reasons: their tendency to aspirate pharyngeal flora, poor functioning of bronchial clearance mechanisms, and impaired leukocyte response (hypogammaglobulinemia generally is not a contributing factor). Pneumococcal pneumonia frequently precedes pneumococcal meningitis. Pneumococci cause pharyngitis extremely rarely.

72. The answer is A-Y, B-N, C-N, D-Y, E-Y. *(Braunwald, ed 11, chap 95.)* Streptococcal M protein is the factor most strongly associated with virulence—strains rich in M protein resist phagocytosis. On the other hand, T protein, which also serves as a basis for typing, is not related to virulence. Titers of antistreptolysin O (ASLO) are elevated in some individuals who have poststreptococcal glomerulonephritis, particularly those who have had pharyngitis; individuals with streptococcal pyoderma generally do not have elevated ASLO titers. The erythrogenic toxin causing scarlet fever is produced in bacteria infected with a lysogenic bacteriophage; several types of streptococci as well as staphylococci can be so infected. Streptococcal pyoderma may lead to acute glomerulonephritis but not to acute rheumatic fever. The reason for this phenomenon remains unexplained.

73. The answer is A-N, B-Y, C-Y, D-Y, E-N. *(Braunwald, ed 11, chap 124.)* Leptospirosis can be transferred from infected animals directly to humans who contact contaminated tissue or urine. Leptospirosis often is confused with influenza because of its initial manifestations: fever, headache, and myalgias. It causes hepatitis often associated with very elevated serum bilirubin levels, probably a result of both intravascular hemolysis and impaired bilirubin excretion. Leptospiral meningitis resembles a viral, or aseptic, meningitis; cerebrospinal fluid has a normal glucose concentration, and although a few neutrophils may be present, lymphocytes are the predominant cell type observed. The diagnosis of acute leptospirosis is made best by blood cultures; dark-field microscopy too often gives false-positive or false-negative results.

74. The answer is A-N, B-Y, C-Y, D-Y, E-N. *(Braunwald, ed 11, chap 104.)* Gonococcemia tends to be a problem of menstruating women, although men also are affected. The characteristic skin lesions are small pustules that usually occur first on the fingers and feet. The arthritis associated with gonococcemia is rarely symmetrical, a clinical finding that is often helpful in making the diagnosis. Gonococci producing β-lactamase are resistant to penicillin and ampicillin but are sensitive to the newer cephalosporins, such as cefotaxime and ceftriaxone. Treatment with spectinomycin is also effective; this agent usually is recommended as the first choice for treatment failures attributed to penicillinase production by the organism. Gonococci with pili are more virulent than gonococci without pili (pili may help the organism stick to epithelial cells to initiate infection).

75. The answer is A-Y, B-N, C-Y, D-N, E-N. *(Braunwald, ed 11, chap 105.) Acinetobacter,* previously called *Mimae herellae* and *Bacterium anitratum,* is a ubiquitous commensal organism that is an important cause of bacteremia, pneumonia, and other serious infections. It is a gram-negative rod that can be confused with *Neisseria* on Gram stain because of its pleomorphic appearance. It is also confused with Enterobacteriaceae species in cultures because of its simple growth requirements. Unlike *Neisseria,* it is resistant to penicillin and ampicillin but sensitive to gentamicin and tobramycin; this difference in antibiotic sensitivity makes it very important to distinguish this organism from *Neisseria* in clinical isolates from patients with serious illnesses.

76. The answer is A-N, B-N, C-N, D-Y, E-Y. *(Braunwald, ed 11, chap 106.)* Melioidosis is caused by *Pseudomonas pseudomallei,* a gram-negative bacillus ubiquitous in many tropical areas of Asia and Africa. Infection occurs from contact with contaminated soil. Pulmonary infections are most frequent; in patients acutely ill with pneumonia, many organisms can be detected in sputum. The organisms can be grown on routine culture media. Serologic tests are used largely for epidemiologic studies. Melioidosis, particularly the chronic form, may be mistaken for tuberculosis; granulomas may develop, but calcification of cavitary lung lesions does not occur. In acute melioidosis, therapy with tetracycline and chloramphenicol plus either trimethoprim-sulfamethoxazole, sulfisoxazole, kanamycin, or novobiocin is recommended. Although the organism is usually sensitive to each of these agents, the high fatality rate of this disease (greater than 50 percent) has led to the use of a multiple antibiotic regimen.

77. The answer is A-Y, B-Y, C-Y, D-N, E-Y. *(Braunwald, ed 11, chap 112.)* Brucellosis is an important veterinary disease in those parts of the world from which it has not yet been eradicated. It is still a problem in cattle-rearing areas of the United States. The disease usually presents with low-grade fever and constitutional symptoms; affected individuals have lymphadenopathy, splenomegaly, and, sometimes, hepatomegaly. During the early bacteremic phase of the illness, *Brucella* can be isolated using routine cultures, provided they are kept long enough (i.e., up to 4 weeks). The diagnosis also is made using agglutination tests. Therapy with streptomycin and tetracycline still is best.

78. The answer is A-Y, B-N, C-Y, D-Y, E-N. *(Braunwald, ed 11, chap 115.) Vibrio cholerae* enterotoxin causes a diffuse, noninflammatory secretion of isotonic intestinal fluid without injury to the absorptive surface. Early diagnosis is aided by dark-field microscopy or immobilization of organisms with type-specific antisera; definitive diagnosis, however, depends on culturing the organisms. Oral therapy with solutions containing sodium bicarbonate and either glucose or sucrose is recommended. This therapy usually is begun on the basis of a presumptive diagnosis in endemic areas. Oral tetracycline also is useful, because it can shorten the symptomatic period. Infection confers some immunity, so that, in endemic areas, children are usually the ones affected. Cholera vaccine is not particularly effective and is now not ordinarily recommended for travelers to endemic areas.

79. The answer is A-Y, B-Y, C-Y, D-N, E-Y. *(Braunwald, ed 11, chap 100.)* The most potent of all poisons, the toxins produced by *Clostridium botulinum* are partially degraded then absorbed in the upper gastrointestinal tract. They block presynaptic transmission, probably by inhibiting acetylcholine release, and cause progressive descending muscle paralysis and, frequently, death. Guanidine hydrochloride pharmacologically enhances acetylcholine release and thus may be useful in treating persons with botulism. Edrophonium (Tensilon) may reverse slightly the weakness of botulism, but the effect is transient and generally less than that associated with its use in persons who have myasthenia gravis.

80. The answer is A-Y, B-Y, C-N, D-Y, E-Y. *(Braunwald, ed 11, chap 122.)* Syphilis causes few symptoms in its earliest phases, especially in pregnant women. The newborn infants of infected women will be reactive serologically, because maternal IgG antibodies cross the placenta and circulate in the fetal blood. In untreated syphilis, the VDRL test often becomes nonreactive; however, the more sensitive fluorescent *Treponema pallidum* antibody-absorption (FTA-ABS) test remains reactive. Untreated individuals are more likely to die of a ruptured aortic aneurysm or other cardiovascular event than from neurosyphilis or any other cause. Treatment with at least 6 million units of penicillin G is usually sufficient to prevent the development of symptomatic neurosyphilis.

INFECTIOUS DISEASES

81. The answer is A-Y, B-Y, C-N, D-Y, E-Y. *(Braunwald, ed 11, chap 146.)* Amphotericin B is an effective systemic antifungal medication associated with rather troublesome side effects. It is best to give a test dose of 1 mg of amphotericin and then gradually increase the dose to about 0.3 (mg/kg)/day; with severe infections, the dose is increased rapidly. Because hydrocortisone may decrease drug fever and phlebitis associated with use of amphotericin, it is recommended that hydrocortisone be added to the intravenous infusion. Alternate-day treatment is as effective as, and much more convenient than, daily therapy and helps to spare veins for future intravenous infusions; however, the incidence of fever is increased with alternate-day therapy. In fungal meningitis, intrathecal amphotericin usually is given into the cisternal or ventricular cerebrospinal fluid—lumbar injections are more likely to cause pain and adhesive arachnoiditis.

82. The answer is A-N, B-Y, C-N, D-Y, E-Y. *(Braunwald, ed 11, chap 146.)* The molds *Mucor* and *Rhizopus*, the main causes of mucormycosis, are more often seen in than grown from pathologic specimens—the reasons why they are so hard to grow have not been identified. Fungal hyphae tend to invade blood vessels, leading to hemorrhagic necrosis. Sinusitis is the predominant illness in infected persons who have diabetes mellitus; in persons with hematologic malignancies, pulmonary disease is more common. Diagnosis is best accomplished by biopsy and histologic examination (serology is still in the investigative stages). Amphotericin is the only known treatment of mucormycosis.

83. The answer is A-N, B-Y, C-N, D-Y, E-Y. *(Braunwald, ed 11, chap 148.)* Rocky Mountain spotted fever is a tick-borne disease caused by *Rickettsia rickettsii*, a gram-negative organism. The disease is associated with severe headache, myalgias, arthralgias, but not frank arthritis. The characteristic rash is at first macular and confined to the extremities; after several days, the rash spreads to involve the buttocks, trunk, axilla, neck, and face and becomes maculopapular, then hemorrhagic, and finally ulcerative. Treatment with chloramphenicol or tetracycline, which are rickettsiostatic agents, is most effective if begun before the rash has become hemorrhagic. Ticks found on household pets should be removed carefully with tweezers, and not by hand, in order to prevent infection through minor skin abrasions.

84. The answer is A-N, B-Y, C-N, D-Y, E-Y. *(Braunwald, ed 11, chap 149.)* *Mycoplasma pneumoniae* is an important cause of pneumonia, particularly in young adults. The organism cannot be seen by Gram stain, because it does not retain the dye-iodine complex. The cold-agglutinin test is nonspecific; firm serologic evidence of mycoplasma infection usually comes from a complement-fixation test (other specific serologic tests also are available). Treatment with either tetracycline or erythromycin is effective. In nonepidemic situations in which it is often difficult to know whether a person has a pneumococcal or *Mycoplasma* infection, erythromycin is the better choice of treatment.

85. The answer is A-Y, B-N, C-Y, D-Y, E-N. *(Braunwald, ed 11, chap 94.)* Toxic shock syndrome (TSS) is a toxin-mediated disorder that has been linked to the ability of hyperabsorbent tampons to bind magnesium, promoting toxin production. Though the patients may appear to be in shock, with refractory hypotension, blood cultures are almost uniformly negative. With the increased recognition and prevention of menstruation-associated TSS, the relative frequency in nonmenstruating women and in men is increasing. In the severe form of the syndrome, gastrointestinal, hepatic, renal, muscular, and CNS involvement occurs not infrequently. The diagnosis of TSS in a postsurgical patient may be a clinical challenge since the signs of infection are usually minimal and occur as soon as two days after the operation.

86. The answer is A-Y, B-Y, C-Y, D-Y, E-N. *(Braunwald, ed 11, chap 134.)* Characteristically, all the lesions in smallpox vesiculate at the same time. Skin lesions remain infectious until they have healed and the crusts are gone. Examination of vesicle fluid by either electron microscopy or immune precipitation of virus particles is helpful in making the diagnosis of variola. Thiosemicarbazone is not effective for treatment, only for prophylaxis. The eradication of smallpox and the risk of untoward complications of vaccination have resulted in the lifting of all requirements for smallpox vaccination by the U.S. government.

87. The answer is A-N, B-Y, C-Y, D-N, E-N. *(Braunwald, ed 11, chap 142.)* With the development of progressively less toxic rabies vaccines, such as the currently available duck embryo vaccine (DEV) and human diploid cell vaccine (HDCV), the indications for prophylactic vaccination are widening. Spelunkers (cave explorers), in addition to veterinarians, animal pathologists, and laboratory technicians who work with potential sources of rabies virus, should be considered for vaccination. With HDCV, preexposure prophylaxis would consist of three intramuscular injections on days 0, 7, and 21 to 28. If DEV is used, two 1-mL subcutaneous injections should be given 1 month apart, followed by a booster in about 7 months. Antibody titers should be checked periodically to ensure that an adequate level of immunity persists.

88. The answer is A-Y, B-Y, C-Y, D-Y, E-Y. *(Braunwald, ed 11, chap 138.)* The most common features of infectious mononucleosis are fever, sore throat, and lymphadenopathy. Sore throat, the most commonly described symptom, is observed in about 80 percent of young adults with this infection. Atypical lymphocytes, identified as T cells with suppressor and cytotoxic action, appear in the peripheral blood during the first week of illness. Heterophil antibodies, which are sheep red-cell agglutinins associated with the immunoglobulin M serum fraction, usually persist in the serum for a few months. On the other hand, antibodies to Epstein-Barr virus often can be detected for years in the serum of persons who have had infectious mononucleosis. The incubation period in young adults is thought to be 30 to 50 days; in children, the incubation period is much shorter.

89. The answer is A-N, B-N, C-N, D-N, E-N. *(Braunwald, ed 11, chap 118.)* Cat-scratch disease, as the name implies, is transmitted to humans chiefly by cat scratches. Other animal vectors have not been recognized. Lymphadenopathy often persists for weeks; examination of a lymph-node biopsy specimen may show granulomas, abscess formation, or generalized reticulum cell hyperplasia. Splenomegaly generally does not develop. Antibiotics are ineffective in treating persons with cat-scratch disease.

90. The answer is A-Y, B-Y, C-N, D-N, E-Y. *(Braunwald, ed 11, chap 153.)* Although *Entamoeba histolytica* can infect some animals, the principal hosts are humans. Even in the presence of large or multiple amebic liver abscesses, defervescence usually occurs in 1 to 3 days with appropriate medical therapy. The abscess cavity in amebic liver abscess usually contains no neutrophils or amebas; the infection does not evoke a typical acute inflammatory response, and amebas are found only at the edge of the advancing infection. Amebic serologic tests stay positive for months to years despite therapy. Deaths from amebiasis are uncommon; however, failure to make the diagnosis in a timely fashion is among the most important causes of these deaths.

91. The answer is A-Y, B-Y, C-Y, D-Y, E-N. *(Braunwald, ed 11, chap 154.)* One of the most intriguing recent findings in malarial research is the fact that there are strain-specific receptors for attachment of the malarial merozoites. For example, the Duffy antigen on red blood cells is a site of attachment for *Plasmodium vivax*. Immune-complex nephritis is a feature of acute malaria; intraglomerular globulin deposits can be detected by immunofluorescent staining. The development of specific antibodies leads to a reduction in parasitemia; however, infection continues because the antibodies do not affect the residual intracellular organisms. "Tropical splenomegaly," which appears to occur because of excessive, persistent immune stimulation, responds to antimalarial treatment. One of the most important causes of malaria in the United States is too-hasty discontinuation of prophylaxis after travelers return home from an endemic area (6 weeks is recommended).

92. The answer is A-Y, B-N, C-Y, D-Y, E-Y. *(Braunwald, ed 11, chap 157.)* Toxoplasmosis is a relatively common infection; serologic data indicate that possibly as many as two-thirds of the U.S. adult population have had some form of the infection. The most serious manifestations appear to arise when the disease is acquired during pregnancy. Infection during the first trimester can result in spontaneous abortion, stillbirth, prematurity, or severe disease in any of several organ systems; infection during the third trimester more commonly leads to neonatal disease, which, however, tends to be asymptomatic. Infections acquired before pregnancy generally are of little consequence to the offspring. Immunocompromised individuals usually have recrudescent disease. Diagnosis in these individuals is often difficult to make, in part because the serologic responses are blunted by the disease process. Serologic screening of asymptomatic immunocompromised patients may be helpful for recognizing toxoplasmosis at a later date.

93. The answer is A-Y, B-N, C-N, D-Y, E-Y. *(Braunwald, ed 11, chap 158.)* The onset of *Pneumocystis carinii* pneumonia is characterized by a paucity of physical findings. Sputum, which is produced in scant amounts, usually contains normal flora and very few, if any, leukocytes. Pleural effusions are rare, and because there is little cellular reaction the lung usually is not damaged permanently. However, fully developed *P. carinii* pneumonia can lead to marked tachypnea and dyspnea, massive consolidation, and extensive changes on chest x-ray. Systemic dissemination is rare. The infection generally arises as a result of a serious underlying disease; consequently, the prognosis is poor. Trimethoprim-sulfamethoxazole and pentamidine are equally efficacious; however, trimethoprim-sulfamethoxazole is preferred because it can be given orally and has fewer side effects.

94. The answer is A-N, B-N, C-Y, D-N, E-N. *(Braunwald, ed 11, chap 164.)* *Schistosoma mansoni* infection of the liver causes cirrhosis from vascular obstruction but relatively little hepatocellular injury. Hepatosplenomegaly, hypersplenism, and esophageal varices develop quite commonly, and schistosomiasis usually is associated with eosinophilia. Spider nevi, gynecomastia, jaundice, and ascites are uncommon.

95. The answer is A-Y, B-N, C-Y, D-Y, E-N. *(Braunwald, ed 11, chap 108.)* *Shigella sonnei* is the most common isolate in developed countries while *S. dysenteriae* and *S. flexneri* predominate in tropical areas. Fewer than 100 organisms can cause disease irrespective of gastric acidity. Transmission by the fecal-oral route is the most important and occurs most frequently in areas of crowding and poor sanitation. Bacteremia with *Shigella* organisms is distinctly unusual, probably because the organism is sensitive to complement-mediated lysis. Unlike infection with *Salmonella* organisms, antibiotic therapy of shigellosis can shorten both symptoms and fecal shedding.

96. The answer is A-N, B-Y, C-Y, D-Y, E-N. *(Braunwald, ed 11, chap 119.)* Pleural effusions occur most frequently in young patients with primary infection associated with an abrupt onset of symptoms. Effusions are being noted more frequently in older individuals with reactivation disease, but they still account for less than one third of patients in North America with pleurisy. Laryngeal and bronchitic tuberculosis are very infectious because the bacilli are readily aerosolized. Response to therapy is usually good. In the absence of neurologic abnormalities, extensive bony involvement by tuberculosis usually requires chemotherapy alone. Involvement of the basilar meninges is very common in meningeal tuberculosis resulting in cranial nerve abnormalities. Gastrointestinal infection usually occurs in association with cavitary disease with large numbers of organisms. The terminal ileum and cecum are the most common sites, resulting in disease that can be difficult to differentiate from Crohn's disease. The stomach is very resistant to infection.

97. The answer is A-N, B-Y, C-N, D-N, E-Y. *(Braunwald, ed 11, chap 127.)* The complete clinical spectrum of Lyme disease was first identified in the northeastern United States, but it is now recognized to have a worldwide distribution. Erythema chronicum migrans usually starts as an erythematous macule at the site of the tick bite and eventually forms a characteristic annular lesion with central clearing which is present in approximately 90 percent of patients within a month. Constitutional symptoms including headache, fever, chills, and fatigue are common at the time of onset of skin lesions. Approximately 10 to 15 percent of patients have neurologic involvement with Lyme disease which can be manifested as meningitis (with a lymphocytic pleocytosis), cranial neuritis, chorea, mononeuritis multiplex, or motor and sensory radiculoneuritis. Parenteral therapy with penicillin is recommended for patients with significant neurologic or cardiac involvement.

98. The answer is A-N, B-Y, C-Y, D-N, E-Y. *(Braunwald, ed 11, chap 101.) Clostridium* species are present in high numbers in normal intestinal flora and soil, and it is not surprising that they are frequent isolates from wound cultures. The presence of necrotic tissue and a low oxidation reduction potential are necessary to establish severe disease. Treatment is based on the clinical setting, and a culture positive for clostridia alone does not warrant therapy. *Clostridium perfringens* produces at least 12 toxins, one of the most important of which is the alpha toxin. It has been associated with hemolysis and capillary and platelet damage. *C. perfringens* is a common cause of food poisoning associated with contaminated meats and poultry. The serous discharge from the overlying skin in a patient with gas gangrene has many gram-positive rods but few inflammatory cells, emphasizing the importance of an early Gram stain when the diagnosis is suspected. More than 70 percent of cases of *C. septicum* septicemia reported in the literature are associated with malignant neoplasms, especially of the gastrointestinal tract.

99. The answer is A-N, B-Y, C-Y, D-N, E-N. *(Braunwald, ed 11, chap 102.)* Anaerobic pulmonary infections most often develop in the setting of aspiration. The sudden development of a bacterial pneumonia in a healthy teenager would most likely be caused by *Streptococcus pneumoniae*. Both anaerobic and aerobic organisms are implicated in Ludwig's angina, an infection originating from the third molar which can rapidly spread through soft tissues of the mandible and pharynx. Pharyngeal anaerobic bacteria, including *Bacteroides melaninogenicus, Fusobacterium* sp., and anaerobic cocci, cause bacterial aspiration pneumonia in a patient who has a diminished gag reflex, such as with a seizure disorder. It is important to differentiate bacterial aspiration, which requires antibiotic therapy, from aspiration of stomach contents, which usually occurs after general anesthesia and resolves with symptomatic therapy. Anaerobic bacteria are a very unusual cause of endocarditis which, like aerobic gram-negative organisms, may in part be explained by a failure to adhere to damaged valves.

100. The answer is A-N, B-N, C-Y, D-Y, E-N. *(Braunwald, ed 11, chap 136.)* Less than 5 percent of patients will have a second recurrence of herpes zoster unless they are immunosuppressed. Acute cerebellar ataxia is the most common form of neurologic involvement in children. It usually develops three weeks after the rash and resolves spontaneously. Chickenpox is one of the most contagious diseases, infecting up to 90 percent of seronegative persons, presumably via the respiratory route. Varicella pneumonia can cause fever and severe hypoxia, complicating the course of chickenpox infection in up to 20 percent of adults. Varicella-zoster immune globulin is recommended only for immunodeficient patients under the age of 15 years who have been exposed to varicella.

101. The answer is A-N, B-Y, C-Y, D-N, E-Y. *(Braunwald, ed 11, chap 137.)* Perinatal transmission of CMV occurs by passage through an infected birth canal or through the breast milk of a seropositive mother. Though such transmission is very common, symptomatic infection is distinctly unusual except in premature infants in whom interstitial pneumonitis may develop. Congenital infection with CMV occurs in approximately 1 percent of births in the United States, but detectable disease develops in less than 0.05 percent of births, almost exclusively in association with primary maternal infections. CMV produces a syndrome very similar to mononucleosis with Epstein-Barr virus. Cervical lymphadenopathy and exudative pharyngitis are usually not present, however, and heterophile antibodies are absent. CMV pneumonia can prove fatal in greater than 80 percent of bone marrow transplant patients. Salivary excretion of the virus or positive sputum cultures do not implicate CMV as the cause of pulmonary infiltrates. Definitive diagnosis rests on the demonstration of the characteristic pathologic findings—intranuclear inclusions in enlarged epithelial cells—on lung biopsy. Diagnosis of CMV infection rests on characteristic pathologic findings, a four-fold rise in serology titer, or culture of CMV, usually from urine, saliva, or buffy coat. Because viral excretion can continue for weeks to months, isolation of CMV does not always implicate acute infection.

102. The answer is A-N, B-Y, C-N, D-Y, E-Y. *(Braunwald, ed 11, chap 140.)* Both Norwalk virus and rotavirus infect the small intestinal epithelium causing malabsorption and osmotic diarrhea. Worldwide, rotavirus is the most important cause of dehydrating diarrhea in infants. Rotavirus is shed in large quantities in the stool allowing for easy diagnosis by culture or immunoassays to detect viral antigens. Norwalk virus is presumably spread by the fecal-oral route and has also been implicated in food-borne

INFECTIOUS DISEASES

and water-borne epidemics. The clinical manifestations of infection by both viruses are characterized by vomiting, diarrhea, and occasionally, low-grade fewer. Rotavirus is a major cause of diarrhea in children under three years of age while Norwalk virus causes disease more often in older children and adults.

103. The answer is A-N, B-N, C-Y, D-N, E-Y. *(Braunwald, ed 11, chap 130.)* Major epidemics are associated only with influenza A and have been attributed to "antigenic shifts" or reassortment of genomic segments possibly with animal strains. Between pandemics, minor antigenic variations occur through point mutations. Antibodies against the hemagglutinin are most important, presumably preventing viral attachment. Influenza B tends to cause smaller outbreaks, with less severe disease, because there is no animal reservoir and major antigenic shifts do not occur. Prolonged fatigue or "postinfluenzal asthenia" may occur, but the etiology is not known. Viral shedding usually stops 2 to 5 days after symptoms in uncomplicated influenza. Both amantadine and rimantadine can either prevent or attenuate infection with influenza A. In major outbreaks, therapy may be useful until immunity can be established by immunization.

104. The answer is A-N, B-Y, C-N, D-Y, E-Y. *(Braunwald, ed 11, chap 99.)* Neonatal tetanus is associated with a more than 60 percent mortality rate. It is caused by infections of the umbilical stump. In third world countries the infection is often associated with practices of applying dirt or feces to the umbilical stump to speed sloughing. Human immune globulin cannot affect tetanus toxin that is already bound in the central nervous system, but it can be helpful if given early to bind any free toxin. Such small amounts of tetanospasmin are present that no immunity develops and active immunization must be initiated. Trismus or lockjaw is the most common manifestation of tetanus, caused by neuromuscular blockade and central disinhibition of motor neurons. Immune globulin provides protective antibody levels for up to four weeks and should be given along with toxoid for serious wounds if fewer than two previous doses of toxoid have been given.

105–108. The answers are: 105-B, 106-D, 107-A, 108-C. *(Braunwald, ed 11, chap 84.)* Several distinct infectious syndromes have been linked to specific deficits in host defenses. Complement appears to be critical in the defense against neisserial infections since patients with deficiencies in the late components have recurrent *N. gonorrhoeae* and *meningitidis* infections. The spleen is one of the most important sites for phagocytosis of opsonized organisms. After splenectomy, whether surgical or functional as in sickle cell diseases, patients are at risk for development of bacteremia with organisms where antibody forms the major host defense: *S. pneumoniae, Haemophilus influenzae*, and *N. meningitidis*. Patients with AIDS are susceptible to multiple infections against which intact cellular immunity is required. *Pneumocystis carinii* is the most frequent infection, but cytomegalovirus, *Mycobacterium avium-intracellulare*, and cryptococcal infections are also common. In chronic granulomatous disease, neutrophils are able to phagocytize but not kill bacteria resulting in recurrent infections with staphylococci and gram-negative bacteria.

109–113. The answers are: 109-E, 110-B, 111-A, 112-C, 113-D. *(Braunwald, ed 11, chap 89.)* In addition to the need for fluid replacement and symptomatic therapy, the management of acute diarrhea should always include consideration of stool examination and culture to guide selection of specific treatment. Usually, fluid replacement and symptomatic therapy are begun immediately, based on the clinical exam. The decision to begin specific antibiotic therapy in persons with invasive bacterial diarrhea depends on finding leukocytes in the stool and culturing pathogenic bacteria or protozoa from the stool. In enterotoxigenic *Escherichia coli* diarrhea, fecal leukocytes are not present; therapy with bismuth subsalicylate should relieve symptoms. In *Yersinia, Shigella*, and *Campylobacter* infections, fecal leukocytes are present and the organisms can be cultured. Antibiotic therapy, especially indicated when symptoms are severe, is with trimethoprim-sulfamethoxazole, ampicillin, and erythromycin, respectively. *Giardia*, which can be seen in a wet mount of infected stool, should be treated with quinacrine or metronidazole.

114–118. The answers are: 114-D, 115-C, 116-A, 117-B, 118-B. *(Braunwald, ed 11, chap 128.)* Steady progress is being made in the prevention and treatment of viral infections. Inactivated virus vaccines are available for influenza, rabies, polio, and several arboviruses causing encephalitis. Attenuated virus vaccines are available for rubella, mumps, measles, polio, and yellow fever. Passive immunization is used for hepatitis, varicella, and Lassa fever; broader application is hampered because the procedure is cumbersome and expensive. Transfer of the slow virus that causes Creutzfeldt-Jakob disease is prevented by careful sterilization of surgical equipment used for neurosurgical procedures. Chemoprophylaxis with methisazone (*N*-methylisatin 3-thiosemicarbazone) for smallpox and amantidine for influenza has been useful; however, vaccination is a more effective preventive measure for both diseases. The development of antiviral agents—e.g., acyclovir and vidarabine (adenine arabinoside, ara-A)—has been significant.

119–123. The answers are: 119-B, 120-C, 121-E, 122-D, 123-D. *(Braunwald, ed 11, chap 128.)* A host can mobilize several defense mechanisms for protection against viral infection. Skin and mucous membranes serve a barrier function. Intracellular, secreted, and circulating proteins have numerous functions. For example, immunoglobulin A prevents viruses from entering the body, and immunoglobulin G prevents viruses from entering host cells once they are within the body. Interferon, which blocks replication of viruses once they enter host cells, is produced by many types of cells, chiefly monocytes of the reticuloendothelial cell system and T lymphocytes. Plasma cells and B lymphocytes manufacture antibody proteins—namely, immunoglobulins A, D, E, G, and M. Patients with impaired humoral or cellular immunity are particularly apt to develop viral infections.

124–127. The answers are: 124-B, 125-C, 126-A, 127-D. *(Braunwald, ed 11, chap 166.)* Each of the helminths listed in the question causes a different kind of human disease. *Enterobius vermicularis* (pinworm) infects the gastrointestinal tract and causes rectal itching. Itching is worse at night, when female pinworms journey outside the intestine to lay eggs in the perianal region. *Necator americanus* (hookworm) also infects the gastrointestinal tract. Infected individuals tend to present with weakness and fatigue, manifestations of the anemia that results from intestinal blood loss. *Clonorchis sinensis*, the Chinese liver fluke, causes vascular obstruction in the liver and, as a consequence, jaundice and cirrhosis. *Schistosoma haematobium* infects the bladder and causes bleeding and urinary tract obstruction, which promotes secondary bacterial infection.

DISORDERS OF THE HEART AND VASCULAR SYSTEM

DIRECTIONS: Each question below contains five suggested answers. Choose the **one best** response to each question.

128. A 48-year-old man is admitted to the coronary care unit with an acute inferior myocardial infarction. Two hours after admission, his blood pressure is 86/52 mmHg; his heart rate is 40/min with sinus rhythm. Which of the following would be the most appropriate initial therapy?

(A) Immediate insertion of a temporary transvenous pacemaker
(B) Intravenous administration of atropine sulfate, 0.6 mg
(C) Administration of normal saline, 300 mL over 15 minutes
(D) Intravenous administration of dobutamine, 0.35 mg/min
(E) Intravenous administration of isoproterenol, 5.0 µg/min

129. All of the following are features of captopril EXCEPT that it

(A) decreases plasma renin activity
(B) retards the degradation of circulating bradykinin
(C) inhibits formation of angiotensin II
(D) can be used safely in combination with a beta-blocking agent
(E) is contraindicated in patients with bilateral renal artery stenosis

130. All of the following statements regarding beta-blocking agents are true EXCEPT

(A) pindolol has partial beta-agonist activity
(B) metoprolol is a selective beta-1 antagonist
(C) labetelol is both an alpha- and a beta-receptor blocking agent
(D) atenolol can be administered safely in large doses to asthmatic patients
(E) nadolol can be administered effectively once a day

131. Which of the following physical findings is associated with the chest x-ray shown below?

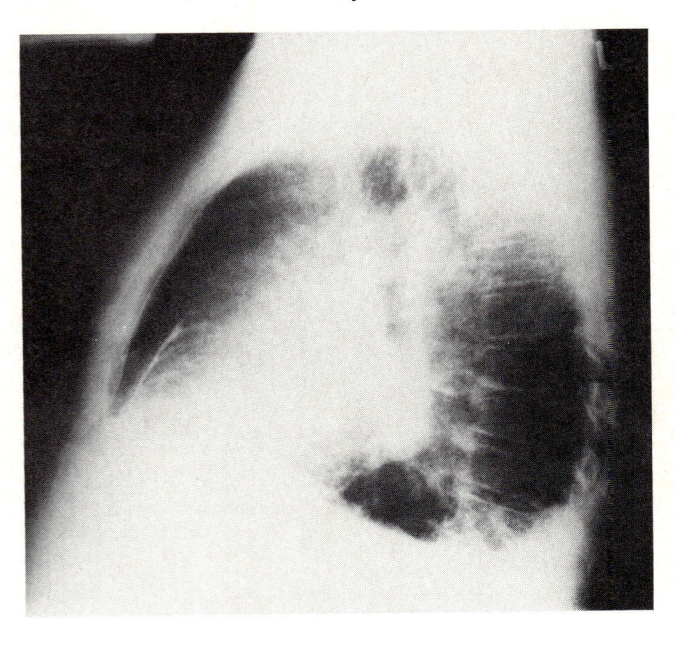

(A) Wide splitting of the second heart sound
(B) Opening snap and diastolic rumble
(C) Pericardial knock
(D) Late-peaking systolic ejection murmur
(E) Central cyanosis

132. Combined echocardiographic and Doppler echocardiographic studies are useful in the evaluation of all of the following disorders EXCEPT

(A) aortic stenosis
(B) atrial septal defect
(C) tricuspid regurgitation
(D) mitral stenosis
(E) calcification of the left coronary artery

133. A 73-year-old man recently began having frequent syncopal episodes upon rising from recumbency. Associated complaints include constipation, difficulty voiding, and dry skin. Evaluation reveals orthostatic hypotension in the absence of compensatory tachycardia while the man is standing, but no evidence of degeneration of the central nervous system, including the extrapyramidal tracts and basal ganglia. Glucocorticoid and mineralocorticoid secretion is normal; plasma norepinephrine concentration, measured while the man is supine, is low.

The treatment LEAST likely to benefit this man is

(A) high salt intake
(B) elastic supportive hose
(C) fludrocortisone acetate (Florinef)
(D) ephedrine sulfate
(E) tyramine

134. All of the following statements regarding percutaneous transluminal coronary angioplasty (PTCA) are true EXCEPT

(A) restenosis resulting after successful dilation develops in approximately 20 percent of patients within 6 months
(B) stenoses within saphenous vein bypass grafts can be dilated using this technique
(C) a recent complete *occlusion* of a coronary artery can be successfully dilated using this technique
(D) A 65 percent stenosis of the left main coronary artery is a contraindication to this procedure
(E) If restenosis develops several weeks after a successful dilation, repeated PTCA is unlikely to be successful

135. The echocardiogram shown below was recorded during a bout of chest pain in a 35-year-old woman. A murmur is present on physical examination. The echo study is diagnostic of

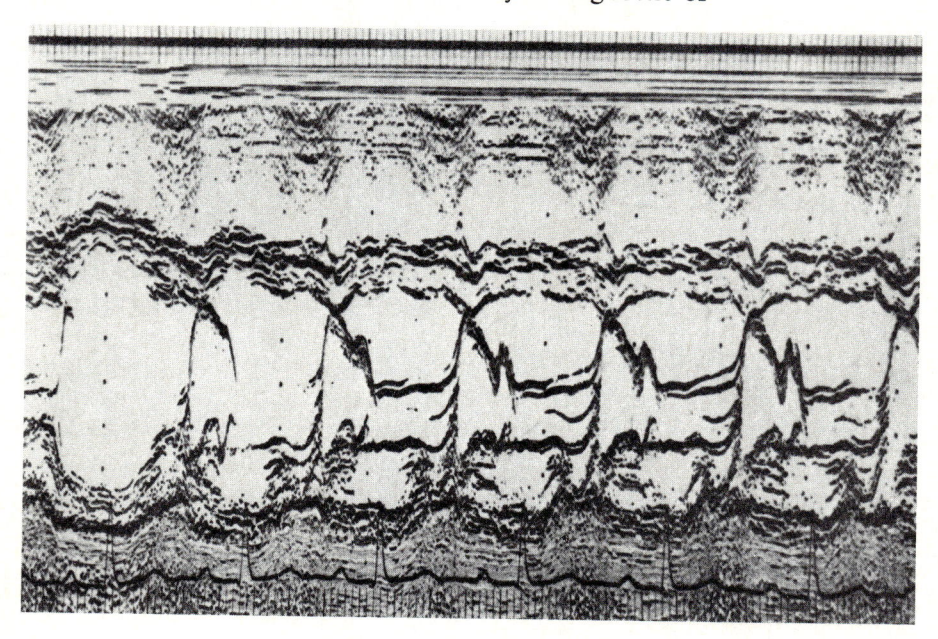

(A) papillary muscle dysfunction
(B) ruptured chordae tendineae
(C) mitral stenosis
(D) mitral regurgitation
(E) mitral valve prolapse

136. A 42-year-old woman has bilateral ankle edema of recent onset. On examination, jugular venous pulse is 5 cmH$_2$O and the hepatojugular reflux is negative. The woman's ankle edema would NOT be explained by which of the following conditions?

(A) Pelvic thrombophlebitis
(B) Venous varicosities
(C) Cyclic edema
(D) Hypoalbuminemia
(E) Right heart failure

137. Which of the following causes of congestive heart failure is NOT associated with a widened arterial–mixed venous oxygen difference?

(A) Tricuspid stenosis
(B) Alcoholic cardiomyopathy
(C) Paget's disease
(D) Constrictive pericarditis
(E) Right ventricular infarction

138. Digitalis glycosides enhance myocardial contractility primarily by which of the following mechanisms?

(A) Opening of calcium channels
(B) Release of calcium from the sarcoplasmic reticulum
(C) Stimulation of myosin ATPase
(D) Stimulation of membrane Na$^+$-K$^+$-ATPase
(E) Inhibition of membrane Na$^+$-K$^+$-ATPase

139. An elderly individual who has been taking digitalis for heart failure is brought to the hospital because of anorexia and nausea. On examination, ventricular bigeminy is noted. Digoxin level is 1.5 ng/mL. Which of the following factors would NOT be expected to contribute to digitalis intoxication?

(A) Chronic obstructive lung disease with hypoxemia
(B) Addition of quinidine to the therapeutic regimen
(C) Diuretic therapy with loop diuretics
(D) Hyperthyroidism
(E) Hyperparathyroidism

140. Clues to the presence of atrioventricular nodal block (as opposed to trifascicular block) would include all the following EXCEPT

(A) clinical evidence of inferior myocardial infarction
(B) Wenckebach periodicity to conduction
(C) escape-focus rate faster than 50 beats/min
(D) a narrow QRS complex at the escape focus
(E) unresponsiveness of the escape focus to atropine

141. A 79-year-old woman has daily episodes of lightheadedness. A rhythm strip shows sinus bradycardia at 52/min, and 2.5-second sinus pause that produces no symptoms. The next step in this woman's management should be

(A) implantation of a permanent demand ventricular pacemaker
(B) trial of a temporary transvenous pacemaker
(C) institution of sublingual isoproterenol therapy
(D) continuous 24-hour Holter monitoring
(E) exercise tolerance testing

142. A 60-year-old man is admitted to a hospital because of respiratory failure and tachycardia. His rectal temperature is 38.3°C (101°F), respiratory rate 32/min and blood pressure 100/60 mmHg. His admission electrocardiogram is shown below. Which of the following measures would constitute the most appropriate management for this man?

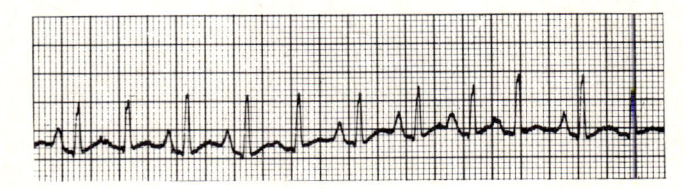

(A) Administration of digitalis
(B) Supplemental oxygenation or mechanical ventilation
(C) Electrical cardioversion after the blood pressure is raised
(D) Administration of quinidine after digitalization
(E) Administration of verapamil

143. A 57-year-old previously healthy woman develops atrial flutter, 2:1 atrioventricular conduction, and a ventricular rate of 150/min. Her ventricular rate could be decreased safely with the use of all the following EXCEPT

(A) digoxin
(B) verapamil
(C) propranolol
(D) quinidine
(E) carotid sinus message

144. All the following statements regarding secundum atrial septal defect are true EXCEPT

(A) it is more frequent in females than in males
(B) affected individuals are usually asymptomatic in childhood
(C) electrocardiography shows a leftward axis
(D) echocardiography shows abnormal ventricular septal motion
(E) atrial arrhythmias are common

145. A 64-year-old man is examined because of episodes of exertional chest pain. An M-mode echocardiogram is shown below. A continuous-wave Doppler signal across the aortic valve showed a peak systolic velocity of 5 m/sec; no diastolic turbulence was detected.

Which of the following statements concerning this patient is true?

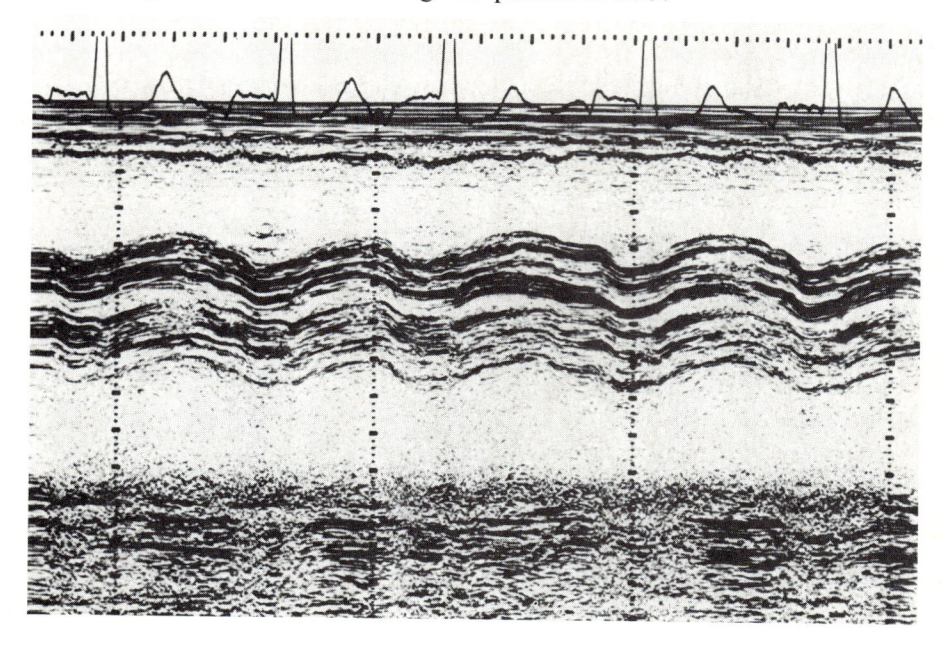

(A) Significant aortic regurgitation is most likely present
(B) The peak gradient across the aortic valve is approximately 100 mmHg
(C) The gradient across the aortic valve cannot be determined from the information given
(D) Coronary arteriography is unnecessary in this patient; immediate aortic valve replacement is indicated
(E) The Doppler findings rule out important aortic stenosis. An exercise test should be performed to evaluate this man's chest pain

---

146. A 20-year-old woman has mild pulmonic stenosis (transvalvular gradient is 20 mmHg). All the following statements regarding this situation are true EXCEPT

(A) heart size on chest x-ray is likely to be normal
(B) electrocardiogram is likely to be normal
(C) her jugular *a* wave is likely to be prominent
(D) compared to other valvular defects, the risk of endocarditis is relatively low
(E) frequent monitoring for progression of the stenosis is indicated

147. Which of the following findings would NOT be expected in a person with coarctation of the aorta?

(A) A systolic murmur across the anterior chest and back and a high-pitched diastolic murmur along the left sternal border
(B) A higher blood pressure in the right arm than in the left arm
(C) Inability to augment cardiac output with exercise
(D) Rib notching on chest x-ray
(E) Persistent hypertension despite complete surgical repair

148. The chest x-ray shown below would most likely have been taken of which of the following individuals?

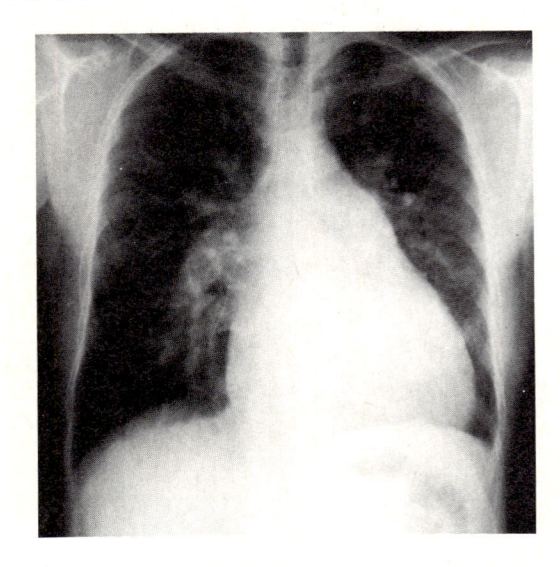

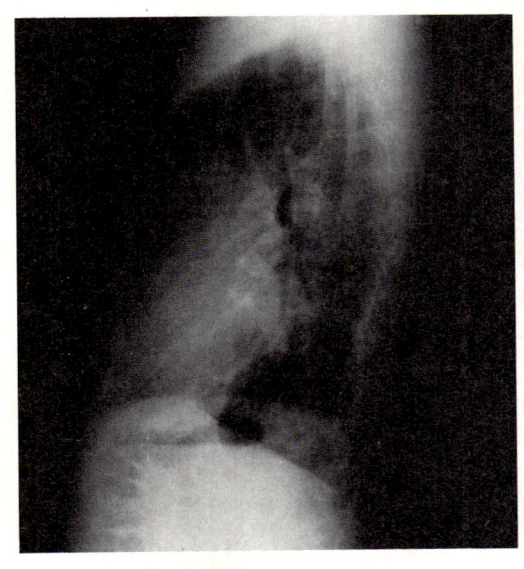

(A) A 38-year-old woman who has hemoptysis, dyspnea on exertion, and fatigability
(B) A 36-year-old woman who has a heart murmur but is asymptomatic
(C) A 32-year-old woman who has a continuous murmur, widened systemic pulse pressure, and dyspnea on exertion
(D) A 40-year-old woman who has a loud first heart sound, a diastolic rumble, a large *v* wave in her jugular pulse, and ascites
(E) None of the above

149. Which of the following statements regarding acute rheumatic fever is NOT true?

(A) Joint deformities are not present
(B) Serum assay for rheumatoid factor is frequently positive
(C) Acute carditis usually produces no symptoms referable to the heart
(D) Incidence is higher in overcrowded areas
(E) Urticaria and angioneurotic edema rarely occur

150. Embolism to the lower extremities most commonly arises from

(A) an abdominal aortic aneurysm
(B) an ulcerated plaque along the thoracic aorta
(C) the heart
(D) localized femoral artery thrombosis
(E) none of the above

151. Which of the following statements best describes long-acting nitrate preparations?

(A) They are almost completely degraded in the liver
(B) Their effect can be blocked by high doses of $beta_2$ selective inhibitors
(C) Nitroglycerin ointment is most effective pharmocologically when applied to the anterior chest
(D) Oral preparations are more effective than sublingual ones
(E) Oral administration of isosorbide should not exceed 15 mg every 3 to 4 hours

152. A previously healthy 58-year-old man is admitted to the hospital because of an acute inferior myocardial infarction. Within several hours, he becomes oliguric and hypotensive (blood pressure is 90/60 mmHg). Insertion of a pulmonary artery (Swan-Ganz) catheter reveals the following pressures: pulmonary capillary wedge, 4 mmHg; pulmonary artery, 22/4 mmHg; and mean right atrial, 11 mmHg.
This man would best be treated with

(A) fluids
(B) digoxin
(C) norepinephrine
(D) dopamine
(E) intraaortic balloon counterpulsation

153. A 62-year-old woman was started on a regimen of quinidine sulfate because of asymptomatic ventricular couplets. One week later, she was admitted to the hospital after a syncopal episode. Serum electrolyte concentrations were normal. The arrhythmia shown below appeared transiently on her cardiac monitor.

The recommended course at this time is to

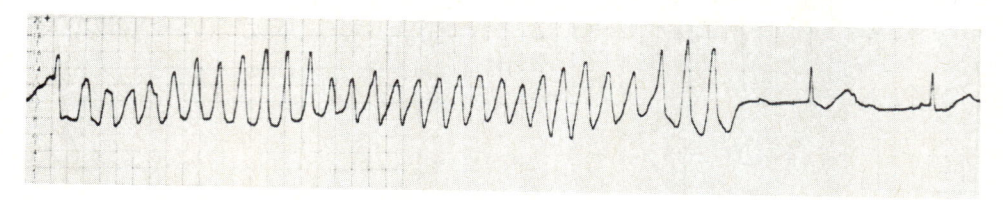

(A) increase the quinidine dose
(B) discontinue administration of quinidine and observe
(C) begin intravenous administration of procainamide 2 mg/min
(D) administer sodium bicarbonate, 70 meq, intravenously
(E) administer potassium chloride, 10 meq, intravenously over one hour

---

154. This 2-dimensional echocardiogram was most likely recorded in which of the following patients?

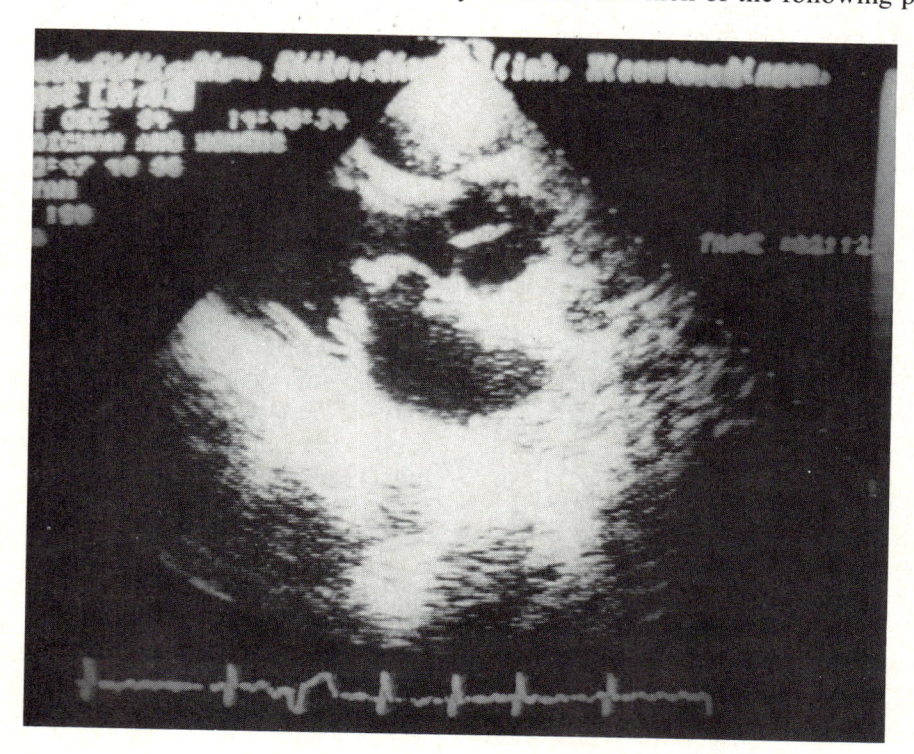

(A) A 54-year-old man with syncopal episodes when bending forward
(B) A previously healthy 68-year-old man with sudden onset of pulmonary edema and a new holosystolic murmur
(C) A 17-year-old girl with atypical chest pain and a midsystolic click
(D) A 42-year-old woman with palpitations, exertional dyspnea, and episodes of hemoptysis
(E) An asymptomatic 32-year-old cardiologist

155. A 68-year-old man who has had a recent syncopal episode is hospitalized with congestive heart failure. His blood pressure is 160/80 mmHg, his pulse rate is 80/min, and there is a grade III/VI harsh systolic murmur. An echocardiogram shows a disproportionately thickened ventricular septum and systolic anterior motion of the mitral valve.

Which of the following findings, would most likely be present in this man?

(A) Radiation of the murmur to the carotid arteries
(B) Decrease of the murmur with hand grip
(C) Delayed carotid upstroke
(D) Reduced left ventricular ejection fraction
(E) Signs of mitral stenosis

156. For the last 6 hours, a 33-year-old man has had sharp, pleuritic, substernal chest pain that is relieved when he sits upright. His electrocardiogram shows diffuse ST-segment elevation. Which of the following observations would LEAST support a diagnosis of acute pericarditis?

(A) Frequent atrial premature beats
(B) PR-segment depression
(C) Diffuse T-wave inversion with ST-segment elevation
(D) Twice-normal serum creatine phosphokinase concentration
(E) No rub

157. All the following are indications for surgical intervention in the treatment of dissection of the aorta EXCEPT

(A) compromised femoral pulse
(B) new murmur of aortic regurgitation
(C) persistent chest pain
(D) involvement of the ascending aorta
(E) involvement of the descending aorta

158. True statements describing dissection of the aorta include all the following EXCEPT

(A) nearly all cases involve medial necrosis
(B) spontaneous intimal tears almost always occur 2 to 5 cm above the aortic valve or just distal to the origin of the left subclavian artery
(C) all false aneurysms begin with rupture of the aorta
(D) dissection associated with Marfan's syndrome (type II dissection) stops before the great vessels arising from the aortic arch
(E) patients treated with trimethaphan (Arfonad) should be kept upright

DIRECTIONS: Each question below contains five suggested answers. For **each** of the five alternatives of **each** item, you are to respond either YES (Y) or NO (N). In a given item all, some, or none of the alternatives may be correct.

159. A 62-year-old man loses consciousness in the street, and resuscitative efforts are undertaken. In the emergency room an electrocardiogram is obtained, part of which is shown below. Which of the following disorders could account for this man's presentation?

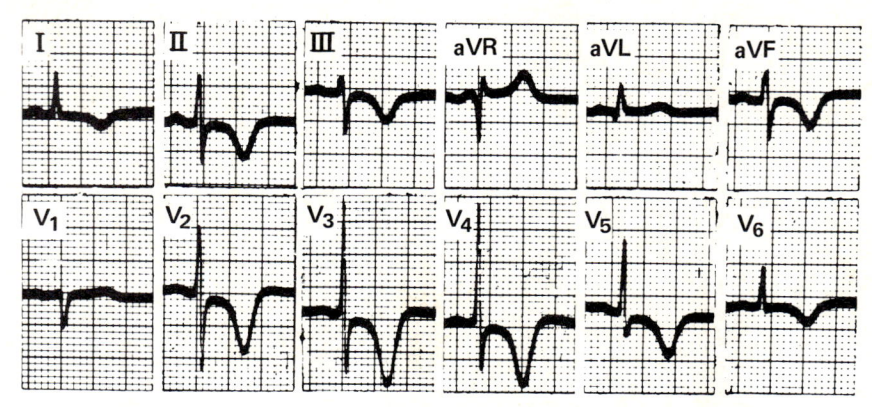

Reprinted with permission from Marriott HJL: *Practical Electrocardiography.* Baltimore, Williams & Wilkins, 7th ed, 1983, p. 400.

(A) Subendocardial infarction
(B) Hyperkalemia
(C) Intracerebral hemorrhage
(D) Myocardial ischemia
(E) Hypocalcemic tetany

---

160. Ebstein's anomaly is correctly described by which of the following statements?

(A) Most affected individuals die in infancy
(B) Wide splitting of S_1 and S_2 is frequent
(C) Giant P waves on electrocardiography are typical
(D) The right ventricle is characteristically dilated and hypertrophied
(E) The tricuspid valve is redundant

161. A loud first heart sound is associated frequently with

(A) hypothyroidism
(B) Lown-Ganong-Levine syndrome
(C) mitral stenosis
(D) mitral regurgitation
(E) fever

162. Acute hyperkalemia is associated with which of the following electrocardiographic changes?

(A) QRS widening
(B) Prolongation of the ST segment
(C) Decrease in the P wave
(D) Prominent U waves
(E) Peaked T waves

163. Bifascicular block commonly is associated with

(A) anteroseptal myocardial infarction
(B) inferior myocardial infarction
(C) prolonged HV interval on a His bundle electrogram
(D) calcific aortic stenosis
(E) mitral valve surgery

164. A 62-year-old woman, who has been fine except for occasional headaches, is found to have a blood pressure of 165/105 mmHg and a systolic bruit in the left upper abdomen during her routine yearly physical examination. Repeat blood pressure 2 weeks later is the same. Evaluation at this point should include

(A) serum potassium concentration
(B) blood urea nitrogen concentration
(C) 24-hour urine collection for vanillylmandelic acid
(D) electrocardiography
(E) rapid-sequence intravenous pyelography

165. Which of the following conditions warrant antibiotic prophylaxis against infective endocarditis in a patient experiencing invasive dental work?

(A) Atrial septal defect
(B) Ventricular septal defect
(C) Coronary artery bypass grafts
(D) Permanent transvenous pacemaker
(E) Mitral regurgitation associated with mitral valve prolapse

---

166. The rhythm shown on the electrocardiogram below can be associated with

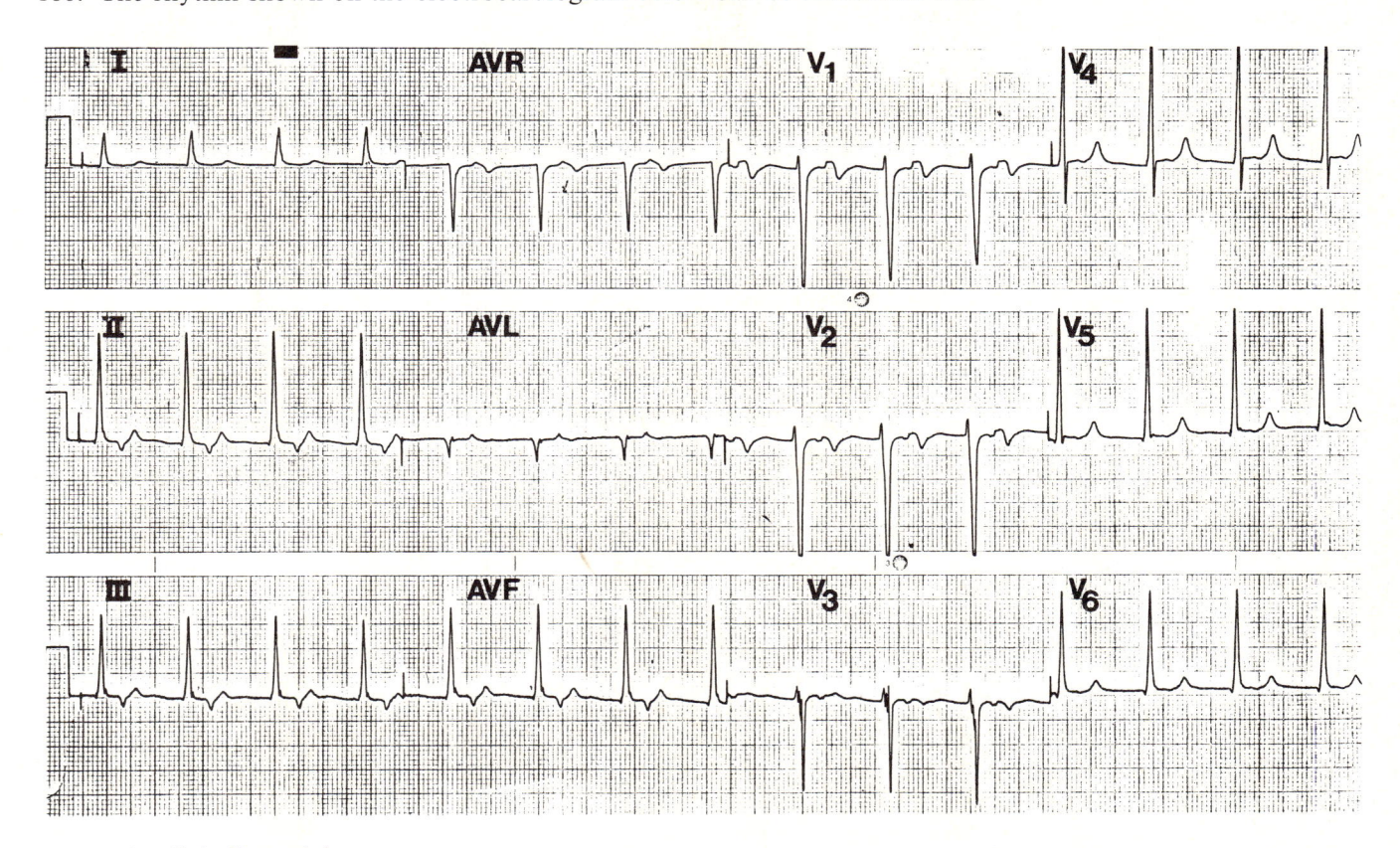

(A) digitalis toxicity
(B) acute myocarditis
(C) anterior myocardial infarction
(D) mitral valve surgery
(E) hypercalcemia

167. Which of the following statements accurately describe mild heart failure due to left ventricular dysfunction?

(A) Cardiac output would be depressed at rest
(B) Plasma norepinephrine levels would be higher than in normal controls during exercise
(C) Myocardial norepinephrine content would be high
(D) Left ventricular end-diastolic pressure would rise more during exercise than in normal controls
(E) Cardiac output would fail to rise appropriately when oxygen consumption is increased during exercise

168. Which of the following statements regarding radionuclide cardiac scans are true?

(A) On radionuclide ventriculography, a fall in the global ejection fraction in an exercising patient with congestive heart failure suggests underlying coronary artery disease
(B) Technetium pyrophosphate scanning is useful in diagnosing myocardial contusion
(C) A "cold spot" present during exercise but not present several hours later on a thallium 201 scan suggests past myocardial infarction
(D) A defect on a thallium 201 scan in a resting patient with chest pain and ST-segment elevation on electrocardiography implies an evolving myocardial infarction
(E) A persistently abnormal technetium pyrophosphate scan is associated commonly with left ventricular aneurysm

169. Which of the following statements are true regarding streptokinase (SK) thrombolysis in acute myocardial infarction?

(A) Successful reperfusion and salvage of jeopardized myocardium is possible when SK is administered between 6 and 8 hours after the onset of chest pain
(B) Intravenous and intracoronary administration of SK are equally effective
(C) Successful clot thrombolysis prevents development of myocardial necrosis in virtually all patients
(D) Intravenous administration of SK produces a systemic lytic state that may result in hemorrhagic complications
(E) Percutaneous transluminal coronary angioplasty (PTCA) is contraindicated for 1 week after an SK infusion

170. A 40-year-old woman with asthma has been taking terbutaline and aminophylline. She comes to the emergency room with palpitations, light-headedness, and shortness of breath. The electrocardiogram shown below is obtained. The rhythm disturbance evident on the ECG can be described by which of the following statements?

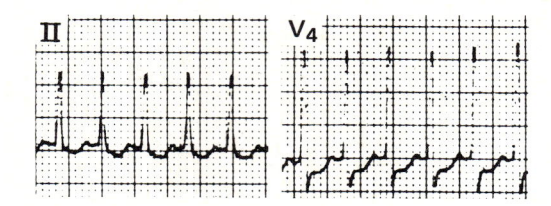

Reprinted with permission from Marriott HJL: *Practical Electrocardiography*. Baltimore, Williams & Wilkins, 7th ed, 1983, p. 164.

(A) It arises from sustained reentry, probably through the atrioventricular (AV) junction
(B) It is dependent upon delayed conduction and unidirectional block
(C) It involves concealed conduction within the AV junction
(D) It may be reliably terminated by administration of nifedipine
(E) Intravenous edrophonium (Tensilon), 10 mg, would be appropriate therapy for affected, normotensive individuals

171. A 37-year-old man with Wolff-Parkinson-White syndrome develops a broad-complex tachycardia at a rate of 200/min. He appears comfortable and has little hemodynamic impairment. Useful treatment at this point might include

(A) digoxin
(B) quinidine
(C) propranolol
(D) verapamil
(E) direct-current cardioversion

172. A 17-year-old girl has an atrial septal defect of the sinus venosus type, with a 3:1 pulmonary-to-systemic blood flow ratio. Which of the following statements concerning her condition are true?

(A) She is probably asymptomatic
(B) She probably has partial anomalous connection of the pulmonary veins
(C) The magnitude of the shunt is a function of the amount of total blood flow
(D) A systolic murmur would likely be due to flow across the defect
(E) A diastolic rumble would strongly suggest coexistence of mitral stenosis (Lutembacher's syndrome)

173. For which of the following individuals would cardiac surgery be appropriately recommended?

(A) An asymptomatic 18-year-old woman who has an atrial septal defect with a 2:1 pulmonary-to-systemic flow ratio
(B) An asymptomatic 19-year-old man who has a loud murmur and a ventricular septal defect with a 1.5:1 pulmonary-to-systemic flow ratio
(C) A 33-year-old man who has chest pain, fatigue, cyanosis, a large ventricular septal defect, a 2:1 right-to-left shunt, and a normal pulmonary outflow tract and pulmonic valve
(D) A 52-year-old man who has chronic mitral regurgitation and has recently developed pulmonary edema associated with the onset of rapid atrial fibrillation
(E) A 54-year-old man who has aortic stenosis and has chest pain on moderate to strenuous exertion

174. Which of the following statements accurately describe acute rheumatic fever?

(A) Group A streptococcal skin infections can initiate an attack
(B) Recurrent rheumatic fever occurs more frequently in individuals who have preexisting rheumatic heart disease than in other individuals
(C) Large numbers of macrophages are found commonly in the first drop of blood extracted from the earlobe
(D) Diagnosis of acute rheumatic fever in a young person presenting with migratory arthritis and congestive heart failure is unlikely if group A streptococci cannot be isolated from a throat culture
(E) All affected individuals, even those without carditis, should receive antibiotic prophylaxis for at least 5 years

175. A 64-year-old man with aortic stenosis is admitted to the hospital because of the recent onset of congestive heart failure. Which of the following statements characterizing his condition are true?

(A) The development of atrial fibrillation (ventricular response of 70/min) could explain the deterioration of his condition
(B) His effective aortic orifice is likely to be less than $0.7 \text{ cm}^2/\text{m}^2$
(C) Absence of aortic valve calcification on chest x-ray rules out severe aortic stenosis
(D) Once his congestive heart failure is treated, he may do well for several more years
(E) If an echocardiogram shows cusp calcification, then his aortic stenosis is likely to be severe

176. A 32-year-old woman who has rheumatic mitral valve disease but has been relatively free of symptoms now presents with pulmonary edema. Conditions that could have been responsible for this woman's clinical presentation include

(A) pregnancy
(B) atrial fibrillation
(C) anemia
(D) hypoxia
(E) bacterial endocarditis

177. A 34-year-old woman is bothered by palpitations and chest pain. On auscultation, the first heart sound is normal, but there is a midsystolic click and a late systolic murmur. Her electrocardiogram shows T-wave inversions in leads II, III, and aVF. Which of the following statements concerning her condition are true?

(A) An exercise stress test would most likely be positive
(B) An echocardiogram may show abrupt posterior displacement of both mitral leaflets
(C) The woman's chest pain could be due to excessive stress on the papillary muscles
(D) The click and murmur would be expected to occur later in systole when the woman stands
(E) Prophylactic measures should be taken to prevent subacute bacterial endocarditis

178. In individuals who have endocarditis, which of the following factors would **adversely** affect the prognosis?

(A) The presence of congestive heart failure
(B) The absence of demonstrable bacteremia
(C) The isolation of organisms resistant to multiple antimicrobial agents
(D) The isolation of *Staphylococcus epidermidis* after cardiac surgery
(E) A delay in instituting therapy

179. Which of the following statements about prosthetic valve endocarditis are true?

(A) Development of endocarditis more than 2 months postoperatively is usually the result of colonization of the prosthesis at surgery
(B) *Staphylococcus epidermidis* endocarditis in the immediate postoperative period usually responds satisfactorily to a course of antibiotics
(C) There is a greater frequency of valve-ring infections and myocardial abscess with prosthetic valve endocarditis than with other types of endocarditis
(D) Relapse following a course of antibiotics is an indication for valve replacement
(E) Mobitz type II heart block during treatment for prosthetic valve endocarditis is an indication for valve replacement

180. Which of the statements regarding right-heart endocarditis are true?

(A) It is unlikely in the absence of murmur
(B) It occurs frequently in drug addicts
(C) Blood cultures are usually negative
(D) Emboli to organs other than the lungs are rare
(E) Prognosis is generally good

181. A permanent atrioventricular sequential pacemaker (DDD) would be preferred to a standard ventricular pacemaker (VVI) in which of the following patients?

(A) A 64-year-old woman with atrial fibrillation and a ventricular rate of 40/min
(B) A 56-year-old man with complete heart block and a global left ventricular ejection fraction of 36 percent
(C) An active 46-year-old man with high-grade atrioventricular block
(D) An 80-year-old woman with symptomatic bradyarrhythmias and normal left ventricular function
(E) A 50-year-old man with hypertrophic cardiomyopathy and infranodal second-degree atrioventricular block

182. Which of the following conditions should be treated with insertion of a temporary transvenous pacemaker?

(A) Acute anterior myocardial infarction and a new left bundle-branch block
(B) Acute anterior myocardial infarction and a new right bundle-branch block
(C) Acute anterior myocardial infarction and a new right bundle-branch block and left anterior hemiblock
(D) Acute inferior myocardial infarction, periods of Wenckebach second-degree heart block, and no symptoms
(E) Acute inferior myocardial infarction, third-degree heart block, escape nodal rhythm at 40/min, and dizzy spells

183. Which of the following statements regarding coronary artery bypass surgery (CABG) are true?

(A) Between 10 and 20 percent of saphenous venous grafts occlude in the first postoperative year
(B) Approximately 85 percent of patients will have an improvement in angina
(C) CABG is contraindicated in patients with severe 3-vessel coronary disease and an ejection fraction of 35 percent
(D) Saphenous venous coronary grafts to the left anterior descending artery have a higher patency rate than internal mammary artery grafts
(E) In a patient with normal ventricular function, the surgical mortality is approximately 5 percent

184. Which of the following statements regarding serum lipoproteins are true?

(A) HDL cholesterol concentrations increase significantly with age
(B) It is unnecessry to measure serum cholesterol before the age of 30 years since such concentrations do not correlate with future disease
(C) Mortality from ischemic heart disease is decreased when increased serum cholesterol concentrations are reduced by diet and cholestyramine therapy
(D) A low serum concentration of HDL cholesterol is an independent risk factor for the development of ischemic heart disease

185. Blood levels of high-density lipoprotein are increased by

(A) estrogens
(B) androgens
(C) cigarette smoking
(D) alcohol
(E) jogging

186. Which of the following statements regarding the cardiac effects of hyperthyroidism are true?

(A) Cardiac symptoms of angina and congestive heart failure are resistant to treatment
(B) Pericardial effusion is frequent
(C) Atrial fibrillation is frequent
(D) Density of myocardial beta receptors is increased
(E) Voltage typically is low on electrocardiography

187. A 23-year-old man has had recent onset of exertional dyspnea. A grade III/VI systolic murmur is heard at the left sternal border. Electrocardiography shows apical and lateral Q waves and left ventricular hypertrophy. Echocardiography reveals asymmetrical septal hypertrophy without evidence of obstruction.
Which of the following statements regarding this clinical situation are true?

(A) The man's dyspnea is best explained by lateral wall infarction
(B) First-degree relatives should be evaluated
(C) The risk of sudden death is low
(D) Calcium-channel blockers may relieve symptoms
(E) The man's heart is normal histologically, aside from changes of infarction

188. A 54-year-old man has severe hypertension, and studies are undertaken to determine whether his hypertension is secondary to renal disease. Which of the following principles should guide the physician in the workup of this man's hypertension?

(A) Split renal function tests should be performed
(B) Provocative tests should be done if 24-hour urine catecholamine content is equivocal
(C) If renin activity and serum potassium are low but aldosterone excretion is increased, then primary aldosteronism should be considered
(D) Even if rapid-sequence intravenous pyelography is normal, there is at least a 10 percent chance that his hypertension is of renovascular origin
(E) Angiographic visualization of renal artery stenosis would definitively diagnose renovascular hypertension

189. Which of the following statements are true with respect to the use of vasodilator drugs in the treatment of chronic congestive heart failure?

(A) Reflex tachycardia is expected with administration of afterload reducing agents
(B) Afterload reducing agents reduce left ventricular end-diastolic pressure and stroke volume
(C) Nitrates are more potent afterload reducing agents than hydralazine
(D) Captopril dilates both the venous and arterial beds, resulting in elevation of cardiac output and reduction in left ventricular filling pressure
(E) The five year mortality is decreased by approximately 30 percent by treatment with an angiotensin-converting enzyme (ACE) inhibitor

190. A 58-year-old man has tightness in the right calf when he walks. On examination, femoral bruits are present bilaterally and the right dorsalis pedis pulse is absent. Which of the following statements concerning this man's condition are true?

(A) If the pain persists for 15 minutes after exercise or if he must lie down for relief, then multiple occlusions exist
(B) If the systolic pressure at the ankle is greater than one-half the arm systolic pressure, significant stenosis is not present
(C) Blood pressure in the ankles would be expected to fall after exercise
(D) Lumbar sympathectomy may be useful
(E) He should embark upon an exercise program

DIRECTIONS: The groups of questions below consist of four or five lettered headings followed by several numbered items. For each numbered item choose the **one** lettered heading with which it is **most** closely associated. Each lettered heading may be used once, more than once, or not at all.

Questions 191–195

For each description that follows, select the type of pulse pattern with which it is most likely to be associated.

(A) Pulsus paradoxus
(B) Pulsus bisferiens
(C) Pulsus alternans
(D) Pulsus tardus
(E) None of the above

191. Associated with cardiomyopathy
192. Associated with pericardial tamponade
193. Associated with aortic regurgitation
194. Associated with severe asthma
195. Follows a premature ventricular beat

Questions 196–200

For each of the following disorders, select the characteristic hemodynamic pattern.

(A) Equalization of diastolic pressures
(B) Dip-and-plateau pattern
(C) Slow *y* descent
(D) Tall *v* wave
(E) None of the above

196. Pericardial tamponade
197. Amyloidosis
198. Mitral stenosis
199. Acute mitral regurgitation
200. Acute septal rupture

Questions 201–204

For each syndrome below, select the associated cardiovascular abnormality.

(A) Coarctation of the aorta
(B) Pulmonic stenosis
(C) Mitral regurgitation
(D) Endocardial cushion defect
(E) Cor pulmonale

201. Marfan's syndrome
202. Turner's syndrome
203. Congenital rubella
204. Cystic fibrosis

Questions 205–208

For each of the following descriptions, select the drug or class of drugs with which it is most likely to be associated.

(A) Thiazide diuretics
(B) Furosemide
(C) Spironolactone
(D) Triamterene
(E) None of the above

205. Acts at the proximal tubule to inhibit sodium reabsorption
206. Spares potassium by the competitive inhibition of aldosterone
207. Inhibits active chloride reabsorption
208. Is the diuretic most likely to be effective in the presence of azotemia

Questions 209–213

Match each cardiac drug with the side effect most likely to develop with its use.

(A) Thrombocytopenic purpura
(B) Urinary retention
(C) Arrhythmias
(D) Seizures
(E) Postural hypotension

209. Disopyramide phosphate (Norpace)
210. Bretylium tosylate
211. Lidocaine hydrochloride
212. Quinidine sulfate
213. Digoxin

Questions 214–217

Match each of the following descriptions with the most appropriate choice.

(A) Pericardial effusion
(B) Constrictive pericarditis
(C) Both
(D) Neither

214. Causes right-heart and left-heart failure
215. Causes paradoxical pulse
216. Produces a pericardial knock in early diastole
217. Is associated with a prominent *x* trough in the jugular pulse

Questions 218–221

Match each of the following causes of right heart failure with the most characteristic set of hemodynamic measurements.

	Right atrial pressure, mmHg	Pulmonary arterial pressure, mmHg	Pulmonary capillary wedge pressure, mmHg
(A)	16	75/30	11
(B)	16	35/17	16
(C)	16	100/30	28
(D)	16	45/22	20
(E)	16	22/12	10
Normal values	0–5	12–28/3–13	3–11

218. Right ventricular infarction

219. Cor pulmonale from bronchitis

220. Mitral stenosis

221. Constrictive pericarditis

Questions 222–226

For each of the following descriptions, select the drug with which it is most likely to be associated.

(A) Minoxidil
(B) Captopril
(C) Saralasin
(D) Clonidine
(E) Prazosin

222. Is a central alpha-receptor agonist

223. Is probably effective because of blockade of postsynaptic alpha-adrenergic receptors

224. Is a direct-acting peripheral vasodilator

225. Is an angiotensin-receptor antagonist

226. Interferes with the conversion of angiotensin I to angiotensin II

Disorders of the Heart and Vascular System

Answers

128. The answer is B. *(Braunwald, ed 11, chap 190.)* The combination of hypotension and bradycardia suggests a vagal response in the setting of an acute myocardial infarction. Administration of the anticholinergic agent atropine is the treatment of choice. If the bradyarrhythmia and hypotension persist after 2.0 mg of atropine has been administered in divided doses, insertion of a temporary pacemaker is indicated. Isoproterenol should be avoided in patients with acute myocardial infarction since it may greatly increase myocardial oxygen consumption and thereby intensify ischemia. Volume replacement or inotropic support may be required if hypotension persists after correction of the bradyarrhythmia, but they are not indicated as initial therapies.

129. The answer is A. *(Braunwald, ed 11, chap 196.)* Captopril is an inhibitor of angiotensin-converting enzyme, and thus it impairs the production of angiotensin II, a potent vasoconstrictor. Through removal of feedback inhibition, renin secretion is *increased*. Additional antihypertension effects of captopril result from a reduction of bradykinin degradation and stimulation of vasodilating prostaglandin production. Converting enzyme inhibitors can be added to a regimen of beta blockade for an additional antihypertensive effect. Captopril is contraindicated in patients with bilateral renal artery stenosis, since reduction in systemic arterial pressure may lead to progressive renal hypoperfusion.

130. The answer is D. *(Braunwald, ed 11, chap 196.)* The beta-blocking agents are effective antihypertensive and antianginal agents. Beta-1 cardioselective agents include metoprolol and atenolol. Although these two drugs may be safer than the other agents to give to patients with bronchospasm, selectivity is lost with larger doses, and they are relatively contraindicated. Nadolol and atenolol can be administered on a once-a-day regimen by virtue of their long half-lives. Pindolol is a nonselective beta-blocking agent with partial agonist activity, resulting in less marked bradycardia than the other agents. Labetolol has both beta- and alpha-receptor antagonist actions.

131. The answer is C. *(Braunwald, ed 11, chap 194.)* The lateral-view chest film demonstrates calcification of the anterior pericardium, consistent with constrictive pericarditis. This pattern is seen in approximately one half of patients with long-standing constriction, and pericardial thickening can often be confirmed by echocardiography. In patients with this disease, a pericardial knock is often heard 0.06 to 0.12 seconds after aortic valve closure, corresponding to the sudden cessation of ventricular filling. Murmurs are typically absent.

132. The answer is E. *(Braunwald, ed 11, chap 179.)* Two-dimensional and M-mode echocardiograms directly image the intracardiac valves and are extremely useful in the detection of valvular stenosis. Doppler echocardiography permits the calculation of the pressure gradient across the intracardiac valves. Regurgitant lesions, such as those of the tricuspid valve, can be detected and the severity estimated by this technique. Although the echocardiographic findings of atrial septal defect are nonspecific (right ventricular volume overload pattern), Doppler studies can determine the presence of the trans-atrial shunt. Coronary calcification cannot at present be imaged with a high degree of sensitivity.

133. The answer is E. *(Braunwald, ed 11, chap 29.)* Chronic idiopathic orthostatic hypotension, most common among elderly men, is characterized by orthostatic hypotension in the absence of reflex tachycardia. Other autonomic disturbances typically are present, including anhidrosis, difficulty with urination, and constipation. In this condition, peripheral norepinephrine synthesis is deficient and plasma norepinephrine levels are low. Treatment consists of increasing intravascular volume and venous return and administering directly acting sympathomimetic agents. Tyramine and other indirectly acting sympathomimetic agents are not helpful. In a condition related to chronic idiopathic orthostatic hypertension, peripheral norepinephrine stores and plasma levels are normal but release of norepinephrine is deficient; this condition, which has a variety of central nervous system manifestations, may respond to tyramine.

134. The answer is E. *(Braunwald, ed 11, chap 189.)* PTCA is now widely used to revascularize suitable coronary lesions. Although adequate dilation is achieved in more than 85 percent of patients, recurrent stenosis develops in approximately 20 percent within 6 months. Angioplasty has been successfully performed on obstructive lesions within bypass grafts and in patients with recent total occlusion (within 3 months) of native coronaries. Significant left main artery disease ordinarily remains a contraindication to the procedure; coronary artery bypass grafting appears to be safer at present. The success rate of repeated PTCA is actually *better* than that of the first procedure.

135. The answer is E. *(Braunwald, ed 11, chap 182.)* The woman described in the question has mitral valve prolapse, which can cause atypical chest pain. Echocardiography is sensitive and specific in the diagnosis of mitral valve prolapse. Usually, there is late systolic sagging in a posterior direction of one or both mitral valve leaflets. Although a mitral regurgitation murmur following a midsystolic click may be present, these classic findings need not be present to ensure the diagnosis. Holosystolic prolapse is not uncommon and is the usual finding in persons in whom Marfan's syndrome is the underlying disease process. Echocardiography cannot directly diagnose mitral regurgitation or papillary muscle dysfunction, even when there is apparent separation of the mitral leaflets in systole, as is the case in the tracing provided. Chordal rupture often is associated with jagged fluttering of one or both mitral leaflets in diastole, which can be difficult to distinguish from the effect of aortic regurgitation on the mitral valve in diastole. In the echo study shown, diastolic motion of the mitral valve is normal, a finding useful in ruling out mitral stenosis.

136. The answer is E. *(Braunwald, ed 11, chap 182.)* Many persons who have ankle edema are inappropriately diagnosed as having heart failure. In particular, the diagnosis of right heart failure should not be made in the absence of jugular venous distension. Venous varicosities, cyclic edema, thrombophlebitis, and hypoalbuminemia all cause ankle edema and should be considered in the differential diagnosis.

137. The answer is C. *(Braunwald, ed 11, chap 182.)* Congestive heart failure associated with pulmonary and systemic venous congestion may occur either with low cardiac output and widened arterial–mixed venous oxygen difference or with high output and normal or narrowed arterial–mixed venous oxygen difference. High-output states are associated with unusually low systemic vascular resistance and peripheral shunting. If Paget's disease is widespread, increased bony vascularity and overlying cutaneous vasodilation can lead to shunting and a high-output state. Venous congestion occurs when the ventricles are unable to handle the increased venous return.

138. The answer is E. *(Braunwald, ed 11, chap 182.)* Digitalis glycosides augment contractility of the heart and slow atrioventricular conduction and heart rate. The primary mechanism of action is inhibition of Na^+-K^+-ATPase, which is located in the sarcolemmal membrane. This action leads to intracellular accumulation of sodium and, subsequently, calcium by way of a sodium-calcium exchange mechanism.

139. The answer is D. *(Braunwald, ed 11, chap 182.)* Elderly individuals are particularly prone to develop digitalis intoxication at relatively low doses and apparently normal serum levels (<2.0 ng/mL). Exacerbating factors in the development of toxicity are hypoxemia and hypercalcemia. Potassium wasting and, perhaps, hypomagnesemia from potent loop diuretics also can foster toxicity. By mechanisms not yet elucidated, quinidine can increase the serum levels of digoxin, thereby inducing toxicity. Hyperthyroidism tends to decrease the efficacy of digitalis, while hypothyroidism enhances the likelihood of toxicity.

140. The answer is E. *(Braunwald, ed 11, chap 183.)* The escape focus in atrioventricular nodal block is relatively high in the conduction system, in an area of vagal innervation. Thus, a beneficial response to vagolytic drugs, such as atropine, is usually apparent. Rate at the escape focus is relatively rapid, and the QRS complex is narrow. Unless complete heart block persists, some Wenckebach periodicity can be observed. Inferior myocardial infarction, mitral valve surgery, and digitalis toxicity can lead to atrioventricular nodal block.

141. The answer is D. *(Braunwald, ed 11, chap 183.)* Sinus bradycardia and a long sinus pause raise the possibility of sick sinus syndrome, not an infrequent cause of lightheadedness among the elderly. It is important that the relationship between symptoms and the arrhythmias documented by Holter monitoring be clarified before implantation of a permanent pacemaker is considered. An exercise tolerance test, though it may strengthen the suspicion of sick sinus syndrome by showing an inadequate heart rate response, cannot prove that the condition is responsible for the patient's symptoms. Sublingual isoproterenol has little usefulness in the management of chronic bradyarrhythmias.

142. The answer is B. *(Braunwald, ed 11, chap 184.)* The rhythm demonstrated in the electrocardiogram presented is multifocal atrial tachycardia, which is characterized by variable P-wave morphology and PR and RR intervals. Control of multifocal atrial tachycardia, usually associated with severe pulmonary disease, comes with improved ventilation and oxygenation. Carotid sinus massage, electrical cardioversion, and administration of digitalis, verapamil, or quinidine are of little benefit, although verapamil may temporarily slow the ventricular rake.

143. The answer is D. *(Braunwald, ed 11, chap 184.)* The ventricular rate in atrial flutter can be decreased by interfering with atrioventricular conduction and slowing the atrial rate. Quinidine slows the rate but enhances conduction; the net result is 1:1 conduction at a somewhat slower atrial rate and a more rapid ventricular rate. Quinidine thus should not be used to treat atrial flutter without the addition of digoxin, verapamil, or propranolol to block atrioventricular conduction.

144. The answer is C. *(Braunwald, ed 11, chap 185.)* Atrial septal defect (ASD) is usually asymptomatic in childhood. Clinical presentation occurs in the third or fourth decade of life and results from atrial arrhythmias and pulmonary hypertension. A frequent cause of symptoms and of right heart failure is coexistent left ventricular dysfunction—even mild left atrial pressure elevation is not tolerated well when transmitted into the systemic venous circulation. Secundum atrial septal defect is associated with a rightward axis on electrocardiography; the axis is leftward in primum defects. Echocardiography also reveals evidence of right ventricular volume overload, including abnormal motion of the ventricular septum (i.e., right-to-left movement) during diastole.

145. The answer is B. *(Braunwald, ed 11, chaps 179, 187.)* The echocardiographic studies demonstrate thickening and calcification of the aortic valve, with minimal leaflet separation in systole, consistent with aortic stenosis. Doppler echocardiography can be useful in estimating the severity of the aortic disease as follows:

$$\text{Peak gradient across the valve} = 4 \times (\text{peak velocity})^2$$

DISORDERS OF THE HEART AND VASCULAR SYSTEM

In this case, the peak velocity distal to the valve is 5 m/sec, yielding a peak gradient of 100 mmHg, suggesting significant aortic stenosis. No diastolic turbulence was detected, ruling against aortic regurgitation. Although severe aortic stenosis may be the cause of this patient's exertional chest pain, coronary arteriography is indicated to rule out significant coronary arterial disease, which may require coronary artery bypass grafting along with aortic valve replacement.

146. The answer is E. *(Braunwald, ed 11, chap 185.)* Adults with mild pulmonic stenosis are generally asymptomatic. Unlike congenital aortic stenosis, this condition usually does not progress; thus, follow-up need not be frequent. The risk of endocarditis is somewhat lower for pulmonic valves than for the other heart valve, whether normal or stenotic. Clinical signs of mild pulmonic stenosis include prominent *a* wave on jugular venous pulse, normal electrocardiogram, and normal cardiac size on chest x-ray.

147. The answer is C. *(Braunwald, ed 11, chap 185.)* Coarctation of the aorta usually occurs just distal to the origin of the left subclavian artery; if it arises above the left subclavian, blood pressure elevation may only be evident in the right arm. The associated murmur is continuous only if obstruction is severe; otherwise, a systolic ejection murmur is heard anteriorly and over the back. Coarctation of the aorta commonly is accompanied by a bicuspid aortic valve, which can produce the diastolic murmur of aortic regurgitation. X-ray findings include the "3" sign, caused by aortic dilation just proximal and distal to the area of stenosis, and rib notching, caused by increased collateral circulation through dilated intercostal arteries. Hypertension is the major clinical problem and may persist even after complete surgical correction. Unless hypertension is very severe, or left ventricular failure has ensued, cardiac output responds normally to exercise.

148. The answer is B. *(Braunwald, ed 11, chaps 185, 187.)* The chest x-ray presented in the question shows enlargement of the right ventricle and main pulmonary artery and pulmonary vascular plethora, or "shunt" vasculature—classic findings for an atrial septal defect, which could well be asymptomatic in a 36-year-old woman. The chest x-ray of an individual with mitral stenosis and hemoptysis and dyspnea would show left atrial enlargement, even in the presence of primary or secondary tricuspid regurgitation, ascites, and a large jugular venous *v* wave. Continuous murmur, widened systemic pulse pressure, and dyspnea on exertion combine to suggest patent ductus arteriosus, which would produce x-ray evidence of left ventricular and perhaps left atrial enlargement and shunt vasculature without right ventricular enlargement.

149. The answer is B. *(Braunwald, ed 11, chap 186.)* Rheumatic fever can be differentiated from rheumatoid arthritis by the absence of rheumatoid factor in the serum and lack of joint deformities on physical examination. It can be differentiated from penicillin-related serum sickness by the absence of urticaria and angioneurotic edema. The incidence of rheumatic fever is higher in areas of high population density. Most affected persons with acute rheumatic carditis display no symptoms referable to the heart.

150. The answer is C. *(Braunwald, ed 11, chap 198.)* Although each of the items listed is a potential source of peripheral embolism, the most common source is the heart. The lesions that predispose to this development include mural left ventricular thrombus (associated with recent myocardial infarction or cardiomyopathy), left atrial thrombus associated with atrial fibrillation or mitral valve disease, and valvular thrombus, especially of a prosthetic valve.

151. The answer is A. *(Braunwald, ed 11, chap 189.)* Nitrates are generalized smooth-muscle dilators whose direct effect on the vasculature is not blocked by any agents presently available. Long-acting preparations of nitroglycerin may be completely degraded by the liver in some individuals and thus are generally less effective than sublingual forms. Because individual variability in metabolism is considerable, dosages should be titrated against side effects and should not conform to a rigidly standardized regimen. Nitroglycerin ointment is absorbed well through any noncornified skin; application to the chest only adds a placebo effect to the therapeutic one.

152. The answer is A. *(Braunwald, ed 11, chap 190.)* The man described in the question probably has a right ventricular infarction complicating his inferior myocardial infarction, because right atrial pressure is elevated out of proportion to the left atrial (pulmonary capillary wedge) pressure. Cardiac output is probably depressed, given the low left-heart filling pressure. The best treatment consists of administration of fluids.

153. The answer is B. *(Braunwald, ed 11, chap 184.)* The rhythm strip shows polymorphic ventricular tachycardia characteristic of torsades de pointes ("twisting of the points"). This life-threatening rhythm is associated with prolongation of the QT interval, resulting, in this case, from the administration of quinidine. The appropriate therapy is to discontinue the offending agent and to withhold other agents that prolong the QT interval, such as procainamide. Hypokalemia can also prolong the QT interval and result in this rhythm; however, this patient had normal serum electrolyte concentrations.

154. The answer is D. *(Braunwald, ed 11, chap 187.)* The echocardiogram shows that the left atrium is enlarged, and there is calcification and thickening of the mitral valve and chordal apparatus. The mitral leaflets show diastolic doming, resulting from fusion of the valve commissures. These are the typical findings of rheumatic mitral stenosis, exemplified by this 42-year-old woman. The aortic leaflets are also mildly thickened, consistent with rheumatic disease. The symptoms of the patient described in Option A are suggestive of a left atrial myxoma. The patient in Option B has acute mitral regurgitation. The patient in Option C has mitral valve prolapse.

155. The answer is B. *(Braunwald, ed 11, chap 192.)* Echocardiographic evidence of a disproportionately thickened ventricular septum and systolic anterior motion of the mitral valve strongly suggests idiopathic hypertrophic subaortic stenosis (IHSS). The typical harsh systolic murmur does not usually radiate to the carotid arteries and decreases when ventricular volume enlarges with isometric exercise (e.g., hand grip). The carotid upstroke is brisk, often bifid. Congestive failure often occurs because of reduced ventricular compliance despite normal ventricular systolic function. Malposition of the mitral apparatus, a result of the distorted septum, often leads to some degree of mitral regurgitation.

156. The answer is C. *(Braunwald, ed 11, chap 194.)* Acute pericarditis is associated with ST-segment elevation and, frequently, PR-segment depression. Usually, reciprocal ST-segment depression is not present. T waves begin to invert only **after** the ST segment becomes isoelectric. Elevations in serum creatine phosphokinase levels to twice normal may be associated with uncomplicated pericarditis.

157. The answer is E. *(Braunwald, ed 11, chap 197.)* Complications of dissection of the aorta include loss of a major pulse, dissection into the pericardial or pleural space, and acute aortic regurgitation. When these events occur, surgical intervention is required. Because the risk of these complications is higher in persons with dissection of the ascending aorta, these persons usually are treated surgically. In contrast, persons with dissection of the descending aorta often can be treated medically. Persistence of pain, which suggests that dissection is continuing, is another indication for surgery.

158. The answer is D. *(Braunwald, ed 11, chap 197.)* Dissection of the aorta is a disease of the media, either from arteriosclerosis or cystic medial necrosis. The associated intimal tear that initiates the dissection almost always begins in the ascending aorta (2 to 5 cm above the valve) or just distal to the left subclavian artery; at these two points the aorta is relatively fixed, so that shear forces are increased. Type I dissections extend around the aortic arch and can affect the abdominal aorta; most type II dissections proceed variably into the arch or reach the left subclavian artery. Dissection can result in aortic rupture, which can result in a false aneurysm (an "aneurysm" contained within the adventitia or a clot) or, if the dissection is of the ascending aorta, in hemopericardium. Patients treated with an infusion of trimethaphan, a ganglionic blocking agent, should be kept in an upright position to achieve optimal lowering of blood pressure. This precaution is not necessary for patients receiving intravenous nitroprusside, a vasodilator.

DISORDERS OF THE HEART AND VASCULAR SYSTEM

159. The answer is A-Y, B-N, C-Y, D-Y, E-N. *(Braunwald, ed 11, chap 178.)* The electrocardiographic T wave represents myocardial repolarization, and its configuration can be altered nonspecifically by metabolic abnormalities, drugs, neural activity, and ischemia by a dispersion effect on the activation or repolarization of action potentials. Although myocardial ischemia and subendocardial infarction can produce deep, symmetric T-wave inversions, which would result in tachyarrhythmias and syncope, such noncardiac phenomena as intracerebral hemorrhage can similarly affect ventricular repolarization. Hyperkalemia is manifested by tall, peaked T waves, not inverted ones. Hypocalcemia is manifested by prolonged QT intervals.

160. The answer is A-N, B-Y, C-Y, D-N, E-Y. *(Braunwald, ed 11, chap 185.)* In Ebstein's anomaly, the tricuspid leaflets are redundant and positioned lower and further into the right ventricle than usual. Hence, the right atrium appears giant, while the right ventricle is small and hypoplastic. Tricuspid regurgitation is frequent. Most affected persons survive to middle age.

161. The answer is A-N, B-Y, C-Y, D-N, E-Y. *(Braunwald, ed 11, chap 177.)* The intensity of S_1 is determined by the contractility of the left ventricle ("slamming the door shut"), the degree of separation of mitral leaflets at the onset of contraction, and the thickness and pliability of the mitral leaflets. Contractility increases with fever but is diminished in hypothyroidism. Lown-Ganong-Levine syndrome is associated with a short PR interval, so that atrial contraction just precedes ventricular contraction; S_1 tends to be loud. Mitral regurgitation may lead to poor leaflet apposition and a soft S_1; on the other hand, mitral stenosis is associated with a loud S_1, unless the thickened valve leaflets are restricted in motion by heavy calcification.

162. The answer is A-Y, B-N, C-Y, D-N, E-Y. *(Braunwald, ed 11, chap 178.)* Hyperkalemia leads to partial depolarization of cardiac cells. As a result, there is slowing of the upstroke of one action potential as well as reduced duration of repolarization. The T wave becomes peaked, the QRS complex widens and may merge with the T wave (giving a sine-wave appearance), and the P wave becomes shallow or disappears. Prominent U waves are associated with hypokalemia; ST-segment prolongation is associated with hypocalcemia.

163. The answer is A-Y, B-N, C-N, D-Y, E-N. *(Braunwald, ed 11, chap 183.)* Anterior myocardial infarction and calcification arising from the aortic valve ring may damage the fascicular conduction system and thus lead to bifascicular block. Inferior myocardial infarction and mitral valve surgery are more likely to interfere with conduction at the level of the atrioventricular node. On a His bundle electrogram, prolongation of the HV interval (i.e., the time in which an impulse is conducted from the common His bundle to the ventricular myocardium) occurs only when all three fascicles are damaged.

164. The answer is A-Y, B-Y, C-N, D-Y, E-N. *(Braunwald, ed 11, chaps 29, 196.)* The basic laboratory evaluation of persons with newly diagnosed hypertension should consist of hematocrit, urinalysis, and BUN and serum potassium levels. Electrocardiography and chest x-ray also should be performed. More comprehensive testing is warranted if secondary hypertension seems likely (based on history, physical examination, and laboratory results) and, more important, if the hypertension has progressed rapidly or has been refractory to initial treatment. Systolic abdominal bruits in the absence of diastolic bruits do not suggest renovascular hypertension; thus, intravenous pyelography would not be indicated. Screening for pheochromocytoma in the absence of a suggestive history has a very low yield.

165. The answer is A-N, B-Y, C-N, D-N, E-Y. *(Braunwald, ed 11, chap 188.)* After transient bacteremia, subacute endocarditis may develop at endocardial sites at which a jet of blood flows from a high-pressure to a low-pressure area. Such lesions include ventricular septal defects and mitral regurgitation. Blood flow velocity across an isolated atrial septal defect is much lower and endocarditis is extremely uncommon in this condition. Similarly, long-standing permanent pacemakers and coronary bypass grafts very rarely result in the degree of turbulent blood flow necessary to incite endocardial infection.

166. The answer is A-Y, B-Y, C-N, D-Y, E-N. *(Braunwald, ed 11, chap 184.)* The electrocardiogram presented in the question demonstrates nonparoxysmal junctional tachycardia. The junctional rhythm is at a rate of 82/min, which is faster than the usual escape nodal rhythm. Retrograde P waves can be seen. This rhythm can occur following mitral-valve surgery and in association with digitalis toxicity, acute myocarditis, and inferior myocardial infarction. These processes all can irritate the atrioventricular node and accelerate its action.

167. The answer is A-N, B-Y, C-N, D-Y, E-Y. *(Braunwald, ed 11, chap 181.)* Stroke volume and cardiac output at rest are not sensitive indexes of myocardial dysfunction. Stroke volume is often normal, though at the expense of higher end-diastolic volume (Frank-Starling mechanism). Even when stroke volume begins to diminish, cardiac output can be maintained by increases in heart rate. However, when the heart is stressed by exercise, cardiac output does not rise proportionately to oxygen consumption, and left ventricular end-diastolic pressure rises more than in normal controls. Although plasma norepinephrine levels are elevated in persons with left ventricular dysfunction, myocardial levels are typically low.

168. The answer is A-N, B-Y, C-N, D-N, E-Y. *(Braunwald, ed 11, chap 179.)* A fall in the global ejection fraction during exercise radionuclide ventriculography occurs in association with coronary artery disease, valvular heart disease, and cardiomyopathy. Regional wall-motion abnormalities more specifically suggest coronary artery disease. Technetium pyrophosphate scans show a "hot spot" within several days of myocardial necrosis, regardless of the etiology. This scan thus would give evidence of myocardial contusion; however, persistence of abnormalities beyond several days would imply more extensive damage and carry a worse prognosis. A left ventricular aneurysm can also result in a persistently abnormal scan. A resting thallium-scan defect occurs in myocardial infarction and coronary artery spasm; a defect present during exercise but not at rest implies reversible ischemia.

169. The answer is A-N, B-N, C-N, D-Y, E-N. *(Braunwald, ed 11, chap 190.)* Most transmural myocardial infarctions are associated with thrombus formation at the site of coronary atherosclerotic plaque, and thrombolytic therapy can result in reperfusion of the ischemic zone. To be effective in salvaging ischemic myocardium, however, it must be administered as early as possible, within 3 to 4 hours of the onset of chest pain. There is little evidence of myocardial salvage in patients treated more than six hours after the onset of chest pain. Even though the thrombus can be lysed in 75 percent of patients, prevention of myocardial necrosis distal to the obstruction is not assured. Intravenous administration of SK is not as effective as intracoronary administration. The major limitations of SK arise from the development of a systemic lytic state and associated hemorrhagic complications; agents with fibriolytic activity only at the site of fresh thrombus, such as tissue plasminogen activator, may prove preferable in the future. Thrombolytic therapy does not preclude immediate PTCA, although the role of the latter is not yet clear in this setting.

170. The answer is A-Y, B-Y, C-N, D-N, E-N. *(Braunwald, ed 11, chap 184.)* The rhythm demonstrated in the electrocardiogram presented in the question is supraventricular tachycardia, a reentry tachycardia probably involving longitudinal stratification in the atrioventricular (AV) junction. Delayed conduction in one limb of the reentry pathway with unidirectional block allows perpetuation of the arrhythmia. Vagal stimuli and carotid sinus massage often terminate the arrhythmia. Although some calcium-channel antagonists (e.g., verapamil) would terminate the arrhythmia predictably by decreasing AV nodal conduction, nifedipine is only rarely effective. Edrophonium (Tensilon), a parasympathomimetic drug, is also useful in treating supraventricular tachycardia but is contraindicated in individuals who have asthma.

171. The answer is A-N, B-Y, C-N, D-N, E-Y. *(Braunwald, ed 11, chap 184.)* Persons who have Wolff-Parkinson-White syndrome are predisposed to developing two major types of atrial tachyarrhythmias. The first, which resembles paroxysmal supraventricular tachycardia (SVT) with reentry, involves the atrioventricular node in anterograde conduction and the bypass tract in retrograde conduction. This tachycardia typically has a nrrow QRS complex and can be treated similarly to other forms of SVT. The other, more dangerous tachyarrhythmia (present in the man described in the question) is atrial fibrillation, which usually is conducted anterograde down the bypass tract and has a wide QRS configuration. The ventricular rate is quite rapid, and cardiovascular collapse or ventricular fibrillation may result. Usual treatment is direct-current cardioversion, though quinidine may also be of use in slowing conduction through the bypass tract. Verapamil and propranolol have little effect on the bypass tract and may further depress ventricular function, which already is compromised by the rapid rate. Digoxin may accelerate conduction down the bypass tract and lead to ventricular fibrillation.

172. The answer is A-Y, B-Y, C-N, D-N, E-N. *(Braunwald, ed 11, chap 185.)* Atrial septal defects (ASD) of the sinus venosus type are located high in the atrial septum and commonly are associated with anomalous pulmonary venous return. The magnitude of the shunt depends upon defect size, relative ventricular compliance, the relative resistances in the pulmonary and systemic circuits, but **not** upon total blood flow. The systolic ejection murmur associated with ASD arises from increased flow across the pulmonic valve; a diastolic rumble due to increased flow across the tricuspid valve is common and should not necessarily be attributed to mitral stenosis, which is associated with ASD in a disorder known as Lutembacher's syndrome. Most individuals even with a large ASD are asymptomatic until late in adult life.

173. The answer is A-Y, B-N, C-N, D-N, E-Y. *(Braunwald, ed 11, chaps 185, 187.)* The risks of cardiac surgery always must be weighed against the potential benefits. The risk is extremely low in the correction of atrial septal defects, and surgery may prevent the development of atrial arrhythmia and pulmonary hypertension, complications that can arise later in life. Small ventricular septal defects, on the other hand, almost never cause hemodynamic problems later in life. The presence of Eisenmenger's reaction—cyanosis and a right-to-left shunt from pulmonary hypertension—is a contraindication to surgery, regardless of the underlying lesion. Individuals with symptomatic aortic stenosis warrant consideration for surgery, because hemodynamic deterioration can ensue quickly. Chronic mitral regurgitation, however, is far more indolent, and mild symptoms or acute decompensation from a correctable cause does not necessarily require surgical intervention.

174. The answer is A-N, B-Y, C-N, D-N, E-Y. *(Braunwald, ed 11, chap 186.)* Acute rheumatic fever is a later complication of pharyngeal streptococcal infections. It is often difficult to isolate group A streptococci by a throat culture at the onset of acute rheumatic fever, though past streptococcal infection can be documented by serologic studies. Recurrences, which are common after the initial episode, are most common in individuals who have rheumatic heart involvement. As a result, all affected individuals should receive prophylactic antibiotic treatment for at least 5 years. Earlobe macrophages are associated with subacute bacterial endocarditis, not acute rheumatic fever.

175. The answer is A-Y, B-Y, C-N, D-N, E-N. *(Braunwald, ed 11, chap 187.)* Although aortic stenosis may be present in affected individuals for several decades, survival for more than 2 years is unlikely once symptoms of heart failure occur. Atrial fibrillation with the loss of synchronized atrial systole can precipitate clinical deterioration. Stenosis of the aortic valve becomes of critical importance when the effective orifice is reduced to less than 0.7 cm^2/m^2. Absence of calcification in aortic valve cusps studied by fluoroscopy or echocardiography essentially rules out severe aortic stenosis in adults; this relationship, however, does not apply to plain chest x-ray. Normal boxlike separation of the aortic cusps on echocardiography excludes the presence of severe aortic stenosis; however, cusp calcification and poor mobility may not necessarily indicate significant valvular stenosis.

176. The answer is A-Y, B-Y, C-Y, D-Y, E-Y. *(Braunwald, ed 11, chap 187.)* A precipitating cause and the presence of an underlying structural heart disorder should be sought in all individuals who present with congestive heart failure. The increased demand for cardiac output associated with such processes as fever, anemia, pregnancy, hypoxia, and infection can overburden a heart that has a limited reserve but operates well when not stressed. Arrhythmias such as atrial fibrillation reduce ventricular filling time while depriving the ventricle of the usual augmentation to filling provided by atrial systole. Individuals with valvular disease are at risk for endocarditis, which can exacerbate heart failure. If the precipitating factor is reversible and preventable, affected individuals may not require valvular surgery.

177. The answer is A-N, B-Y, C-Y, D-N, E-Y. *(Braunwald, ed 11, chap 187.)* The systolic click-murmur syndrome is associated with mitral valve prolapse, which can place excessive stress on the papillary muscles and lead to ischemia and chest pain. Although often associated with inferior T-wave changes, the systolic click-murmur syndrome only occasionally results in an ischemic response to exercise. On standing or during a Valsalva's maneuver, as ventricular volume gets smaller the click and murmur move earlier into systole. Echocardiography reveals midsystolic prolapse of the posterior mitral leaflet, or on occasion both mitral leaflets, into the left atrium. Persons with mitral regurgitation from prolapse are at risk for developing subacute bacterial endocarditis and should be treated accordingly.

178. The answer is A-Y, B-Y, C-Y, D-Y, E-Y. *(Braunwald, ed 11, chap 188.)* Subacute bacterial endocarditis can be treated quite successfully. However, for individuals who have endocarditis and in whom bacteremia cannot be demonstrated, or offending organisms are isolated but are highly resistant to standard antimicrobial agents, the prognosis is less favorable. Delay in therapy also compromises the prognosis. The development of congestive heart failure is a most ominous sign. Endocarditis due to *Staphylococcus epidermidis* carries a poor prognosis if acquired at the time of cardiac surgery or if complicated by the adverse factors mentioned above.

179. The answer is A-N, B-N, C-Y, D-Y, E-Y. *(Braunwald, ed 11, chap 188.)* Individuals who have prosthetic valve endocarditis can be treated adequately with antibiotics, particularly if infection occurs several months after surgery. Endocarditis arising within the first two postoperative months likely is due to colonization of the prosthetic valve at surgery, whereas endocarditis that develops later probably is due to prosthesis colonization by transient bacteremias. Relapse following adequate antimicrobial therapy is an indication for valve replacement, as are valve-ring infections, which are commonly associated with prosthetic valve endocarditis, and myocardial penetration, which can be evidenced by heart block or bundle-branch block. Such situations carry a poor prognosis, as does intraoperative prosthetic infection by such organisms as *Staphylococcus epidermidis*.

180. The answer is A-N, B-Y, C-N, D-Y, E-Y. *(Braunwald, ed 11, chap 188.)* Right-sided endocarditis occurs frequently in persons addicted to parenteral drugs. The usual presentation, aside from such constitutional symptoms as fever, malaise, and anorexia, features septic pulmonary emboli. Blood cultures are positive as frequently in right-heart as in left-heart endocarditis. Heart murmur is often absent. With appropriate treatment the prognosis is generally good.

181. The answer is A-N, B-Y, C-Y, D-N, E-Y. *(Braunwald, ed 11, chap 183.)* The choice of a permanent pacemaker type depends on the underlying conduction disease and the patient's clinical profile. DDD pacing preserves the normal relationship between atrial and ventricular contraction, and physiologic atrial sensing with ventricular pacing improves exercise tolerance in young, active persons. As this form of pacing preserves the normal atrial contribution to cardiac output, it is desired in patients with decreased left ventricular function or hypertrophied ("stiff") left ventricular chambers. DDD pacing is contraindicated in atrial fibrillation or flutter since the ventricular rate response is unpredictable.

182. The answer is A-Y, B-N, C-Y, D-N, E-Y. *(Braunwald, ed 11, chap 190.)* Criteria for insertion of a temporary transvenous pacemaker differ for anterior and inferior myocardial infarctions. In an inferior myocardial infarction complicated by heart block, the escape focus is higher in the conduction system and is more rapid and reliable. A temporary pacemaker is inserted in patients with inferior myocardial infarction and complete heart block primarily if they are symptomatic or have extreme bradycardia. Because the escape focus in patients with an anterior myocardial infarction is unreliable and lower in the conduction system, a temporary pacemaker should be inserted; evidence of new bifascicular conduction defects is enough to warrant pacemaker insertion.

183. The answer is A-Y, B-Y, C-N, D-N, E-N *(Braunwald, ed 11, chap 189.)* The rate of occlusion of saphenous venous grafts is highest in the first postoperative year and declines subsequently. Internal mammary artery grafts to the left anterior descending artery have gained popularity, since the incidence of occlusion is lower than that with venous grafts. Angina is abolished or significantly reduced in the majority (85 percent) of patients after CABG. Impaired left ventricular (LV) function is not a contraindication to CABG; in fact, a reduction in mortality has been found in patients with 3-vessel disease and moderate LV dysfunction. In the hands of an experienced surgical team, surgical mortality associated with CABG should be less than 1 percent.

184. The answer is A-N, B-N, C-Y, D-Y. *(Braunwald, ed 11, chap 195.)* Hypercholesterolemia involving the LDL fraction is a risk factor for the development of ischemic heart disease. Low serum concentrations of HDL are also an independent risk factor. Serum triglyceride and total cholesterol concentrations increase with age, but the increase in the latter is of the LDL fraction. Since atherosclerotic disease begins early in life, it is good practice to measure serum lipid concentrations in persons, 20 to 30 years old, particularly in individuals with a family history of hypercholesterolemia or premature vascular disease. Successful dietary and pharmacologic therapy of hypercholesterolemia has been shown to reduce the morbidity and mortality associated with myocardial infarction.

185. The answer is A-Y, B-N, C-N, D-Y, E-Y. *(Braunwald, ed 11, chap 195.)* The Framingham heart study found that low plasma levels of high-density lipoprotein (HDL) are a potent risk factor for coronary artery disease. HDL levels are increased by exercise, intake of small amounts of alcohol, and administration of estrogens. Cigarette smoking and androgen therapy depress plasma HDL levels.

186. The answer is A-Y, B-N, C-Y, D-Y, E-N. *(Braunwald, ed 11, chap 193.)* Hyperthyroidism is an important, reversible cause of cardiac disease. Some of the manifestations are hyperadrenergic in nature and may in part be related to increased numbers of beta receptors. Atrial arrhythmias are frequent. The diagnosis should be entertained particularly for persons whose cardiac disease is resistant to the usual treatments as well as for the elderly, in whom many of the typical manifestations of hyperthyroidism tend to be lacking. Low-voltage electrocardiograms and pericardial effusion are features of hypothyroidism.

187. The answer is A-N, B-Y, C-N, D-Y, E-N. *(Braunwald, ed 11, chap 192.)* The symptoms of dyspnea in persons with asymmetrical septal hypertrophy are related as much to decreased left ventricular compliance as to the degree of obstruction. Use of calcium-channel blockers often relieves dyspnea by decreasing left ventricular stiffness. Sudden death in affected persons does not correlate with the degree of obstruction and is thought to be due to arrhythmias. On electrocardiography, Q waves commonly are seen and do not imply a coexistent infarction. Histologic abnormalities consist of disorganized arrangements of myocytes in the ventricular septum.

188. The answer is A-N, B-N, C-Y, D-Y, E-N. *(Braunwald, ed 11, chap 196.)* Renal artery stenosis can be diagnosed angiographically, but renal-vein renin measurements are required to assess the functional significance of the stenosis. Although rapid-sequence intravenous pyelography is a good screening test for renovascular hypertension, it is associated with a false-negative rate of 12 percent and a false-positive rate of 11 percent. Split renal function tests and randomly obtained renin levels are not considered reliable. If a pheochromocytoma is suspected, measurement of catecholamines or their metabolites in a 24-hour urine sample collected at a time when the affected person is hypertensive is adequate; provocative tests are not indicated in this condition. Primary aldosteronism should be suspected when hypokalemia accompanies a low serum renin level and high aldosterone excretion.

189. The answer is A-N, B-N, C-N, D-Y, E-N. *(Braunwald, ed 11, chap 182.)* In advanced heart failure, left ventricular afterload is augmented because of increased levels of circulating catecholamines and activation of the renin-angiotensin system. Afterload reducing agents reduce aortic impedance, resulting in elevation of stroke volume and cardiac output, with reduction in the left ventricular filling pressure. As cardiac output increases, reflex sympathetic nerve activity and circulating catecholamine levels decrease, and the heart rate tends to slow. Hydralazine is a potent afterload reducing agent; nitrates primarily dilate the systemic veins and are, therefore, potent *preload* reducing agents. Captopril is a balanced vasodilator. There is, thus far, no compelling evidence that therapy with an ACE inhibitor greatly increases long-term survival in patients with advanced heart failure.

190. The answer is A-N, B-N, C-Y, D-N, E-Y. *(Braunwald, ed 11, chap 198.)* Arteriosclerosis obliterans, an occlusive disease of large and medium-sized arteries, characteristically causes exercise-induced muscle pain. Typically, pain resolves quickly with rest; if it does not, or if recumbency is required for relief, then pseudoclaudication from neurospinal disease should be suspected. When ankle systolic pressure is greater than one-half arm systolic pressure, a single occlusion is usually present; when ankle systolic pressure is less than one-half arm systolic pressure, multiple occlusions usually are found. In exercise-provoked ischemia, ankle pressure falls—often becoming unrecordable—as the ischemic muscle dilates, stealing blood flow away from the foot. Marked symptomatic improvement can occur if affected individuals daily walk 75 percent of the claudication distance. Lumbar sympathectomy should be reserved for those individuals with mild rest pain.

191–195. The answers are: 191-C, 192-A, 193-B, 194-A, 195-C. *(Braunwald, ed 11, chap 177.)* Pulsus paradoxus is an exaggeration of the decrease in systolic arterial pressure normally observed during inspiration. It can be seen in persons with pericardial tamponade as well as in association with conditions featuring large swings in intrathoracic pressure (e.g., asthma). Bisferious pulse, a bifid pulse with two systolic peaks, is associated with aortic regurgitation. A variant of pulsus bisferiens called "spike-and-dome" pulse is seen in persons with hypertrophic obstructive cardiomyopathy. Pulsus alternans refers to variations in the amplitude of the arterial pulse in the face of a regular rhythm. It can occur in persons with severe left ventricular decompensation and, on occasion, following a premature ventricular contraction. Pulsus tardus refers to a slowly rising aortic pressure usually associated with valvular aortic stenosis. The degree of upstroke retardation correlates with the severity of aortic stenosis.

196–200. The answers are: 196-A, 197-B, 198-C, 199-D, 200-D. *(Braunwald, ed 11, chap 180.)* Equalization of diastolic pressures in the four cardiac chambers occurs in pericardial tamponade and constrictive pericarditis. The dip-and-plateau pattern in the ventricles and steep y descent in the atria are features of constrictive pericarditis but not pericardial tamponade.

In persons who have restrictive cardiomyopathy diastolic pressures may be nearly equal. Often, however, a separation of at least 5 mmHg exists or can be brought out by acute volume loading. The dip-and-plateau pattern in ventricular pressures is typical.

Acute mitral regurgitation is associated with tall regurgitant v waves, which reflect regurgitation of blood into a noncompliant left atrium during systole. They are often absent in more chronic mitral regurgitation—a dilated left atrium can accommodate large volumes of blood without a significant increase in pressure. A regurgitant v wave often slightly precedes the usual physiologic v wave, which reflects venous return to the atria while atrioventricular valves are closed. In ventricular septal rupture with left-to-right shunt, venous return to the left atrium increases and the v wave becomes exaggerated.

Slow y descent is due to delayed atrial emptying. This phenomenon occurs in mitral or tricuspid stenosis, atrial myxomas, and cor triatrium.

201–204. The answers are 201-C, 202-A, 203-B, 204-E. *(Braunwald, ed 11, chap 185.)* Many hereditary conditions and exposures to infectious agents during pregnancy result in congenital heart disease. Marfan's syndrome is a disorder of connective tissue in which cardiac abnormalities produce the greatest mortality. Decreased strength of the aortic connective tissue results in dilatation with aortic regurgitation and aortic dissection. Prolapse of the aortic and mitral valves are usually present, the latter associated with mitral regurgitation. Turner's syndrome is a chromosomal abnormality (45 XO) characterized by short stature and hypogonadism. Associated cardiac defects include coarctation of the aorta and bicuspid aortic valve. Maternal rubella during pregnancy can result in deafness, microcephaly, and cataracts in the infant. The most common cardiovascular lesions are pulmonic stenosis, multiple pulmonary artery stenoses, and patent ductus arteriosus. Cystic fibrosis is an autosomal recessive disease primarily affecting exocrine glands, resulting in chronic obstructive lung disease and pancreatic insufficiency. The prominent abnormalities of lung function may result in cor pulmonale. (Also see *Braunwald, ed 11, Chap. 207.*)

205–208. The answers are: 205-A, 206-C, 207-B, 208-B. (*Braunwald, ed 11, chap 182.*) Diuretic therapy is a mainstay in the treatment of persons in heart failure. The thiazide diuretics act in part at the proximal tubule to inhibit sodium reabsorption, while furosemide and ethacrynic acid act at the thick ascending limb of the loop of Henle to inhibit active chloride reabsorption. Spironolactone exerts its potassium-sparing effects by competitive inhibition of aldosterone; triamterene, on the other hand, acts by an unknown mechanism that is independent of the adrenal glands. In the presence of azotemia, thiazides often are ineffective, and spironolactone and triamterene are contraindicated because of possible hyperkalemia. Furosemide may remain effective even if azotemia develops.

209–213. The answers are: 209-B, 210-E, 211-D, 212-A, 213-C. (*Braunwald, ed 11, chap 184.*) Disopyramide phosphate has potent vagolytic effects, including urinary retention, which is especially poorly tolerated by elderly men with prostatic obstruction. It also can intensify myocardial dysfunction as a result of its potent negative inotropic effects. Bretylium tosylate initally causes alpha-adrenergic discharge. This action may lead to transient hypertension and exacerbation of ventricular arrhythmias initially. Chronic side effects may include postural hypotension. Lidocaine mainly produces central nervous system side effects, such as confusion, slurring of speech, and seizures. Persons with underlying central nervous system disease are particularly sensitive; so, too, are persons with hepatic disease and low cardiac output, because metabolism of lidocaine is reduced. Quinidine sulfate on occasion causes autoimmune thrombocytopenic purpura. Its more frequent side effects are diarrhea and excessive QT prolongation. The major side effects of digoxin are cardiac arrhythmias. When not caused by digoxin, many of the same arrhythmias would benefit from digoxin therapy. Thus, whether digoxin should be increased in dosage or discontinued is a frequent clinical dilemma when a new arrhythmia is noted. Nausea, anorexia, and yellow vision also are encountered frequently.

214–217. The answers are: 214-C, 215-C, 216-B, 217-A. (*Braunwald, ed 11, chap 194.*) Constrictive pericarditis and pericardial effusion can cause failure of either side of the heart. Differentiation of these two disorders can best be made clinically by examination of the neck veins: a prominent *x* trough occurs with effusion and *y* descent with constriction. Only constriction produces a pericardial knock in early diastole. A drop of more than 10 mmHg in systolic arterial pressure during inspiration (paradoxical pulse) is associated most commonly with pericardial effusion and resulting cardiac tamponade but also occurs in one-third of all persons with constrictive disease. Kussmaul's sign—inspiratory increase in venous pressure—occurs with pericardial constriction.

218–221. The answers are: 218-E, 219-A, 220-C, 221-B. (*Braunwald, ed 11, chaps 187, 191, 194.*) Right heart failure, or elevated right-heart filling pressure, can develop from many causes. Right heart failure most commonly occurs as a result of pulmonary artery hypertension. Pulmonary artery hypertension, in turn, arises either from increased pulmonary vascular resistance with lung disease, in which case the pulmonary capillary wedge pressure (left atrial pressure) is not elevated, or from left-sided failure or valvular disease, in which case left atrial pressure is increased. Massive right ventricular infarction can cause the right side of the heart to fail at low systolic pressures. With primary myocardial disease, both left and right atrial pressures are elevated; however, when diastolic pressures are **equal** in the left and right cardiac chambers, external compression, such as constrictive pericarditis, must be suspected as the cause.

222–226. The answers are: 222-D, 223-E, 224-A, 225-C, 226-B. (*Braunwald, ed 11, chap 196.*) Clonidine predominantly is an alpha-receptor agonist in the central nervous system. The stimulation of central alpha receptors reduces sympathetic outflow and arterial pressure. Baroreceptor reflexes are usually not particularly altered, and orthostatic hypotension is minimized. Minoxidil is a direct-acting peripheral vasodilator useful in treating patients with severe hypertension and renal failure. Its limiting side effect, especially bothersome in women, is hirsutism. Captopril blocks the conversion of angiotensin I to angiotensin II. However, unlike saralasin it does not block the angiotensin II receptor. Prazosin is an antihypertensive agent that appears to block postsynaptic alpha-adrenergic receptors. Sudden syncopal episodes can occur with use of this drug.

DISORDERS OF THE RESPIRATORY SYSTEM

DIRECTIONS: Each question below contains five suggested answers. Choose the **one best** response to each question.

227. A 27-year-old man says that his physical tolerance for tennis has declined during the last 3 months and that, lately, he has noticed audible wheezing while playing. His doubles partner, an asthmatic, recommended an over-the-counter inhaled bronchodilator, which the man has used without improvement in his symptoms. Two years ago, he required mechanical ventilation for Guillain-Barré syndrome but recovered uneventfully. On pulmonary function testing performed now, he produces the flow-volume curve shown below. As the next step in the workup of this man's illness, his physician should

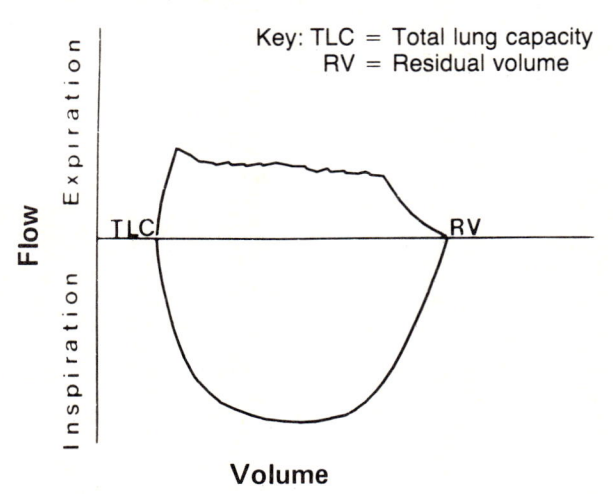

(A) prescribe an oral theophylline preparation
(B) prescribe inhaled sodium cromoglycate
(C) conduct further pulmonary function testing, including a test of a small-airways function
(D) order a chest x-ray
(E) prescribe a course of prednisone, to be tapered over 2 weeks

228. All the following conditions impair the release of oxygen to body tissues EXCEPT

(A) methemoglobinemia
(B) carbon monoxide poisoning
(C) hyperventilation
(D) hypophosphatemia
(E) acidosis

229. A 63-year-old man has pneumococcal pneumonia with extensive air-space consolidation in the left upper and left lower lobes. He complains of extreme shortness of breath when positioned with his left side down. An arterial blood sample drawn in this position shows a P_{O_2} of 46 mmHg; 10 minutes earlier, an arterial blood sample drawn while his right side was dependent had revealed a P_{O_2} of 66 mmHg. The most likely explanation for the drop in P_{O_2} when the man was lying on his left side is

(A) increased blood flow to the dependent lung
(B) reduced ventilation to the dependent lung
(C) increased airway resistance in the dependent lung
(D) accumulation of interstitial edema in the dependent lung
(E) increased stiffness of the chest wall on the dependent side

230. Asthmatic attacks may be precipitated in susceptible persons by a wide variety of stimuli. All the following have been demonstrated to produce airway obstruction in certain asthmatic subjects EXCEPT

(A) viral respiratory infections
(B) cold air
(C) sodium salicylate
(D) exercise
(E) airborne allergens

231. Although asthma is a heterogeneous disease, a given individual with asthma would be most likely to

(A) relate a personal or family history of allergic diseases
(B) conform to a characteristic personality type
(C) display a skin-test reaction to extracts of airborne allergens
(D) demonstrate nonspecific airway hyperirritability
(E) have supranormal serum immunoglobulin E

232. A diagnosis of allergic bronchopulmonary aspergillosis in a person who has asthma, recurrent pulmonary infiltrates, and eosinophilia would be supported by all the following findings EXCEPT

(A) delayed, tuberculin-type skin test reaction to *Aspergillus fumigatus*
(B) sputum culture positive for *A. fumigatus*
(C) presence of serum precipitins to *A. fumigatus*
(D) marked elevation of serum immunoglobulin E level
(E) radiographic evidence of bronchiectasis

233. Upper-lobe bronchiectasis in a person who is wheezing and has eosinophilia suggests the presence of

(A) Loeffler's syndrome
(B) polyarteritis nodosa
(C) drug hypersensitivity to nitrofurantoin
(D) allergic bronchopulmonary aspergillosis
(E) *Strongyloides stercoralis* infection

234. Bronchospasm may be produced by exposure in the workplace to all of the following EXCEPT

(A) cotton dust
(B) toluene diisocyanate
(C) fluorocarbons
(D) flax
(E) silica

235. Cavity formation is a common complication of pneumonia caused by

(A) anaerobic bacteria
(B) *Legionella pneumophila*
(C) *Streptococcus pneumoniae*
(D) *Mycoplasma pneumoniae*
(E) influenza virus

236. A 46-year-old woman complains of sudden anxiety and breathlessness. She has been at bed rest for 2 weeks for back pain. She uses oral contraceptives. All of the following findings would support further testing to diagnose pulmonary embolism EXCEPT

(A) subsegmental atelectasis on chest x-ray
(B) a P_{O_2} of 90 mmHg
(C) a temperature of 39.5°C (103.1°F)
(D) sinus tachycardia on electrocardiogram
(E) normal findings on examination of the lower extremities

Questions 237–238

A 60-year old man with emphysema and bronchitis is brought to an emergency room by an ambulance crew that has been giving him oxygen by mask. Three days ago, he noted that his sputum had changed color and increased in amount. His wife called the ambulance when he became suddenly short of breath and confused. On arrival at the hospital he is somnolent. Mid-inspiratory crackles and diffuse expiratory wheezes are audible on examination of the chest, and he has marked peripheral edema and ascites. Hemoglobin is 18 g/dL. Arterial blood gases are pH 7.08, P_{O_2} 148 mmHg, and P_{CO_2} 106 mmHg.

237. The most appropriate immediate therapy for the man described above would be

(A) intravenous infusion of sodium bicarbonate
(B) endotracheal intubation and assisted ventilation
(C) administration of isoetharine by air-compressor nebulizer
(D) discontinuation of supplemental oxygen
(E) subcutaneous injection of epinephrine

238. For the man described above, manifestations of right ventricular heart failure would best be treated with

(A) diazoxide
(B) digoxin
(C) hydralazine
(D) oxygen
(E) phlebotomy

239. A 34-year-old man complains of shortness of breath after minimal exertion. He has no systemic symptoms. He developed a nonproductive cough 10 months ago. A chest x-ray which was reportedly normal, was done at that time. Examination now reveals a respiratory rate of 28 breaths per minute, and diffuse end inspiratory crackles are heard over his lower lung fields. His chest x-ray is shown below. An arterial P_{O_2} measured while patient is breathing room air is 55 mmHg, and arterial P_{CO_2} is 26 mmHg. Routine blood counts are normal. The next step in his evaluation should be

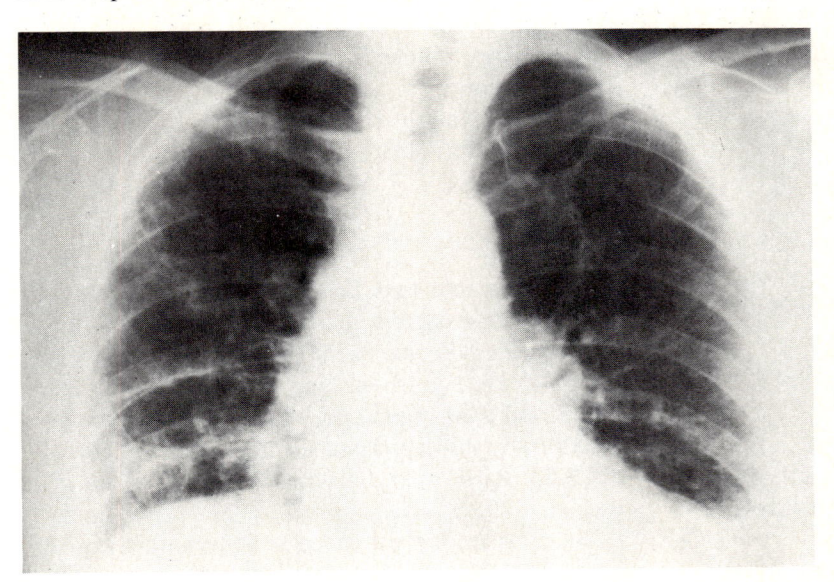

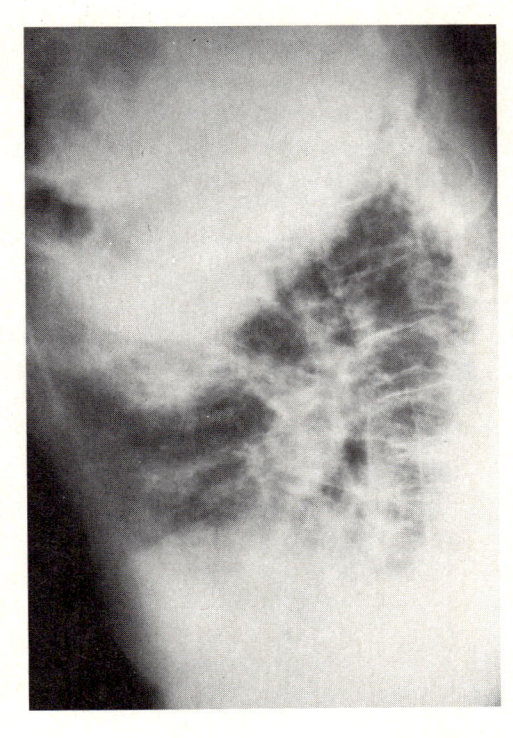

(A) angiotensin-converting enzyme level
(B) open lung biopsy
(C) percutaneous lung biopsy
(D) salivary gland biopsy
(E) serology for rheumatoid factor

240. A 23-year-old woman complains of dyspnea and substernal chest pain on exertion. Evaluation for this complaint 6 months ago included arterial blood-gas testing, which revealed pH 7.48, P_{O_2} 79 mmHg, and P_{CO_2} 31 mmHg. Electrocardiography then showed a right axis deviation. Chest x-ray now shows enlarged pulmonary arteries but no parenchymal infiltrates, and a lung perfusion scan reveals subsegmental defects that are thought to have a "low probability for pulmonary thromboembolism." The most appropriate diagnostic test now would be

(A) open lung biopsy
(B) Holter monitoring
(C) right-heart catheterization
(D) transbronchial biopsy
(E) serum α_1-antitrypsin level

241. A 53-year-old man is noted to be tachypneic and confused 48 hours after suffering multiple orthopedic and internal injuries in an automobile accident. Chest x-ray is interpreted as normal, but arterial blood-gas values are as follows: pH 7.49, P_{O_2} 52 mmHg, and P_{CO_2} 30 mmHg. The course of action most likely to confirm the diagnosis of this man's condition would be to

(A) order a ventilation-perfusion scan
(B) order pulmonary angiography
(C) order impedence plethysmography
(D) order blood testing for fibrin split products
(E) repeat the physical examination

242. A 42-year-old man who is a heavy cigarette smoker develops chills, malaise, and tenderness at the angle of the jaw a week after onset of a sore throat. On examination he is febrile and tachypneic, and a pleural friction rub is audible over the left chest. Chest x-ray reveals several nodular densities in both lung fields. The most likely diagnosis is

(A) osteoma of the tonsil
(B) retropharyngeal abscess
(C) peritonsillar cellulitis
(D) pharyngeal tuberculosis
(E) postanginal sepsis

243. A 52-year-old woman with long-standing rheumatoid arthritis is hospitalized for total knee replacement. On her admission chest x-ray, a 2-cm nodule is noted near the right hilus. She has smoked one pack of cigarettes daily for the last 32 years. The most appropriate management of this woman's pulmonary condition would be

(A) observation with chest x-rays every 4 months
(B) therapy for 2 months with oral corticosteroids
(C) an upper gastrointestinal series
(D) scalene node biopsy
(E) exploratory thoracotomy

244. The most sensitive noninvasive test for bilateral diaphragmatic paralysis is

(A) testing of vital capacity
(B) "sniff test"
(C) chest x-ray
(D) fluoroscopy
(E) physical examination

245. All the following statements about sleep apnea syndrome (SAS) are true EXCEPT

(A) men are affected more often than women
(B) systemic hypertension is a common finding
(C) enuresis occurs in a minority of cases
(D) obesity is a cardinal feature
(E) personality changes may be the presenting complaint

246. A 54-year-old man has a nonproductive cough and exertional breathlessness. He also notes low-grade fever, malaise, and a 7 kg (15 lb) weight loss occurring over six weeks. His white blood cell count is 13,500/mm^3. He has a history of mild asthma. A chest x-ray is obtained. The most likely diagnosis is

(A) idiopathic pulmonary fibrosis
(B) alveolar proteinosis
(C) polymyositis
(D) chronic eosinophilic pneumonia
(E) lymphangiomyomatosis

Questions 247–248

An 18-year-old man develops adult respiratory distress syndrome after a near drowning. Breathing room air, he has the following arterial blood-gas values: pH 7.50, P$_{O_2}$ 48 mmHg, and P$_{CO_2}$ 28 mmHg. Arterial blood gases obtained while he is breathing 80% oxygen by mask (measured in the nasopharynx) are pH 7.50, P$_{O_2}$ 63 mmHg, and P$_{CO_2}$ 29 mmHg.

247. The most important cause of hypoxemia in the man described above would be

(A) a block in alveolar-capillary diffusion
(B) right-to-left shunting
(C) ventilation-perfusion mismatch
(D) hypoventilation
(E) poor cardiac output

248. Due to profound hypoxemia, tracheal intubation is performed on the man described above, and mechanical ventilation is begun. Inspired oxygen concentration is 80%. Initially, the man is agitated and fights the respirator. Arterial blood gases are obtained and show pH 7.21, P$_{O_2}$ 70 mmHg, and P$_{CO_2}$ 56 mmHg. The most appropriate management step at this time would be to

(A) add positive end-expiratory pressure (5 cmH$_2$O)
(B) sedate the man and control his ventilation
(C) infuse sodium bicarbonate intravenously
(D) raise the inspired oxygen concentration
(E) initiate extracorporeal membrane oxygenation

DISORDERS OF THE RESPIRATORY SYSTEM

DIRECTIONS: Each question below contains five suggested answers. For **each** of the five alternatives of **each** item, you are to respond either YES (Y) or NO (N). In a given item all, some, or none of the alternatives may be correct.

249. A 25-year-old woman comes to the hospital because of an acute exacerbation of her long-standing asthma. When examined, she is anxious and tachypneic. She is using accessory muscles of respiration to breathe, and diffuse wheezes are audible on expiration. Which of the following measures would be inappropriate initial therapy for this woman?

(A) Administration of inhaled beclomethasone
(B) Administration of inhaled cromolyn sodium
(C) Administration of inhaled isoproterenol
(D) Intravenous infusion of aminophylline
(E) Intravenous administration of sedatives

250. The diagnosis of cystic fibrosis is best made by measurement of sweat chloride concentration. This measurement should be made in a boy who has chronic airways obstruction and any of the following EXCEPT

(A) intussusception
(B) sinusitis
(C) steatorrhea
(D) dextrocardia
(E) clubbing

251. Which of the following statements about cystic fibrosis are true?

(A) It is unusual for an affected male to live past the age of 20 years
(B) Affected newborns typically have patchy atelectasis due to bronchiolar obstruction
(C) Portal hypertension may occur in affected persons who lack pancreatic function
(D) Affected women are likely to have difficulty conceiving a child
(E) Meconium ileus occurs in approximately 10 percent of cases

Questions 252–253

A 35-year-old man seeks medical attention for breathlessness on exertion. He has never smoked cigarettes and has not been coughing. One sibling died at 40 years of age of respiratory failure. His three children are healthy. Physical examination reveals him to be tachypneic as he exhales through pursed lips. His chest is tympanitic to percussion, and breath sounds are poorly heard on auscultation. Chest x-ray shows flattened diaphragms with peripheral attenuation of bronchovascular markings most noticeable at the lung bases.

252. Expected results of the pulmonary function testing of the man described above would include

(A) increased lung elastic recoil
(B) increased total lung capacity
(C) reduced functional residual capacity
(D) reduced vital capacity
(E) increased diffusing capacity

253. Initial laboratory assessment of the man described above should include

(A) measurement of oxygen consumption during exercise
(B) measurement of sweat chloride concentration
(C) serum protein electrophoresis
(D) complete spirometry
(E) arterial blood-gas determination

254. In persons with chronic airway obstruction, prognosis can be improved by

(A) oxygen therapy
(B) exercise programs
(C) cessation of smoking
(D) phlebotomy
(E) use of oral expectorants

255. Which of the following statements about idiopathic interstitial pneumonitis are true?

(A) Although chest x-ray is not a good screening test for interstitial fibrosis, it is a sensitive marker for following disease activity
(B) Early in the illness, the chest x-ray typically shows a reticular pattern around the periphery of the lung
(C) A gallium scan can be used to distinguish idiopathic interstitial fibrosis from lung involvement associated with rheumatoid arthritis
(D) The most sensitive pulmonary function test for idiopathic interstitial fibrosis is arterial blood-gas measurement during exercise
(E) In the absence of therapy, most individuals with fibrosis but little cellular infiltration progressively worsen

256. Hypoxemia occurring after pulmonary thromboembolism can result from

(A) lowered mixed venous P_{O_2} due to heart failure
(B) perfusion of atelectatic areas
(C) increased dead-space ventilation in the area of vascular occlusion
(D) perfusion of areas poorly ventilated due to airway constriction
(E) inadequate time for oxygen diffusion secondary to a reduction in the capillary bed

257. A middle-aged woman has a large central mass on chest x-ray. Sputum cytology is positive for squamous-cell carcinoma. Which of the following conditions would be considered indications NOT to operate on this woman?

(A) Resting P_{CO_2} above 50 mmHg
(B) Syndrome of inappropriate antidiuretic hormone secretion
(C) Pleural effusion
(D) Recurrent laryngeal nerve paralysis
(E) Metastasis to lobar lymph nodes

258. Which of the following statements about pleural effusions are true?

(A) Although acid-fast bacilli rarely are seen on smears of fluid from postprimary tuberculous effusions, the fluid culture is positive in a majority of cases
(B) If eosinophils comprise more than 10 percent of cells in a pleural effusion, hypereosinophilic syndrome is a likely diagnosis
(C) Pleural effusion following abdominal surgery usually is due to a subphrenic abscess
(D) Low glucose concentration in a rheumatoid pleural effusion is due to impaired glucose transport
(E) Epidemic pleurodynia usually produces small, unilateral pleural effusions

259. Which of the following are health effects of exposure to asbestos fibers?

(A) Pulmonary fibrosis
(B) Pleural effusion
(C) Oat cell carcinoma
(D) Peritoneal mesothelioma
(E) Pleural plaques

260. A 51-year-old man develops pancreatitis associated with the passage of a gallstone. His treatment includes meperidine and intravenous normal saline. Two days later, he becomes anxious, tachypneic, and short of breath. An emergency chest x-ray demonstrates diffuse, bilateral interstitial and alveolar infiltrates. A year ago, he suffered a myocardial infarction, but since then he has no evidence of congestive heart failure. In this case, adult respiratory distress syndrome can be distinguished from cardiogenic pulmonary edema by

(A) measurement of lung water
(B) measurement of edema fluid protein concentration
(C) measurement of pulmonary artery wedge pressure
(D) measurement of lung compliance
(E) calculation of the alveolar-arterial P_{O_2} difference

DISORDERS OF THE RESPIRATORY SYSTEM

DIRECTIONS: The groups of questions below consist of four or five lettered headings followed by several numbered items. For each numbered item choose the **one** lettered heading with which it is **most** closely associated. Each lettered heading may be used once, more than once, or not at all.

Questions 261–264

For each condition listed below, select the set of pathologic findings from open lung biopsy with which it is most likely to be associated.

(A) Diffuse alveolar hemorrhage with many hemosiderin-laden alveolar macrophages; thickened alveolar septae; linear deposition of immunoglobulin G in alveolar-capillary basement membrane
(B) Necrotizing vasculitis of small arteries and veins; eosinophilic infiltration of vessel walls; extravascular granulomas
(C) Necrotizing granulomas involving bronchial walls; small pulmonary arteries and veins infiltrated with plasma cells and lymphocytes
(D) Interstitial aggregates of atypical histiocytes with an admixture of eosinophils; surrounding alveoli with macrophages and sloughed pneumocytes
(E) Noncaseating granulomas in alveolar walls and interstitium composed of large epithelioid cells without surrounding inflammatory cells

261. Eosinophilic granuloma

262. Wegener's granulomatosis

263. Allergic granulomatosis and angiitis of Churg and Strauss

264. Sarcoidosis

Questions 265–268

For each cell type of pulmonary neoplasm listed below, select the paraneoplastic syndrome with which it is most closely associated.

(A) Hypercalcemia without bone destruction
(B) Excessive secretion of adrenocortical hormones
(C) Gynecomastia
(D) Intermittent flushing
(E) Hypertrophic pulmonary osteoarthropathy

265. Squamous cell carcinoma

266. Large cell carcinoma

267. Adenocarcinoma

268. Small cell carcinoma

Disorders of the Respiratory System

Answers

227. The answer is D. *(Braunwald, ed 11, chap 200. Miller, Am Rev Respir Dis 108:475, 1973.)* Although expiratory wheezing in a young adult usually indicates asthma, numerous conditions can mimic diffuse, reversible airway disease. Upper-airway obstruction should always be considered in an individual who has been wheezing, and a flow-volume study provides a simple, relatively sensitive screening test. The loop shown in the figure demonstrates the "cutoff" of expiratory flow that occurs in variable intrathoracic obstruction. Once a flow-volume curve is obtained, the next diagnostic step should be chest x-ray and then bronchoscopy or cinebronchography.

228. The answer is E. *(Braunwald, ed 11, chap 200.)* The affinity of the hemoglobin molecule for oxygen is altered primarily by blood pH, temperature, red blood cell concentration of 2,3-diphosphoglycerate (2,3-DPG), and arterial carbon dioxide tension. Increased affinity, such as is produced by a rise in pH or a drop in 2,3-DPG, temperature, or P_{CO_2}, favors the transport of oxygen to body tissue. That is, under these conditions, at a given P_{O_2} a greater percentage of hemoglobin will be saturated with oxygen and more oxygen can be carried by the blood. Reduced affinity for oxygen favors unloading of oxygen from the hemoglobin molecule to the tissues—or, at a given P_{O_2} less oxygen will be bound to hemoglobin. Carbon monoxide causes hemoglobin to bind oxygen more avidly. Hyperventilation, by lowering P_{CO_2} and raising pH, and hypophosphatemia, by reducing levels of 2,3-DPG, both increase affinity. Methemoglobin binds oxygen more avidly than hemoglobin, therefore impairing the release of oxygen to the tissues.

229. The answer is A. *(Braunwald, ed 11, chap 200.)* In a person standing erect, blood flow per unit volume increases from the apex of the lung to the base. Ventilation also increases from apex to base, but the gradient is less than that for blood flow, making the ventilation-perfusion ratio less at the bottom of the lung than at the top. Both ventilation and perfusion are affected by posture; as a general rule, the dependent regions are better ventilated and perfused and have the lowest ratio of ventilation to perfusion. Thus, an individual with unilateral air-space disease may have an increase in venous admixture when the diseased lung is dependent. In that situation, blood flow increases to the diseased lung, perfusing atelectatic and poorly ventilated alveoli, and hypoxemia ensues.

230. The answer is C. *(Braunwald, ed 11, chap 202.)* Respiratory infections, particularly those that are viral in origin, are common precipitants of acute asthmatic attacks. Bacterial infections are relatively less common precipitants; in fact, they may be implicated wrongly in acute asthma if purulent sputum due to sputum eosinophilia is mistakenly attributed to bacterial disease. Hyperventilation with cold air is now used as a bronchoprovocation test in some pulmonary function laboratories to identify asthmatic subjects. Heat loss across the respiratory mucosa is believed to be the stimulus producing airway narrowing in asthmatic individuals who breathe cold air and who have exercise-induced asthma. Although some persons with asthma develop bronchospasm after ingestion of acetylsalicylic acid or tartrazine dye, they tolerate sodium salicylate without symptoms. In allergic asthma subjects, inhalation challenge testing with appropriate antigens causes reproducible bronchospasm.

231. The answer is D. *(Braunwald, ed 11, chap 202.)* The importance of immune mechanisms in the pathogenesis of asthma is suggested by the common association between the disease and the presence of allergic diseases, skin-test sensitivity, and increased serum IgE levels. In addition, many susceptible persons develop bronchospasm after inhalation challenge with airborne allergens. A large proportion of asthmatic subjects, however, have none of these markers of immunologic activity and are classified as having idiosyncratic asthma. When tested for bronchial hyperirritability with various nonantigenic bronchoprovocational agents (e.g., histamine or cold air), asthmatic subjects are found to be more sensitive than normal; the reason for this airway hyperirritability, which is a common feature of all asthmatic individuals, is unknown. Although psychologic factors certainly influence the expression of asthma, no single personality type is considered "asthmatic."

232. The answer is A. *(Braunwald, ed 11, chap 203.)* Allergic bronchopulmonary aspergillosis is a hypersensitivity pneumonitis involving an allergic reaction to antigens from *Aspergillus* species, most commonly *A. fumigatus*. The diagnosis should be suspected in asthmatic persons who have recurrent pulmonary infiltrates associated with peripheral blood or sputum eosinophilia. Suggestive laboratory findings include serum immunoglobulin E levels elevated many times normal and the presence of aspergilli in the sputum. Antigenic skin testing is positive both in immediate (type I, wheal and flare) reaction and reaction evident after 4 to 6 hours (type III, erythema and induration). Delayed, tuberculin-type (type IV, cell-mediated) reactions, however, do not occur. Serum precipitins to aspergilli are found in a majority of affected persons. The inflammatory response leads to dilatation of central airways and often is evident radiographically as mucoid impaction.

233. The answer is D. *(Braunwald, ed 11, chap 203.)* Allergic bronchopulmonary aspergillosis involves a hypersensitivity reaction to antigens from the fungus *Aspergillus*, which colonizes airways of certain asthmatic individuals. Usually most intensive in upper-lobe airways, the reaction leads to mucous impaction, inflammation, and, ultimately, dilatation of the involved bronchi. Loeffler's syndrome, or simple pulmonary eosinophilia, consists of transient pulmonary infiltrates and peripheral blood eosinophilia and is usually associated with cough, not wheezing. It often produces no symptoms and is usually benign. The airways are not involved. Polyarteritis nodosa may be associated with asthma and eosinophilia when it involves the lung, although most clinicians now believe such involvement is rare. Pathologically, it involves vessels and not the bronchial wall. Nitrofurantoin produces primarily interstitial inflammation of lower lobes. Infection with *Strongyloides stercoralis* may lead to cough, hemoptysis, and wheezing associated with eosinophilia as the filariform larvae pass through the lungs; however, this infection does not produce bronchiectasis.

234. The answer is E. *(Braunwald, ed 11, chap 204.)* Occupational respiratory illness resulting from inhalation of cotton dust or flax is first evident as a drop in airflow, with chest tightness and wheezing occurring on the first day of the work week. If exposure continues, symptoms may persist through the week. Persons exposed for ten years or more may have irreversible airflow obstruction. Toluene diisocyanate exposure during production of polyurethane may produce persistent asthma in susceptible individuals. Fluorocarbons, transmitted by a worker's hands to his or her cigarettes, are volatilized as the cigarette burns and may cause polymer fume fever, characterized by fever, malaise, and wheezing. Intense exposure to silica may produce acute silicosis with extensive pulmonary fibrosis that often terminates in respiratory failure in less than 2 years. Long-term exposure to lower levels of silica will cause nodular pulmonary fibrosis with hilar adenopathy. The fibrosis is usually greatest in the upper lobes. However, silica does not cause bronchospasm.

235. The answer is A. *(Braunwald, ed 11, chap 205.)* Anaerobic organisms often cause pneumonia that features a gradually developing, almost indolent course characterized by weight loss and fever. However, single or multiple cavities are common complications usually occurring in lung segments that were dependent at the time of the initial aspiration. In contrast, cavitation is uncommon in pneumococcal pneumonia, rare in *Mycoplasma* pneumonia and in pneumonia due to *Legionella pneumophila*. Viral infections usually do not produce cavitation.

236. The answer is C. *(Braunwald, ed 11, chap 211.)* Although radiographic findings such as a pleural-based infiltrate, focal oligemia, or "cutoff" of a vessel should suggest pulmonary thromboembolism, the most common radiographic finding is subsegmental atelectasis. Often the chest x-ray shows entirely normal findings, especially in the 24 to 36 hours after formation of the embolus. Pulmonary embolism almost invariably widens the alveolar-arterial oxygen tension gradient. By hyperventilating and lowering carbon dioxide tension, however, normal arterial P_{O_2} may be preserved. Pulmonary infarction may cause temperature elevations, but the oral temperature rarely rises above 38.5°C (101.3°F). Temperature elevations above this level should suggest an alternative diagnosis or a complication of pulmonary embolism such as an infected pulmonary infarction. Sinus tachycardia is the most common electrocardiographic finding associated with pulmonary embolism. Other ECG findings that are consistent with pulmonary embolism are rightward shift of the QRS axis, peaking of the P wave, and ST-T changes of right ventricular strain. Ninety-five percent of pulmonary thromboemboli arise in the deep veins of the legs, but fewer than 50 percent of patients have clinical signs or symptoms to suggest deep venous thrombosis.

237. The answer is B. *(Braunwald, ed 11, chap 208.)* Certain persons with severe obstructive lung disease appear to respond to uncontrolled oxygen therapy by dangerously reducing their minute ventilation. Because they are relatively insensitive to changes in arterial P_{CO_2}, hypoxemia is the major ventilatory stimulus in these persons. When hypoxemia is suddenly treated with supplemental oxygen therapy given in an uncontrolled fashion, ventilation drops, arterial P_{CO_2} rises, acidosis results, and coma may develop. However, abrupt removal of supplemental oxygen may precipitate life-threatening hypoxemia. Because acidosis must nevertheless be rapidly reversed by increasing ventilation, endotracheal intubation should be performed, followed by mechanical ventilation of sufficient amount to return arterial pH to physiologic range. Inhaled bronchodilators cannot be given to comatose, unintubated persons. Epinephrine is relatively ineffective in persons with acute or chronic respiratory failure and is dangerous in elderly, acidemic individuals.

238. The answer is D. *(Braunwald, ed 11, chaps 191 and 208.)* Right-heart failure in persons with chronic pulmonary disease is usually evident as edema and ascites—that is, signs of increased extravascular water. Evidence also suggests that increased right-heart filling pressures contribute to increases in lung water. Treatment should be aimed at reducing the afterload of the right ventricle. This goal can be accomplished most physiologically by increasing alveolar oxygen tension with supplemental oxygen therapy. Although hydralazine and diazoxide are vasodilators with important effects on the pulmonary circulation, they would not be needed in the case described and may, in fact, worsen gas exchange. Although the usefulness of digoxin therapy in cor pulmonale is debated, the drug generally is reserved for treating persons who have coexisting left ventricular disease. Phlebotomy, although it may improve oxygen delivery in persons with right-heart failure and elevated hemoglobin concentrations (> 20 g/dL), would not be a reliable remedy for the ascites and edema in the patient presented.

239. The answer is B. *(Braunwald, ed 11, chap 209. Crystal, Ann Int Med 85:769–788, 1976.)* The chest x-ray presented shows diffuse, severe interstitial infiltrates without hilar adenopathy. Although sarcoidosis may produce this radiographic picture, it is also compatible with idiopathic interstitial pneumonitis, hypersensitivity pneumonitis, collagen vascular disease, inhalation of inorganic dusts, and many other processes. The degree of respiratory system dysfunction demonstrated by this patient necessitates rapid evaluation and a definitive histologic diagnosis so that appropriate therapy can be initiated. Angiotensin-converting enzyme levels, although elevated in many patients with sarcoidosis, are not sufficiently sensitive or specific to replace tissue biopsy in the workup of persons with interstitial infiltrates. Although biopsy of extrapulmonary tissue may demonstrate noncaseating granulomas in patients with sarcoidosis, such biopsies may be negative in individuals with active disease. Percutaneous and transbronchial biopsies rarely yield sufficient tissue for specific diagnosis in a patient such as the one presented, and most often an open lung biopsy is required. For this reason, an open procedure should be done without delay in a patient who presents for initial evaluation with extensive interstitial lung disease.

240. The answer is C. *(Braunwald, ed 11, chap 210.)* Primary pulmonary hypertension is an uncommon disease that usually affects young women. Early in the illness affected individuals often are diagnosed as psychoneurotic because of the vague nature of presenting complaints—for example, dyspnea, chest pain, and evidence of hyperventilation without hypoxemia on arterial blood-gas testing. However, progression of the disease leads to syncope in approximately one-half of cases and signs of right-heart failure on physical exam. Chest x-ray typically shows enlarged central pulmonary arteries with or without attenuation of peripheral markings. The diagnosis of primary pulmonary hypertension is made by documentation of elevated pressures by right-heart catheterization and by exclusion of other pathologic processes. Lung disease of sufficient severity to cause pulmonary hypertension would be evident by history and on exam. Major differential diagnoses include thromboemboli and heart disease; outside the United States, schistosomiasis and filariasis are common causes of pulmonary hypertension, thus necessitating a careful travel history.

241. The answer is E. *(Braunwald, ed 11, chap 211. Moylan, Annu Rev Med 28:85, 1977.)* The clinical triad of dyspnea, confusion, and petechiae in a person who has had recent long-bone fractures establishes the diagnosis of fat embolism syndrome. This disorder, which usually occurs within 48 hours of injury, may lead to respiratory failure and death. Petechiae most often are found across the neck, in the axillae, and in the conjunctivae; however, their appearance is often evanescent. No laboratory test is specific for fat embolism.

242. The answer is E. *(Braunwald, ed 11, chap 212.)* Postanginal sepsis is a complication of acute bacterial pharyngitis in which a tonsillar abscess leads to infection of the ipsilateral carotid sheath and suppurative thrombophlebitis of the jugular vein. Anaerobic organisms are most commonly cultured from the blood and metastatic foci of infection. At the time of dissemination of infection the pharynx may not be painful, so the origin of the infection may be unsuspected.

243. The answer is E. *(Braunwald, ed 11, chap 213.)* A solitary lung nodule in a middle-aged person who is a cigarette smoker requires surgical resection. Although a rheumatoid nodule would be in the differential diagnosis of the lesion described in the case, such nodules are usually subpleural and are more common in men than in women. The central location and small size of the lesion described make it relatively inaccessible to nonsurgical biopsy techniques. Because 95 percent of malignant solitary nodules originate in the lung, an undirected search for a primary source is likely to be fruitless. Mediastinoscopy has largely replaced scalene node biopsy in most centers, but because the incidence of mediastinal metastases in malignant solitary nodules is less than 10 percent, surgical exploration would be indicated for the woman described in the question.

244. The answer is E. *(Braunwald, ed 11, chap 214.)* When the diaphragm is completely paralyzed, it behaves as a floppy membrane. With inspiration, the intercostal and other accessory muscles of respiration contract, causing intrathoracic pressure to become more negative. A floppy diaphragm would then be drawn upward into the chest, and the anterior abdominal wall would move inward. This "paradoxical" motion of the abdominal wall, which is best seen while an affected person is supine, is the most sensitive sign of bilateral diaphragmatic paralysis. Other disorders, such as severe obstructive lung disease, may also produce paradoxical motion of the anterior abdominal wall; however, the paradoxical motion usually improves when a person with this disorder is supine.

245. The answer is D. *(Braunwald, ed 11, chap 215. Guilleminault, Annu Rev Med 27:465, 1976.)* Sleep apnea syndrome (SAS) is a complex entity that involves intermittent upper-airway obstruction during sleep. Most of the manifestations, such as hypertension, cor pulmonale, chronic fatigue, personality changes, and disordered sleep behavior, resolve when obstruction is bypassed by a tracheostomy or endotracheal tube. Although the syndrome is more common in men, the prevalence increases in women after menopause. Obesity was once believed to be the most important risk factor; now, however, large numbers of affected persons who are of normal weight have been identified.

246. The answer is D. *(Braunwald, ed 11, chap 209.)* Chronic eosinophilic pneumonia is an interstitial lung disorder of unknown cause that produces a systemic illness characterized by fever, weight loss, and malaise. Although lung biopsy shows an eosinophilic infiltrate involving both the interstitium and the alveolar space, there may not be an associated eosinophilia in the peripheral blood. The diagnosis should be suggested by the "photonegative pulmonary edema" pattern, with central sparing and nonsegmental, patchy infiltrates in the lung periphery. This disorder often responds dramatically to corticosteroid therapy. Idiopathic pulmonary fibrosis and polymyositis produce diffuse reticular, nodular, or reticulonodular infiltrates on chest x-ray. Alveolar proteinosis is a rare disorder that most often produces a diffuse air-space filling pattern on chest x-ray, often with air bronchograms. Alveolar proteinosis does not cause fever unless complicated by infection such as nocardiosis. Lymphangiomyomatosis is also rare. It occurs exclusively in women of childbearing age. The chest x-ray shows reticulonodular infiltration but the lungs often appear hyperinflated. Lymphangiomyomatosis is complicated by pleural effusion and pneumothorax, but not fever.

247. The answer is B. *(Braunwald, ed 11, chap 216.)* With mild respiratory distress syndrome, or early in the clinical picture, ventilation-perfusion abnormalities are primarily responsible for hypoxemia; therefore, modest increases in the inspired oxygen tension would produce significant increases in arterial oxygenation. As the disease becomes fully developed, however, diffuse alveolar collapse occurs, and right-to-left shunts are created. Under these circumstances, hypoxemia would be insensitive to small changes in inspired oxygen concentration.

248. The answer is B. *(Braunwald, ed 11, chap 216.)* Some persons who become agitated or anxious while on a mechanical ventilator receive inadequate ventilation, because they are breathing out of phase with the machine. The man described in the question has adequate oxygenation—a P_{O_2} of 70 mmHg means his hemoglobin is more than 90% saturated. However, he is hypoventilating and has developed an acute respiratory acidosis. Positive end-expiratory pressure (PEEP) improves oxygenation by raising the lung volume and reducing shunting but it does not have a large effect on carbon dioxide clearance. Therefore, the appropriate first step in management would be to administer a sedative and control the man's ventilation, in order to reduce arterial P_{CO_2} and raise pH.

249. The answer is A-N, B-N, C-Y, D-Y, E-N. *(Braunwald, ed 11, chap 202.)* Immediate drug therapy for a severe asthmatic attack consists primarily of intravenous administration of aminophylline and administration by inhalation or subcutaneous injection of a beta-adrenergic agent. Isoproterenol is a potent beta agonist highly effective when given by inhalation during an acute attack. Both the steroid beclomethasone and the mast-cell inhibitor cromolyn sodium are often effective when given by inhalation to asthmatic individuals during periods of relative remission; however, both preparations actually can worsen airway function when administered during an acute attack. Because of the danger of respiratory depression, sedatives should not be used during acute exacerbations of asthma. Oral or parenteral steroids are useful in treating acute episodes of asthma but are not effective until several hours after initial administration.

250. The answer is A-N, B-N, C-N, D-Y, E-N. *(Braunwald, ed 11, chap 207.)* Although the majority of patients with cystic fibrosis receive their diagnosis in childhood, a significant number of patients will not be identified until their late teens, twenties, or even thirties. Accurate diagnosis requires that the sweat chloride test be utilized in all individuals with clinical features of cystic fibrosis. Airway obstruction resulting from bronchiectasis is associated with sinusitis and infertility in males with both cystic fibrosis and the immotile cilia syndrome, but only males with immotile cilia have Kartagener's syndrome (bronchiectasis, sinusitis, and dextrocardia). Patients with cystic fibrosis may have any of several gastrointestinal manifestations including intussusception, fecal impaction, volvulus, portal hypertension, and steatorrhea. Steatorrhea is a manifestation of pancreatic insufficiency. Nearly all patients with cystic fibrosis show clubbing.

251. The answer is A-N, B-N, C-Y, D-Y, E-Y. *(Braunwald, ed 11, chap 207.)* Since 1948, the life expectancy of persons who have cystic fibrosis has improved from 2 years to more than 19 years. This rise can be attributed to two factors. First, due to increased physician awareness and more aggressive screening programs, a population of older persons with slowly developing disease has now been identified. Second, meticulous treatment regimens, including regular pulmonary toilet and nutritional support with pancreatic enzymes, are improving survival. The lungs of affected individuals are normal at birth, but poor clearance of secretions leads to chronic airway infections and destruction. Only 20 percent of persons with cystic fibrosis have persistent pancreatic function; the others are subject to malabsorption and may also develop portal hypertension. Nearly all men with cystic fibrosis (97 percent) are infertile due to structural defects in the reproductive system. Women with cystic fibrosis are likely to have difficulty conceiving a child, but a number of pregnancies have occurred and been carried to term. Meconium ileus occurs in 10 percent of cases and is a common mode of presentation.

252. The answer is A-N, B-Y, C-N, D-Y, E-N. *(Braunwald, ed 11, chap 208.)* The man described in the question presents physical signs (pursed lip breathing, chest hyperexpansion) and radiographic evidence (flattened diaphragms, attenuated markings) suggestive of obstructive lung disease with loss of lung tissue. Reduced expiratory air-flow rates are produced by narrowing of airways (e.g., in asthma), by loss of airways (e.g., in bronchiolitis obliterans), or by loss of elastic tissue (e.g., in emphysema). Pathophysiologically, these conditions cause increased resistance as airways are narrowed or collapse, as well as decreased driving pressure, representing loss of elastic recoil. Air-trapping and reduced lung recoil lead to an increase in both total lung capacity (TLC) and functional residual capacity (FRC), which is the volume at which the tendency of the lung to recoil inward is just balanced by the tendency of the chest to recoil outward. Although TLC is increased, vital capacity, the maximum amount of gas that can be exhaled from the lungs with a single breath, is reduced due to the great increase in residual volume produced by gas trapping. Not only is vital capacity reduced, but it takes longer to empty the lungs; thus, forced expiratory volume in one second (FEV_1) is reduced as a percent of vital capacity. When alveolar capillaries are destroyed due to emphysema, the diffusing capacity, which reflects in part the surface area of alveolar membrane available for gas exchange, is reduced.

253. The answer is A-N, B-N, C-Y, D-Y, E-Y. *(Braunwald, ed 11, chap 208.)* To establish baseline information in persons who have emphysema, spirometry should be performed, and for those persons with significant complaints or physical findings, arterial blood gases also should be checked. Although cigarette smoking accounts for the vast majority of cases of emphysema, a small percentage of affected individuals who develop this illness have had no exposure to tobacco products. A subset of this nonsmoking, emphysematous population is deficient in α_1-antitrypsin, which is a protease inhibitor normally found in the serum. It is currently believed that release of proteolytic enzymes from inflammatory cells accounts for the lung destruction that typifies emphysema, and α_1-antitrypsin deficiency, a familial disorder diagnosed by serum electrophoresis, permits this destruction to occur unimpeded. Exercise testing is not necessary as an initial screening test for emphysema but should be considered before oxygen therapy is prescribed. A male individual who has emphysematous respiratory failure, gives no history of respiratory infections, and who has children would not have cystic fibrosis (affected men are sterile); therefore, a sweat chloride test would not be a useful procedure.

254. The answer is A-Y, B-N, C-Y, D-N, E-N. *(Brunwald, ed 11, chap 208.)* All persons suffer a gradual decline in expiratory flow rates with age, but smoking can cause some persons to lose function three or more times faster than in nonsmokers. Although lost function cannot be restored, cessation of smoking can reduce the rate at which function is lost, thereby improving the prognosis for persons who have chronic airway obstruction. In a subset of individuals with air-flow obstruction—those whose resting P_{O_2} is less than 60 mmHg on room air—oxygen therapy has been shown to improve prognosis (this effect is not attributable to cessation of smoking). These two interventions, oxygen therapy and abstinence from smoking, can thus prolong life expectancy in selected persons. Exercise programs, phlebotomy, and use of oral expectorants may improve exercise performance and provide symptomatic relief, but none has a positive impact on survival in chronic airway obstruction.

255. The answer is A-N, B-N, C-N, D-Y, E-Y. *(Braunwald, ed 11, chap 209.)* Idiopathic interstitial fibrosis is a diffuse infiltrative lung disease that usually is first manifested as dyspnea on exertion but may progress to full respiratory failure. In the early stages of the disease, radiographic signs may be absent in up to 10 percent of affected persons, and usual tests of lung function, such as total lung capacity, may fall above the lower limit of normal. In such persons, an increased alveolar-to-arterial oxygen tension gradient is evident on exercise, so that arterial blood-gas testing done during exercise may be abnormal. More typically, symptoms occur in conjunction with abnormal pulmonary function testing, which shows the typical pattern of restrictive lung disease and a bibasilar reticulonodular picture on chest x-ray. Changes on chest x-ray correlate poorly with changes in disease activity. Recently, use of the gallium scan has been advocated to assess the degree of inflammation present in the lung; moreover, because more "active" cellular infiltrates may respond more favorably to steroid therapy, the gallium scan also might be helpful in predicting therapeutic response. Neither noninvasive tests nor special pathologic studies distinguish idiopathic interstitial fibrosis from lung involvement associated with collagen vascular disease. Although the course of interstitial fibrosis usually is progressive deterioration and death, recent studies have suggested that up to 20 percent of persons with active cellular inflammation on lung biopsy have a spontaneous remission and that the presence of inflammation on biopsy suggests longer survival.

256. The answer is A-Y, B-Y, C-N, D-Y, E-N. *(Braunwald, ed 11, chap 211.)* Hypoxemia occurs commonly after massive pulmonary thromboembolism, although normal arterial oxygen tension does not exclude the diagnosis. The most important mechanism producing hypoxemia in this setting is an increase in venous admixture due to continued perfusion of poorly ventilated areas. Ventilation may be decreased by atelectasis or by airway constriction in response to the release of bronchoactive mediators. A fall in cardiac output producing a low mixed venous P_{O_2} can increase the effect of venous admixture. Increased dead-space ventilation would not be a cause of hypoxemia.

257. The answer is A-Y, B-N, C-N, D-Y, E-N. *(Braunwald, ed 11, chap 213. Mittman, Am Rev Respir Dis 116:477, 1977.)* Although persons with pulmonary lesions often require sophisticated pulmonary function testing to determine their suitability for surgery, hypercapnia at rest usually is considered a contraindication to resection. Obviously, metabolic and other causes of hypoventilation must be excluded. The presence of systemic syndromes, including syndrome of inappropriate antidiuretic hormone secretion (SIADH), does not rule out surgery; in fact, these syndromes often remit following surgical resection of the pulmonary lesion. Pleural effusion in the absence of cytologic or histologic evidence of pleural metastasis also is not a contraindication to surgery. Paralysis of either the recurrent laryngeal nerve or the phrenic nerve indicates that the affected person has nonoperable disease. Although metastatic invasion of mediastinal lymph nodes usually is considered an indication not to operate, metastatic spread to lobar lymph nodes that could be included in the surgical block resection does not rule out surgery.

258. The answer is A-N, B-N, C-N, D-Y, E-N. *(Braunwald, ed 11, chap 214.)* Pleural fluid culture is positive in less than 20 percent of cases of postprimary tuberculous pleural infection. For this reason, a closed pleural biopsy should be performed in suspected cases of tuberculous pleuritis. Eosinophils are a nonspecific finding in pleural effusion, often occurring in large numbers after thoracentesis. Eosinophils also may be found in effusions associated with viral or bacterial pneumonias, pancreatitis, and carcinomatous involvement of the pleura. Glucose concentration less than 20 mg/dL is characteristic of rheumatoid pleural effusion. This low glucose concentration is due to a defect in glucose transport across the pleural surface and is not sensitive to changes in serum glucose levels. Pleural effusions occur commonly after abdominal surgery but usually are benign and resolve without treatment. However, the occurrence of fever postoperatively in association with pleural effusions and pleuritic pain should prompt a search for a subdiaphragmatic abscess. Epidemic pleurodynia, a viral infection involving the intercostal muscles, is not associated with inflammation of the pleural surface or lung parenchyma.

259. The answer is A-Y, B-Y, C-N, D-Y, E-Y. *(Braunwald, ed 11, chap 204.)* Inhalation of asbestos fibers for 10 years or more may lead to interstitial fibrosis that typically begins in the lower lobes, later spreading to mid and upper lung fields. This fibrosis is associated with a restrictive pattern on pulmonary function testing. The chest x-ray shows linear densities, thickening or calcification of the pleura (pleural plaques), and, in severe cases, honeycombing. Exposure to asbestos may also cause exudative pleural effusions. These effusions are often blood-stained and may be painful. The diagnosis may be elusive if a careful occupational exposure is not obtained. These effusions are benign, but affected persons may later sustain malignant mesotheliomas of the pleura or peritoneum. Unlike pulmonary fibrosis, pleural effusions and mesotheliomas may develop after brief exposures to asbestos, often of one to two years. Mesotheliomas are not associated with cigarette smoking, but the combination of exposure to asbestos and cigarette smoking has a multiplicative effect on the risk of development of lung cancer. Exposure to asbestos increases the risk for both adenocarcinoma and squamous cell (but not oat cell) carcinoma of the lung, suggesting that lung cancer screening may be useful in selected individuals.

260. The answer is A-N, B-Y, C-Y, D-N, E-N. *(Braunwald, ed 11, chap 216. Staub, Am Rev Respir Dis 109:358, 1974.)* The adult respiratory distress syndrome (ARDS) is a descriptive label for the clinical triad of hypoxemia, diffuse lung infiltrates, and reduced lung compliance not attributable to congestive cardiac failure. This syndrome has many causes, suggesting its complex pathogenesis. However, the pathologic outcome is the same: an increase in lung water due to an increase in alveolar capillary permeability. This noncardiogenic pulmonary edema is identical to congestive cardiac pulmonary edema in its effect on the mechanical properties of the lung and on gas exchange. Just as in cardiac pulmonary edema, the increase in lung water associated with ARDS produces interstitial edema and alveolar collapse, so the affected lung becomes still and the alveolar-arterial oxygen tension difference widens. Unlike cardiac edema, however, the increase in lung water in ARDS occurs as a result of an increase in alveolar capillary permeability and not due to an increase in hydrostatic forces. Edema fluid in ARDS, therefore, often contains macromolecules, such as serum proteins, and measurement of pulmonary artery wedge pressure is normal or low. In clinical practice, determination of pulmonary artery wedge pressure is the most helpful discriminant between ARDS and cardiac failure.

261–264. The answers are: 261-D, 262-C, 263-B, 264-E. *(Braunwald, ed 11, chaps 209 and 270.)* Eosinophilic granuloma is a chronic infiltrative disease involving lung, bone, and, occasionally, other tissues. The disease is classed with Letterer-Siwe disease and Hand-Schüller-Christian disease as a histiocytic reticulosis and is characterized by aggregates of atypical histiocytes in the lung interstitium and other tissues. Men are affected slightly more commonly than women; the usual age of onset is from 20 to 40 years. Manifestations of the disease range from asymptomatic lung involvement noted on chest x-ray, to an acute cellular infiltration with weight loss and fever, to chronic scarring of the pulmonary parenchyma with progressive respiratory insufficiency.

Wegener's granulomatosis is characterized by necrotizing vasculitis and granulomatous inflammation of the upper respiratory tract, the lower respiratory tract, and the kidneys. Although the mean age of onset is 40 years, it may present at any age. The typical chest x-ray pattern is one of single or multiple nodules and cavities, and improvement may be seen in one lesion while another lesion worsens. No laboratory test is specific for Wegener's granulomatosis.

Allergic granulomatosis and angiitis as described by Churg and Strauss is a necrotizing systemic vasculitis that involves skin, peripheral nerves, the gastrointestinal tract, the genitourinary tract (but usually not the kidneys), as well as the lungs. Although it is a small-vessel vasculitis occurring in asthmatic individuals, extrapulmonary symptoms often predominate. Eosinophilia, which always is present, may be extreme—up to 80 percent of white blood cells on differential count.

Sarcoidosis is a granulomatous disease of unknown etiology. It can involve nearly all organ systems, including skin, heart, lung, and the lymphoreticular, nervous, and gastrointestinal systems. A significant minority (30 percent) of affected persons are asymptomatic and are identified by an abnormal chest x-ray. Pulmonary involvement typically produces a restrictive defect, but abnormalities of airways function also are common. The diagnosis is one of exclusion, although the finding on biopsy of typical noncaseating granulomas in a person with a compatible clinical history is compelling evidence for this diagnosis.

265–268. The answers are 265-A, 266-C, 267-E, 268-B. *(Braunwald, ed 11, chap 213.)* A paraneoplastic syndrome may provide the first, and sometimes most dramatic, evidence of a pulmonary neoplasm. The mechanisms of some of these syndromes are well worked out, but others are poorly understood. Patients with extensive skeletal metastases from many cancers will have increased serum calcium concentrations. Hypercalcemia also occurs with certain cancers in the absence of obvious bone involvement, most often caused by ectopic production of parathyroid hormone. Between 13 and 25 percent of patients with squamous cell carcinoma have increased calcium concentrations without bone disease; a smaller percentage of patients with large cell carcinoma have the same syndrome. Hypercalcemia is *not* caused by small cell carcinoma without extensive bone destruction. Gonadotropin production by pulmonary neoplasms occurs most commonly with large cell undifferentiated carcinomas. Gonadotropin release is associated with the development of gynecomastia. Hypertrophic pulmonary osteoarthropathy (HPO) consists of periosteal new bone formation in the long bones, usually associated with clubbing. There is vasomotor instability, and the ankles are frequently painful, especially when dependent. HPO occurs most commonly in association with adenocarcinoma. Symptoms frequently remit immediately after surgical resection. Small cell carcinoma of the oat cell subtype is associated with several paraneoplastic syndromes. The syndrome of inappropriate secretion of antidiuretic hormone occurs in a significant minority of patients with oat cell carcinoma. Hyponatremia occurs in one third of such patients. Small cell carcinoma is also the tumor most likely to cause excessive secretion of adrenocortical hormones by ectopic secretion of ACTH. This syndrome is associated with hypokalemia, metabolic alkalosis, muscle weakness, and polyuria, but it does not usually produce rounded facies, abdominal striae, and centripetal fat distribution.

DISORDERS OF THE KIDNEY AND URINARY TRACT

DIRECTIONS: Each question below contains five suggested answers. Choose the **one best** response to each question.

269. Laboratory evaluation of a 19-year-old man being worked up for polyuria and polydipsia yields the following results:

> Serum electrolytes (meq/L): Na$^+$ 144; K$^+$ 4.0; Cl$^-$ 107; HCO$_3^-$ 25
> BUN: 18 mg/dL
> Blood glucose: 102 mg/dL
> Urine electrolytes (meq/L): Na$^+$ 28; K$^+$ 32
> Urine osmolality: 195 mosmol/kg

After 12 hours of fluid deprivation, body weight has fallen by 5 percent. Laboratory testing now reveals the following:

> Serum electrolytes (meq/L): Na$^+$ 150; K$^+$ 4.1; Cl$^-$ 109; HCO$_3^-$ 25
> BUN: 20 mg/dL
> Blood glucose: 98 mg/dL
> Urine electrolytes (meq/L): Na$^+$ 24; K$^+$ 35
> Urine osmolality: 200 mosmol/kg

One hour after the subcutaneous administration of 5 units of pitressin, urine values are as follows:

> Urine electrolytes (meq/L): Na$^+$ 30; K$^+$ 30
> Urine osmolality: 199 mosmol/kg

The most likely diagnosis in this case is

(A) nephrogenic diabetes insipidus
(B) osmotic diuresis
(C) salt-losing nephropathy
(D) psychogenic polydipsia
(E) none of the above

270. A 70-year-old woman who has adult-onset diabetes is brought to an emergency room in an unresponsive state. Her family states that several days ago she got a "cold" and then became increasingly weak and finally disoriented. She has not been taking insulin or any other medication. Admission vital signs are temperature 38.3°C (101°F), pulse 100/min, respiratory rate 36/min, and blood pressure 110/70 mmHg. Her weight is 70 kg (154 pounds). Laboratory values include the following:

> Serum electrolytes (meq/L): Na$^+$ 142; K$^+$ 3.2; Cl$^-$ 102; HCO$_3^-$ 26
> Blood glucose: 1200 mg/dL
> BUN: 35 mg/dL
> Serum creatinine: 1.6 mg/dL

A reasonable estimate of this woman's total body water and sodium deficits would be

(A) 5 L water, 50 meq sodium
(B) 5 L water, 150 meq sodium
(C) 5 L water, 350 meq sodium
(D) 10 L water, 150 meq sodium
(E) 10 L water, 350 meq sodium

271. A 70-year-old man with diabetes mellitus and hypertension has the following serum chemistries:

> Electrolytes (meq/L): Na$^+$ 138; K$^+$ 5.0; Cl$^-$ 106; HCO$^-_3$ 20
> Glucose: 200 mg/dL
> Creatinine: 2.0 mg/dL

All of the following may contribute to worsening hyperkalemia EXCEPT

(A) propranolol
(B) indomethacin
(C) captopril
(D) heparin
(E) gentamicin

272. A 35-year-old man with a history of alcoholism and hepatic cirrhosis is hospitalized because of massive ascites and severe pitting edema of the lower extremities and sacrum. Admission laboratory values are as follows:

> Serum electrolytes (meq/L): Na$^+$ 135; K$^+$ 3.0; Cl$^-$ 95; HCO$_3^-$ 28
> Serum chemistries (mg/dL): BUN 15; creatinine 2.0

During the first hospital day the man makes 400 mL of urine with a sodium concentration of 6 meq/L and an osmolality of 638 mosmol/kg. Which of the following measures is likely to be most beneficial in the treatment of the sodium-retaining state described?

(A) Oral furosemide, 120 mg twice daily
(B) Intravenous furosemide, 120 mg twice daily
(C) Intravenous mannitol, 25 g twice daily
(D) Abdominal paracentesis to drain 2 L of fluid daily
(E) Bed rest and a low-sodium diet

273. A 28-year-old woman says she has had generalized weakness and aching in her legs for the last several months. She has taken oral contraceptives for 3 years but has no other record of medical treatment or known illness. Physical examination is normal except for questionable proximal muscle weakness. Laboratory values include the following:

> Serum electrolytes (meq/L): Na$^+$ 138; K$^+$ 2.2; Cl$^-$ 90; HCO$_3^-$ 40
> Urine electrolytes (meq/L): Na$^+$ 40; K$^+$ 10; Cl$^-$ 3
> Arterial blood gases: pH 7.58; P$_{O_2}$ 90 mm Hg; P$_{CO_2}$ 48 mmHg

The most likely explanation for the woman's electrolyte disorder is

(A) oral contraceptive therapy
(B) Bartter's syndrome
(C) surreptitious diuretic abuse
(D) surreptitious vomiting
(E) primary hyperaldosteronism

274. In severe chronic renal failure (serum creatinine greater than 8.0 mg/dL), dose interval should be most prolonged for which of the following antimicrobial agents?

(A) Methicillin
(B) Cefoxitin
(C) Cefazolin
(D) Vancomycin
(E) Gentamicin

275. A 72-year-old man becomes oliguric following surgery for repair of an abdominal aortic aneurysm. He is alert, oriented, and able to take fluids and medications by mouth. Laboratory testing done on the fourth postoperative day reveals the following:

> Serum electrolytes (meq/L): Na$^+$ 139; K$^+$ 5.1; Cl$^-$ 104; HCO$_3^-$ 17
> Serum chemistries (mg/dL): BUN 90; creatinine 8.4; calcium 8.0; phosphorus 10.5; uric acid 18.0; glucose 140
> Urine volume: approximately 400 mL per day (Foley catheter in place)
> Urine electrolytes (meq/L): Na$^+$ 50; K$^+$ 30; Cl$^-$ 40

All the following orders would be appropriate in the management of this man EXCEPT

(A) discontinue Foley catheter drainage
(B) give oral aluminum hydroxide gel (Amphogel), 60 mL four times daily
(C) give oral allopurinol, 300 mg once daily
(D) limit total fluid intake to 800 mL per day
(E) begin a low-protein diet as tolerated

276. All of the folowing are important contributors to renal osteodystrophy EXCEPT

(A) Impaired renal production of 1,25-dihydroxyvitamin D$_3$
(B) hyperphosphatemia
(C) aluminum-containing antacids
(D) loss of vitamin D and calcium via dialysis
(E) metabolic acidosis

277. A 45-year-old woman who has had slowly progressive renal failure begins to complain of increasing numbness and prickling sensations in her legs. Examination reveals loss of pinprick and vibration sensation below the knees, absent ankle jerks, and impaired pinprick sensation in her hands. Serum creatinine concentration, checked during her most recent clinic visit, is 8.9 mg/dL. The woman's physician should now recommend

(A) a therapeutic trial of phenytoin (Dilantin)
(B) a therapeutic trial of pyridoxine (vitamin B$_6$)
(C) a therapeutic trial of cyanocobalamin (vitamin B$_{12}$)
(D) initiation of maintenance hemodialysis
(E) neurologic referral for nerve conduction studies

278. The condition of a 50-year-old obese woman with a five-year history of mild hypertension controlled with a thiazide diuretic is being evaluated because proteinuria was noted on her routine yearly medical visit. Physical examination disclosed a height of 167.6 cm (66 in); weight 91 kg (202 lb); blood pressure 130/80 mmHg; and trace pedal edema. Laboratory values are as follows:

Serum creatinine: 1.2 mg/dL
BUN: 18 mg/dL
Creatinine clearance: 87 mL/min
Urinalysis: pH 5.0; specific gravity 1.018; protein 3+; no glucose; occasional coarse granular cast
Urine protein excretion: 5.9 g/24 hours

A renal biopsy was performed and the results are as shown below. Sixty percent of the glomeruli appeared as shown (by light microscopy); the remainder were unremarkable.

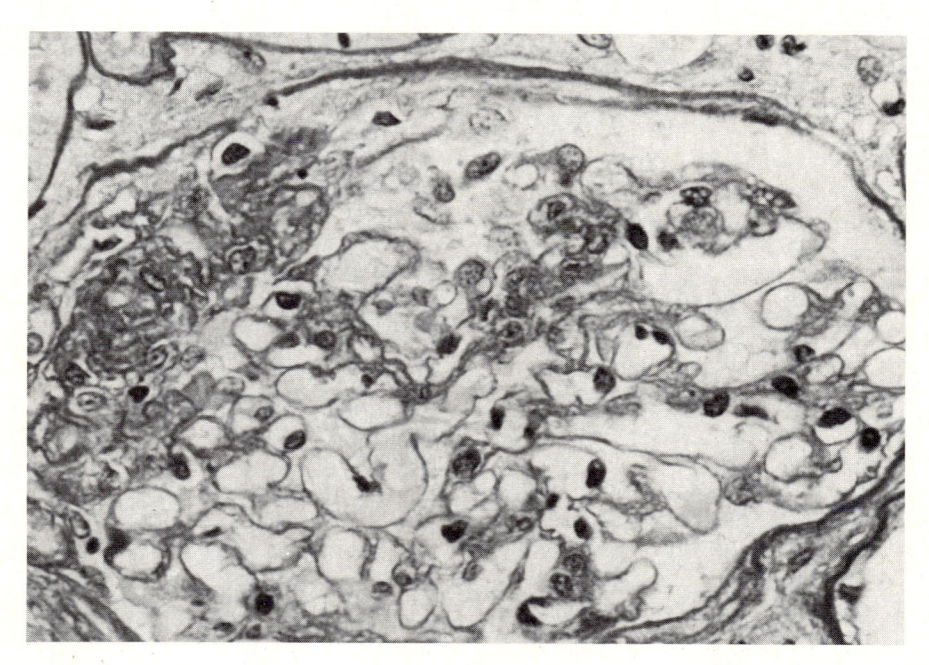

The most likely diagnosis is

(A) hypertensive nephrosclerosis
(B) focal and segmental sclerosis
(C) minimal-change (nil) disease
(D) membranous glomerulopathy
(E) crescentic glomerulonephritis

---

279. Renal biopsy performed on a person who has carcinoma of the lung and typical nephrotic syndrome would most likely show

(A) minimal change disease
(B) diffuse proliferative glomerulonephritis
(C) membranoproliferative glomerulonephritis
(D) membranous glomerulopathy
(E) focal glomerulosclerosis

280. A 19-year-old U.S. Marine, who has had a feeling of malaise for a few hours, begins passing coffee-colored urine. During the next 2 days pedal edema develops. Urinalysis reveals 4+ hematuria, 3+ proteinuria, and a sediment containing many red-cell and white-cell casts. Serum testing shows that the BUN level is 40 mg/dL and creatinine concentration is 4.0 mg/dL. Renal biopsy reveals diffuse endocapillary proliferative lesions with infiltration of glomeruli by polymorphonuclear leukocytes. All the following conditions could produce this clinical picture EXCEPT

(A) infectious mononucleosis
(B) streptococcal infection
(C) heroin abuse
(D) acute viral hepatitis
(E) falciparum malaria

281. Controlled trials have shown that corticosteroid therapy reduces the tendency toward progressive renal failure in which of the following glomerulopathies?

(A) Acute glomerulonephritis
(B) Rapidly progressive glomerulonephritis
(C) Focal and segmental glomerulosclerosis (focal sclerosis)
(D) Membranous nephropathy
(E) Berger's disease (IgA nephropathy)

282. A 40-year-old woman who has never had significant respiratory disease is hospitalized for evaluation of hemoptysis. Urinalysis reveals 2+ proteinuria and microscopic hematuria. BUN concentration is 20 mg/dL, and serum creatinine concentration is 2.0 mg/dL. Serologic findings include normal complement levels, increase immunoglobulin A levels, and a negative assay for fluorescent antinuclear antibodies. Renal biopsy reveals granulomatous necrotizing vasculitis with scattered immunoglobulin and complement deposits. The most likely diagnosis in this case is

(A) allergic granulomatous arteritis (Churg and Strauss syndrome)
(B) Henoch-Schönlein purpura
(C) microscopic polyarteritis
(D) Wegener's granulomatosis
(E) Goodpasture's syndrome

283. A 44-year-old woman with acute myelogenous leukemia and a peripheral white blood cell count of 100,000/mm^3 is treated with hydroxyurea. She subsequently develops oliguria and rising blood urea nitrogen and serum creatinine levels. Which of the following statements is most likely to be true regarding this woman?

(A) Retrograde pyelography probably would demonstrate multiple radiolucent, bilaterally obstructing stones
(B) She is not likely to regain acceptable renal function and faces the prospect of chronic dialysis even if her leukemia is successfully treated
(C) She may have developed acute renal failure due to leukemic infiltration of her kidney
(D) Furosemide would have been useful in forestalling renal damage
(E) Probenecid would have been useful in forestalling renal damage

284. A marked decline in renal function due to acute interstitial nephritis has been reported in association with all of the following drugs EXCEPT

(A) methicillin
(B) cephalothin
(C) heparin
(D) ampicillin
(E) furosemide

285. A patient being examined for acute renal failure has a urine sodium concentration of 15 meq/L and a urine osmolality of 410 mosmol/kg. These findings might be consistent with all of the following conditions EXCEPT

(A) acute poststreptococcal glomerulonephritis
(B) acute partial urinary obstruction
(C) cholesterol embolization of the kidneys
(D) rhabdomyolysis
(E) cirrhosis of the liver with ascites

286. A 30-year-old woman with diabetic nephropathy received a cadaveric renal allograft. On the third postoperative day her serum creatinine concentration was 1.8 mg/dL. She is being treated with cyclosporine and prednisone. On the sixth postoperative day she experiences a decrease in urine output from 1500 mL/day to 1000 mL/day; the serum creatinine concentration increases to 2.2 mg/dL. Her blood pressure remains stable at 170/90 mmHg and her temperature at 37.2°C (99.0°F). The best initial step in management would be to

(A) decrease the dose of cyclosporine
(B) obtain ultrasonography of the renal allograft
(C) obtain a biopsy of the renal allograft
(D) administer pulsed steroid therapy
(E) administer an intravenous bolus of furosemide

287. A 55-year-old man undergoes intravenous pyelography as part of a workup for hypertension. A solitary radiolucent mass, 3 cm in size, is noted in the left kidney; the study otherwise is normal. The man complains of no symptoms referable to the urinary tract, and examination of urine sediment is within normal limits. Which of the following studies should be performed next?

(A) Repeat intravenous pyelography in 6 months
(B) Early-morning urine collections for cytology (three samples)
(C) Selective renal arteriography
(D) Renal ultrasonography and, if warranted, needle aspiration of the mass
(E) CT scanning (with contrast enhancement) of the left kidney

DIRECTIONS: Each question below contains five suggested answers. For **each** of the five alternatives of **each** item, you are to respond either YES (Y) or NO (N). In a given item all, some, or none of the alternatives may be correct.

288. A 43-year-old construction worker is noted to be anuric following a crush injury to the lower extremities. Serum electrolytes (meq/L) obtained 8 hours following admission are Na^+ 138, K^+ 8.8, Cl^- 100, and HCO_3^- 19. Electrocardiography reveals peaked T waves, prolongation of the PR interval, and widening of the QRS complex. Which of the following measures would rapidly lower serum potassium concentration in the man described?

(A) Intravenous infusion of 10 mL of a 10% calcium gluconate solution
(B) Intravenous infusion of 10 mL of a 10% magnesium sulfate solution
(C) Intravenous infusion of 50 mL of a 50% glucose solution with 10 units of regular insulin
(D) Intravenous infusion of 2 ampules of sodium bicarbonate
(E) Administration by nasogastric tube of 60 mL of a potassium-binding resin

289. Rhabdomyolysis or acute myoglobinuric renal failure can develop as a result of

(A) strenuous muscular exercise
(B) barbiturate overdose
(C) ethanol ingestion
(D) hypokalemia
(E) volume depletion

290. A 38-year-old man who has diverticulitis develops azotemia after 7 days of inpatient therapy with gentamicin. His BUN and serum creatinine concentrations, normal on admission, now are 60 mg/dL and 5.1 mg/dL, respectively. His urine output never has been less than 2 L per day. Which of the following statements about this case are true?

(A) About 25 percent of individuals with acute renal failure are not oliguric
(B) Oliguric and nonoliguric renal failure carry similar prognoses
(C) Nonoliguric renal failure is characteristic of gentamicin toxicity
(D) The maximum BUN achieved by this man would be less than that expected if he developed oliguria
(E) Urine sodium concentration would probably be less than 10 meq/L and urine osmolality greater than 400 mosmol/kg

291. A 26-year-old woman is on dialysis because of renal failure due to chronic ureteral reflux and pyelonephritis. Her kidneys have been removed, and she is currently awaiting cadaveric transplantation. On dialysis her hematocrit is routinely 24 percent (volume of cells). The peripheral smear reveals microcytic and hypochromic red blood cells. Appropriate treatment for her anemia would include

(A) splenectomy
(B) folate therapy
(C) iron therapy
(D) androgen therapy
(E) routine transfusions to maintain hematocrit at or above 30 percent

292. Serum complement levels typically are low during the acute or active phase of which of the following diseases?

(A) Diffuse proliferative glomerulonephritis associated with systemic lupus erythematosus
(B) Membranous glomerulopathy
(C) Poststreptococcal glomerulonephritis
(D) Membranoproliferative glomerulonephritis
(E) Immunoglobulin A nephropathy

293. Metabolic abnormalities associated with the nephrotic syndrome include

(A) increased serum lipid levels
(B) increased serum thyroxine levels
(C) reduced serum calcium levels
(D) reduced serum iron levels
(E) increased serum antithrombin III (heparin cofactor) levels

294. Which of the following statements about acute poststreptococcal glomerulonephritis (PSGN) are true?

(A) The latent period appears to be longer when PSGN is associated with cutaneous rather than with pharyngeal infections
(B) Serologic evidence of a streptococcal infection may not be forthcoming if antimicrobial therapy is begun early
(C) Antimicrobial therapy for streptococcal infection is without value once the presence of renal disease is established
(D) Long-term antistreptococcal prophylaxis is indicated following documented cases of PSGN
(E) Lasting and progressive deterioration in renal function is more common in adults than in children with PSGN

295. A 23-year-old woman develops gross hematuria following an upper respiratory tract infection. Urinalysis shows 4+ hematuria and 2+ proteinuria with a sediment containing red-cell casts. Gross hematuria resolves during the next several days. Renal biopsy shows diffuse mesangial deposition of immunoglobulin A (IgA). Which of the following statements about this woman's disease are true?

(A) Elevation of circulating IgA levels would be unusual
(B) IgA deposits are often found in dermal capillaries
(C) Further episodes of gross hematuria typically would be associated with flu-like infections or with exercise
(D) Development of the nephrotic syndrome would be unusual
(E) The disease leads to dialysis or transplantation in 10 percent of cases

296. A 27-year-old woman whose diabetes was diagnosed when she was 9 years old has had 1+ to 2+ proteinuria without abnormality of the urine sediment for the last 3 years. During the last year her serum creatinine concentration has doubled, so that now it is 2.4 mg/dL. Blood pressure has risen from 95/70 to 125/95 mmHg. Presuming the diagnosis of diabetic nephropathy is established, which of the following statements concerning the woman's condition are true?

(A) Ophthalmologic examination would likely reveal retinal microvascular disease
(B) Rigorous control of hypertension would likely slow the progression of renal failure
(C) Rigorous control of blood sugar levels would likely slow the progression of renal failure
(D) Insulin requirement would likely decline with worsening renal failure
(E) Dialysis or transplantation would likely be required within 5 years

297. Which of the following have been found to *recur* in the transplanted kidney?

(A) Rapidly progressive crescentic glomerulonephritis (Goodpasture's syndrome)
(B) Interstitial nephritis
(C) Membranoproliferative glomerulopathy
(D) IgA nephropathy (Berger's disease)
(E) Idiopathic focal and segmental sclerosis

298. A 48-year-old woman is hospitalized for elective knee surgery. Routine preoperative laboratory evaluation reveals the following:

Serum electrolytes (meq/L): Na^+ 142; K^+ 4.3; Cl^- 110; HCO_3^- 20
Blood glucose: 95 mg/dL
Serum creatinine: 1.8 mg/dL
BUN: 20 mg/dL
Urinalysis: pH 6.0; specific gravity 1.005; protein 1+; glucose 2+; 3 to 5 white blood cells per high-power field

This woman says she voids several times during the night but is unaware of any problem with her kidneys. Disorders associated with the findings in this case would include

(A) multiple myeloma
(B) diabetic nephropathy
(C) Sjögren's syndrome
(D) penicillamine-induced nephropathy
(E) analgesic abuse

299. Which of the following statements concerning renal artery stenosis as a cause of hypertension are true?

(A) It is more likely to occur in persons less than 30 years of age or more than 50 years of age than in other persons
(B) It is often associated with a tendency towards hyperkalemia
(C) Captopril is a useful agent in the control of the blood pressure
(D) Administration of captopril may precipitate acute renal failure
(E) Intravenous pyelography is the most sensitive and specific screening procedure

300. Renal involvement in persons with scleroderma can be described correctly by which of the following statements?

(A) Serious renal insufficiency develops in a small minority of persons with scleroderma
(B) Accelerated hypertension is the most common presentation of renal disease in scleroderma
(C) Proliferative glomerulonephritis is the typical morphologic finding
(D) Aggressive antihypertensive therapy has been shown to preserve renal function
(E) Renal transplantation is generally contraindicated because of the risk of recurrent disease in the allograft

301. A 45-year-old woman presents with her third episode of nephrolithiasis. Laboratory studies disclose:

> Serum electrolytes (meq/L): Na$^+$ 134; K$^+$ 2.5; Cl$^-$ 106; HCO$^-_3$ 18
> Serum chemistries (mg/dL): creatinine 1.1; calcium 9.5; albumin 4.0
> Arterial blood gas values: P$_{CO_2}$ 30 mmHg; P$_{O_2}$ 108 mmHg; pH 7.30
> Urine pH: 7.2

A plain film of the abdomen is shown below. Which of the following statements about this clinical picture are true?

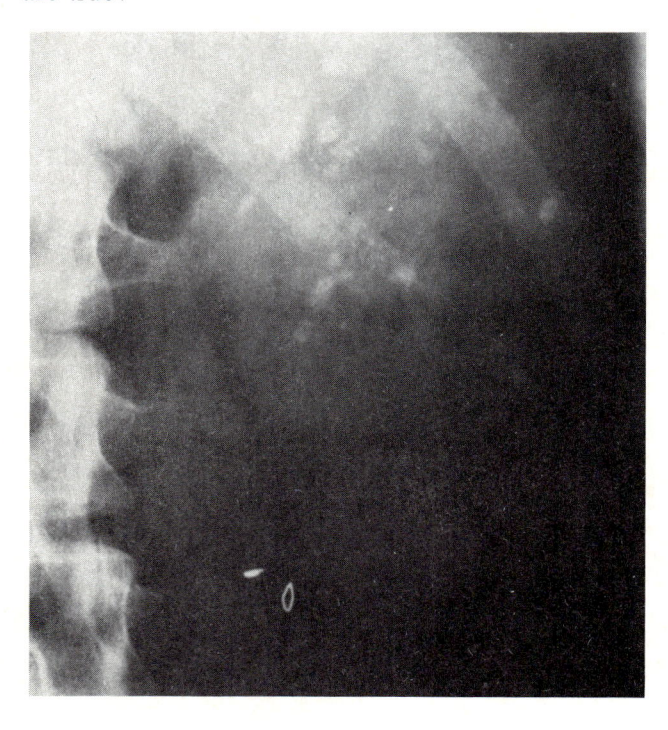

(A) The findings are consistent with the presence of multiple myeloma
(B) The findings are consistent with the presence of medullary sponge kidney
(C) There is evidence for type I distal renal tubular acidosis (RTA)
(D) Family members should be screened for electrolyte disorders
(E) Intravenous pyelography would provide further useful information

302. An 18-year-old man has passed many renal stones since childhood but has so far not required urologic surgery. Serum creatinine and BUN concentrations are within normal limits. Urine sediment is shown below. Which of the following statements regarding this man's condition are true?

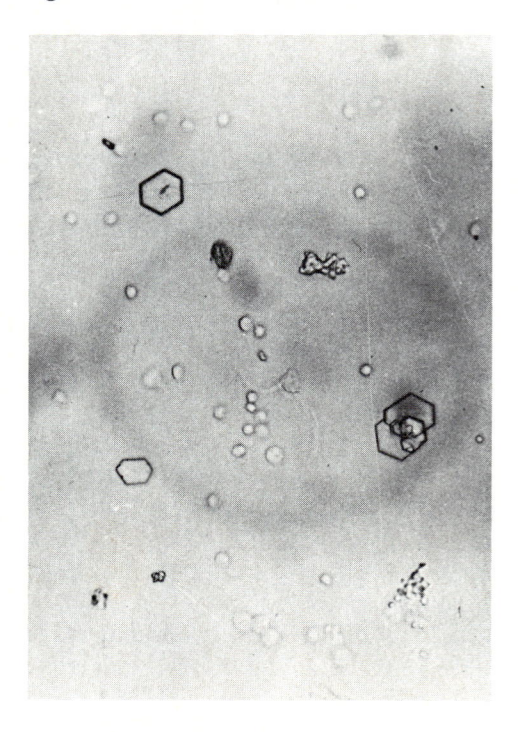

(A) Increased intake of fluid is a useful treatment
(B) Dietary amino acid restriction is a useful treatment
(C) With proper treatment, renal function should remain normal
(D) Moderate mental deficiency may be expected
(E) This man's offspring would be unlikely to suffer from frequent renal stones

DISORDERS OF THE KIDNEY AND URINARY TRACT

DIRECTIONS: The groups of questions below consist of four or five lettered headings followed by several numbered items. For each numbered item choose the **one** lettered heading with which it is **most** closely associated. Each lettered heading may be used once, more than once, or not at all.

Questions 303–305

For each case history that follows, select the set of laboratory serum values with which it is most likely to be associated.

	Na⁺	K⁺	Cl⁻	HCO₃⁻	BUN	Creatinine	Osmolality
			(meq/L)			(mg/dL)	(mosmol/kg)
(A)	122	3.0	90	16	25	1.8	245
(B)	122	3.0	76	30	35	2.0	245
(C)	122	4.2	88	24	8	0.8	245
(D)	122	4.0	90	22	12	1.1	290
(E)	122	6.0	94	18	20	1.4	245

303. A 45-year-old man has developed acute bacterial meningitis following a sinus infection

304. A 55-year-old woman has been hospitalized with newly diagnosed multiple myeloma

305. A 63-year-old man has been given vincristine (Oncovin) as part of a lymphoma treatment protocol

Questions 306–308

For each case history that follows, select the set of laboratory values with which it is most likely to be associated.

	Na⁺	K⁺	Cl⁻	HCO₃⁻	Creatinine	pH (Arterial blood)	(Urine)
		(Serum, meq/L)			(Serum, mg/dL)		
(A)	143	4.8	100	10	3.0	7.25	5.0
(B)	135	4.5	107	21	3.0	7.37	5.0
(C)	140	2.5	114	14	3.0	7.30	6.2
(D)	139	5.1	104	21	3.0	7.37	5.0
(E)	139	6.3	108	19	3.0	7.35	5.0

306. A 28-year-old man, comatose, is believed to have been drinking ethylene glycol

307. A 48-year-old woman has been given amphotericin B for treatment of disseminated coccidioidomycosis

308. A 19-year-old man is recovering from acute poststreptococcal glomerulonephritis

Questions 309–312

For each case history that follows, select the urine sediment most likely to be associated.

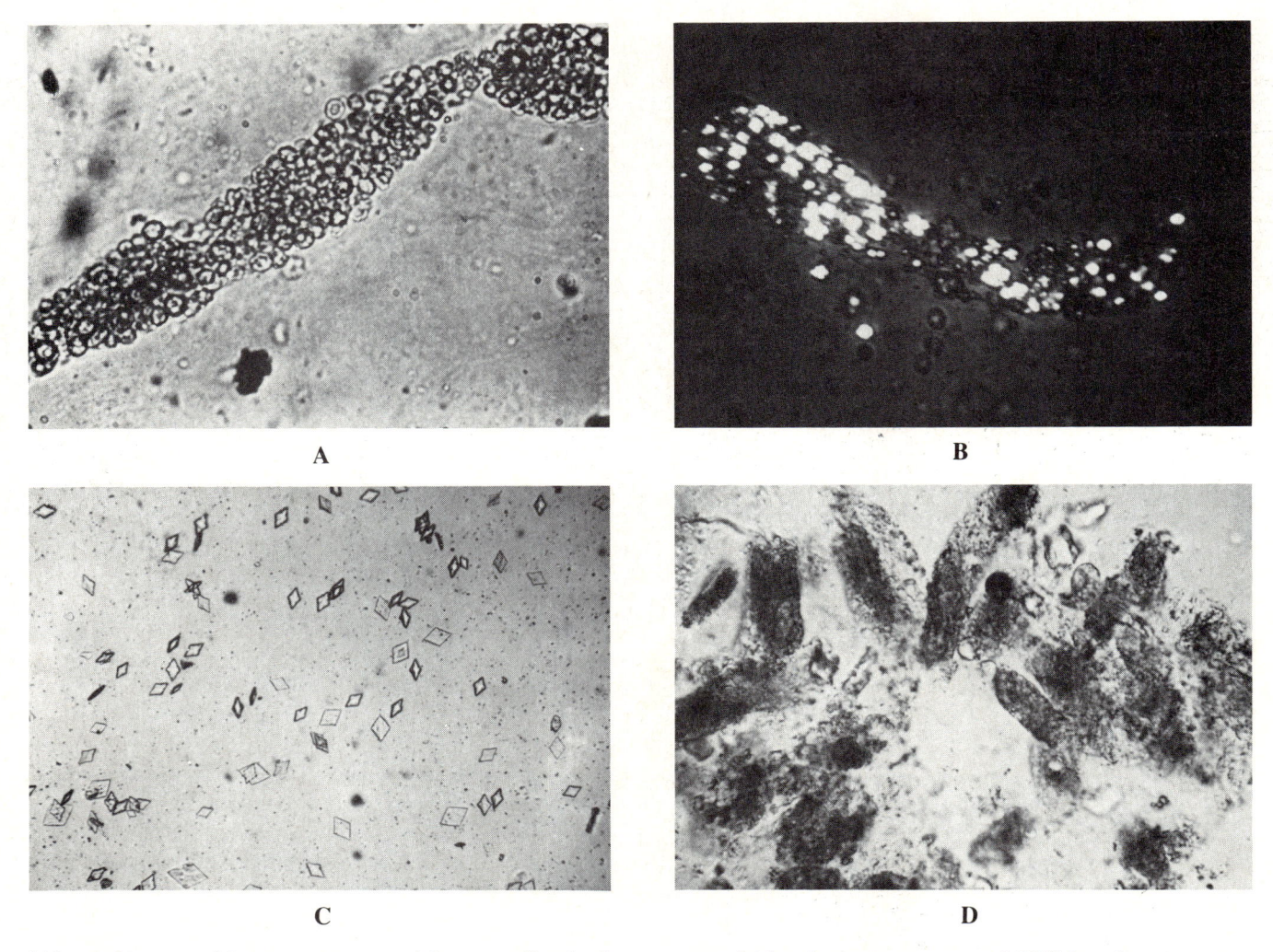

A

B

C

D

309. A 23-year-old man presents with generalized edema, normal blood pressure, normal BUN and serum creatinine concentrations, serum albumin 1.9 g/dL, and proteinuria (4+).

310. A 60-year-old woman with a poorly differentiated lymphoma is noted to have an increasing serum creatinine concentration two days after a chemotherapeutic infusion.

311. An 82-year-old man with a prosthetic aortic valve has had fever for several days and a serum creatinine concentration of 2.5 mg/dL.

312. A 43-year-old man with alcoholism is brought to the emergency room intoxicated, with pressure necrosis noted on his posterior scalp and buttocks; serum creatinine concentration is 3.0 mg/dL.

Disorders of the Kidney and Urinary Tract

Answers

269. The answer is A. *(Braunwald, ed 11, chap 41.)* Failure to concentrate urine despite substantial hypertonic dehydration suggests a diagnosis of diabetes insipidus. A nephrogenic origin would be postulated if there is no response in urine concentration to exogenous vasopressin. The only useful mode of therapy is a low-salt diet and use of a thiazide diuretic agent. The resultant volume contraction presumably enhances proximal reabsorption and thereby reduces urine flow.

270. The answer is E. *(Braunwald, ed 11, chap 41.)* The woman described has nonketotic hyperosmolar coma. The calculated effective extracellular fluid (ECF) osmolality is approximately 350 mosmol/kg [(2 × sodium concentration) + (glucose concentration in mg/L ÷ 180, which is the molecular weight of glucose)]. This calculated ECF osmolality is about 25 percent above normal, meaning that about one-fifth of the woman's intracellular water has been lost. In addition, due to the osmotic diuretic effect of glucose, there have presumably been significant losses of sodium and extracellular water. Loss of extracellular volume is reflected in the elevated BUN/creatinine ratio. A rough estimate of the magnitude of the changes accompanying the development of the hyperosmolar state in the case described would be as follows:

	Prior to illness	In emergency room
Weight (kg)	81	70
Intracellular vol (L)	35	28
Extracellular vol (L)	16	13.5
ECF Na$^+$ (total meq)	2500	2100

271. The answer is E. *(Braunwald, ed 11, chap 41.)* This man's electrolyte pattern is consistent with the "syndrome of hyporeninemic hypoaldosteronism," or type IV renal tubular acidosis. Inhibition of the renin-angiotensin system by nonsteroidal anti-inflammatory agents, converting enzyme inhibitors, and beta-adrenergic blockade can contribute to hyperkalemia. Beta blockade can also interfere with intracellular potassium uptake. Heparin has been associated with a decrease in aldosterone production. Aminoglycosides do not cause hyperkalemia and may be associated with renal K$^+$ wasting.

272. The answer is E. *(Braunwald, ed 11, chap 41, 219.)* In a cirrhotic patient, massive extracellular volume expansion and low urine sodium excretion are evidence of inappropriate sodium retention. If serum creatinine concentration is elevated in addition, the possibility of incipient renal failure—the so-called hepatorenal syndrome—should be entertained. Attempts as rapid volume reduction in this setting can precipitate renal failure and thus are contraindicated. Current treatment recommendations call for rest, observation, a possible trial of plasma expansion, and then gentle diuresis if renal function remains stable.

273. The answer is D. *(Braunwald, ed 11, chap 42.)* The woman described has a prominent metabolic alkalosis. The absence of chloride in the urine indicates the alkalosis is being maintained by volume depletion. Cathartic abuse would produce a similar electrolyte profile except that stool bicarbonate loss would moderate the alkalosis. If volume depletion were the result of diuretic abuse, the urine would contain chloride, reflecting the action of the diuretic. Metabolic alkalosis in Bartter's syndrome and in primary hyperaldosteronism is generally less severe than in the woman presented, and urinary chloride excretion is normal (unusual extrarenal loss does not occur). Thus, of the choices presented the most likely diagnosis of the woman's metabolic alkalosis is surreptitious vomiting.

274. The answer is D. *(Braunwald, ed 11, chap 88.)* Because all the antimicrobial drugs listed in the question are excreted principally by the kidneys, dose interval for them should be significantly prolonged (or individual doses reduced) in persons with severe renal failure. Lengthening of the dose interval should be greatest with vancomycin, which can be given as infrequently as once every 7 days when the glomerular filtration rate is less than 10 mL/min. Consequently, vancomycin is of particular value in persons who are uremic and require antimicrobial therapy, because its use can obviate the need for continuous maintenance of intravenous access.

275. The answer is C. *(Braunwald, ed 11, chap 219.)* The management of oliguric acute renal failure is largely conservative, although some clinicians believe that early dialysis and hyperalimentation lessen morbidity and speed recovery. Fluid intake should match output plus estimated insensible losses; food intake should be encouraged to lessen tissue catabolism. Continuous Foley catheter drainage should not be routinely employed, because it increases the risk of infection; however, if supervening bladder outlet obstruction is suspected, recatheterization should be considered. Reduction of high serum phosphate levels usually is recommended to reduce the risk of soft-tissue calcification. Reduction of high uric acid levels, however, is unnecessary, both because symptomatic gout is very unusual in persons with oliguric renal failure and because there is no evidence that kidneys are damaged by hyperuricemia that develops after an acute reduction in the glomerular filtration rate.

276. The answer is D. *(Braunwald, ed 11, chap 220.)* Impaired renal production of 1,25-dihydroxy-vitamin D_3 leads to decreased calcium absorption from the gut. Impaired renal phosphate excretion contributes to increased calcium entry into bone. The resultant decreased serum calcium concentration leads to secondary hyperparathyroidism. Chronic metabolic acidosis leads to dissolution of bone buffers and decalcification. Aluminum administered in long-term therapy, although useful in controlling hyperphosphatemia and, thereby, controlling hypocalcemia, can be taken up by bone and contribute to altered bone matrix. There is *no* significant loss of vitamin D or calcium associated with presently employed dialysis techniques.

277. The answer is D. *(Braunwald, ed 11, chap 220.)* Development of advancing peripheral neuropathy is an indication for dialysis. Delaying dialysis could allow development of irreversible motor deficits, such as foot drop. Prompt institution of dialysis, on the other hand, usually prevents progression of uremic peripheral neuropathy and may ameliorate early sensory defects. No pharmacologic agent would be of significant benefit in the clinical situation described.

278. The answer is B. *(Braunwald, ed 11, chap 223.)* The characteristic pattern of focal and segmental glomerular scarring is shown. The history and laboratory features are also consistent with this lesion, i.e., some associated hypertension, diminution in creatinine clearance, and a relatively inactive urine sediment. The "nephropathy of obesity" may be associated with this lesion secondary to hyperfiltration. Hypertensive nephrosclerosis exhibits more prominent vascular changes and patchy ischemic, totally sclerosed glomeruli. In addition, nephrosclerosis seldom is associated with nephrotic-range proteinuria. Minimal-change disease is usually associated with symptomatic edema and normal-appearing glomeruli as demonstrated by light microscopy. This patient's presentation is consistent with that of membranous nephropathy but the biopsy is not. With membranous glomerular nephritis all glomeruli are uniformly involved with subepithelial dense deposits. There are no features of crescentic glomerulonephritis present.

DISORDERS OF THE KIDNEY AND URINARY TRACT

279. The answer is D. *(Braunwald, ed 11, chap 223.)* Persons who have solid tumors and develop nephrotic syndrome usually have membranous glomerulopathy. Diagnosis of the nephrotic syndrome may precede the recognition of the primary tumor. In several cases, tumor antigens have been discovered in the glomerular deposits; the nephrotic syndrome may remit following effective tumor therapy.

280. The answer is C. *(Braunwald, ed 11, chap 223.)* The presentation and renal pathology described in the question are typical of acute glomerulonephritis. This syndrome, both when originally described and currently, occurs most often in association with streptococcal infection. Antibodies generated in response to *Streptococcus* are assumed to comprise part of the immune deposits seen in damaged glomeruli. More recently, acute glomerulonephritis has been noted in association with a number of other infectious illnesses, which presumably also give rise to immune complexes capable of damaging glomerular capillaries. Heroin abuse is associated with focal and segmental glomerulosclerosis (focal sclerosis), not acute glomerulonephritis; proteinuria and a decline in renal function usually are the first signs.

281. The answer is D. *(Braunwald, ed 11, chap 223.)* The apparent immunopathologic basis of the major glomerulopathies has led to attempts to influence their course by the use of corticosteroids. The results have in many cases been disappointing. A recent, carefully controlled trial has shown that steroid therapy reduces the tendency toward renal insufficiency in membranous glomerulopathy. Because of the poor prognosis, steroids, often in conjunction with cytotoxic agents and plasmapheresis, are used routinely in treating rapidly progressive glomerulonephritis; however, the benefit of steroids in this setting has not been conclusively demonstrated. Steroids have not been shown to retard progression to renal failure in persons with focal sclerosis or IgA nephropathy. They do not either lessen the severity or shorten the course of acute renal insufficiency caused by acute glomerulonephritis.

282. The answer is D. *(Braunwald, ed 11, chap 224.)* A variety of diseases involve both pulmonary and renal (and, often, also dermal) microvasculature and may present with either prominent pulmonary or renal manifestations. When a firm diagnosis cannot be made serologically or by biopsy of skin or upper respiratory-tract lesions, renal biopsy may be necessary. In the case described in the question, the serologic findings, though not specific, are typical of Wegener's granulomatosis, a diagnosis established by the renal biopsy report. Granulomas are not typical of microscopic polyarteritis or Goodpasture's syndrome.

283. The answer is D. *(Braunwald, ed 11, chap 226.)* Leukemic infiltrates of the kidney, although common in persons with leukemia, rarely impair renal function. In the case described in the question, the more likely diagnosis is acute uric acid nephropathy, which could have developed as a consequence of hydroxyurea therapy as well as of the hyperuricemia associated with leukemia. Acute uric acid nephropathy is predominantly due to intrarenal uric acid deposition and not to bilateral renal obstruction by stones. The large majority of affected persons regain essentially normal renal function with proper supportive care. Diuresis, as achieved by a potent diuretic agent and use of intravenous fluids, may mitigate renal damage if serum uric acid concentration has risen because of inadequate allopurinol prophylaxis. Probenecid, a uricosuric agent, could be harmful in this setting.

284. The answer is C. *(Braunwald, ed 11, chap 226. Linton, Ann Intern Med 93:735, 1980.)* Methicillin therapy is the most frequently reported cause of acute renal failure resulting from interstitial inflammation. This condition usually is associated with prominent eosinophilia and other features of an immune hypersensitivity disorder, although eosinophilia and other common signs such as fever and skin rash need not be present. Cases of interstitial nephritis also have been reported in connection with the use of many other drugs, including some antibiotics (e.g., cephalothin, ampicillin, and penicillin), certain nonsteroidal anti-inflammatory agents, and furosemide. Thus, medication effects must be included in the differential diagnosis of an unexplained decline in renal function. Heparin therapy has not yet been implicated in the development of interstitial nephritis.

285. The answer is D. *(Braunwald, ed 11, chap 40.)* Cholesterol embolization of the kidneys and cirrhosis fit clearly into the "prerenal" azotemia category, with a low urine sodium concentration and high urine osmolality. Cholesterol emboli cause "plugging" of renal arterioles and cirrhosis causes hypoalbuminemia, hypovolemia, and possibly a humorally mediated reduction of renal perfusion. However, it is important to recall that other disorders associated with abrupt decline in renal function but with intact tubular integrity, such as acute partial urinary obstruction and acute glomerulonephritis, can also give urinary solute values similar to those in prerenal states if evaluated early in the process. When rhabdomyolosis causes renal damage it typically produces the picture of acute tubular necrosis, with a urine osmolality less than 400 mosmol/kg and a urinary sodium exceeding 20 meq/L.

286. The answer is B. *(Braunwald, ed 11, chap 221.)* In the first week after renal transplantation, the differential diagnosis of graft dysfunction includes early rejection, hypovolemia, cyclosporine intoxication, acute tubular necrosis, urinary obstruction, and renal artery thrombosis. Cyclosporine can mask many of the classic signs of rejection, such as fever and graft tenderness; renal biopsy is often needed to make the diagnosis. However, renal ultrasonography should precede any manipulation to rule out mechanical outflow obstruction, as it should in any patient with acute deterioration of renal function.

287. The answer is D. *(Braunwald, ed 11, chap 231.)* The most important differential diagnosis in the case presented is between a renal cell carcinoma and a benign cystic lesion. Urinalysis may be normal in the presence of renal cell carcinoma, and urinary cytology is unfortunately of little value in the diagnosis of this lesion. Ultrasonography will reveal whether or not the lesion is cystic. Because cystic necrosis may occur within a carcinoma, needle aspiration of cyst contents for cytologic and chemical examination is generally recommended. (Refinement of diagnostic criteria based on the appearance of the lesion on ultrasonography or computer-assisted tomography may ultimately make aspiration unnecessary.)

288. The answer is A-N, B-N, C-Y, D-Y, E-N. *(Braunwald, ed 11, chap 41, 219.)* Intravenous calcium infusion, although the correct treatment for the cardiac disturbances caused by hyperkalemia, does not lower serum potassium concentration. Sodium bicarbonate infusion, on the other hand, lowers serum potassium levels rapidly by causing potassium to move into cells. Intravenous infusion of glucose and insulin achieves the same result though slightly less rapidly. Potassium-binding resins effectively remove potassium from the body but are slow, particularly when instilled into the stomach. Persons who are in acute renal failure and have a large potassium load due to severe muscle damage may require emergency dialysis.

289. The answer is A-Y, B-Y, C-Y, D-Y, E-Y. *(Braunwald, ed 11, chap 219. Koffler, Ann Intern Med 85:23, 1976.)* Muscle cells may be sufficiently taxed during strenuous exercise (e.g., distance running) to result in cell breakdown and myoglobin release. Muscle breakdown associated with sedative overdose is generally attributed to ischemia caused by muscle compression in immobile, comatose patients. Not only can ethanol ingestion promote muscle breakdown in a similar manner, but also ethanol itself has a direct toxic effect on muscle. Hypokalemia and hypophosphatemia decrease muscle-cell energy production and thus increase the risk of rhabdomyolysis in any setting. Volume depletion can contribute to decrease muscle perfusion and, more importantly, increase the susceptibility of the kidneys to damage from myoglobin and other muscle breakdown products.

290. The answer is A-Y, B-N, C-Y, D-Y, E-N. *(Braunwald, ed 11, chap 219. Anderson, N Engl J Med 296:1134, 1977.)* Nonoliguric acute renal failure (urine volume greater than 800 mL/day) occurs in 25 to 50 percent of cases of acute renal failure and is most commonly associated with the use of nephrotoxic drugs, such as gentamicin. It generally is associated with less severe elevations of blood urea nitrogen and serum creatinine levels than is oliguric renal failure; urine composition, however, is similar to that in the more common oliguric type. Prognosis of nonoliguric renal failure is better than that of oliguric renal failure.

DISORDERS OF THE KIDNEY AND URINARY TRACT

291. The answer is A-N, B-Y, C-Y, D-N, E-N. *(Braunwald, ed 11, chap 220.)* Microcytic hypochromic anemia is typical of uremia and is usually most severe in anephric persons. Hypersplenism contributes significantly to anemia in an occasional person on dialysis, but splenectomy is not routinely of value. Folate, which is removed during dialysis, should be replaced. Iron stores may frequently be depleted due to gastrointestinal bleeding (often subclinical) and blood loss from dialysis. Androgens are not of significant value in treating anephric patients. Although transfusion (a total of 6 to 12 units of blood) has been recommended in preparation for cadaveric transplantation, routine maintenance of the hematocrit above 30 percent is not necessary in young persons who are without established cardiovascular disease.

292. The answer is A-Y, B-N, C-Y, D-Y, E-N. *(Braunwald, ed 11, chap 222.)* Serum complement levels usually are normal in individuals who have membranous and immunoglobulin A nephropathies. The complement level is depressed during the acute phase of acute poststreptococcal glomerulonephritis but returns to normal about 8 weeks after onset of the disease. Serum complement concentration tends to fall during exacerbations of lupus nephritis. Most individuals with membranoproliferative glomerulonephritis have reduced serum levels of complement component C3.

293. The answer is A-Y, B-N, C-Y, D-Y, E-N. *(Braunwald, ed 11, chap 223.)* Persons who have nephrotic syndrome may lose a variety of serum proteins other than albumin. Loss of thyroxine-binding globulin leads to reduced serum thyroxine levels, and loss of cholecalciferol-binding protein may combine with a decrease in albumin-bound calcium to reduce serum calcium levels. Loss of antithrombin III has been implicated in hypercoagulability, which affects some individuals who have nephrotic syndrome. Hyperlipidemia is associated commonly with nephrotic syndrome; the cause remains uncertain.

294. The answer is A-Y, B-Y, C-N, D-N, E-Y. *(Braunwald, ed 11, chap 223.)* Studies during epidemics of streptococcal disease have shown the latent period between symptomatic pharyngitis and the appearance of poststreptococcal glomerulonephritis (PSGN) to be between 6 and 10 days. The latent period following cutaneous infection is more difficult to establish but appears to be longer. Persons who receive early antimicrobial therapy for streptococcal infection may develop glomerulonephritis but not mount the immune response to streptococcal enzymes (e.g., streptolysin O) on which laboratory testing for antecedent streptococcal infection is based. Antimicrobial therapy is recommended for persons who have acute glomerulonephritis and continuing streptococcal infection. Long-term prophylaxis, however, is unwarranted, because affected persons are not markedly predisposed to recurrent episodes of PSGN. For unknown reasons, PSGN leads to permanent, progressive renal insufficiency more often in adults than in children.

295. The answer is A-N, B-Y, C-Y, D-Y, E-N. *(Braunwald, ed 11, chap 223.)* When first described, Berger's disease was thought to be a relatively benign glomerulopathy characterized by episodes of gross hematuria most often associated with viral illness or exercise. More recently, however, it has become apparent that as many as half the persons affected by this disorder progress to end-stage renal failure. The nephrotic syndrome is associated occasionally with immunoglobulin A (IgA) nephropathy; elevated circulating IgA levels and dermal IgA deposition are common. The latter phenomenon has led to the suggestion that a common immunopathologic mechanism may underlie Berger's disease and Henoch-Schönlein purpura.

296. The answer is A-Y, B-Y, C-N, D-Y, E-Y. *(Braunwald, ed 11, chap 224.)* Diabetic nephropathy invariably progresses to end-stage renal failure. Although no available therapy can prevent progression of diabetic nephropathy, careful blood pressure control has been shown to slow the loss of renal function. However, rigorous blood sugar control has unfortunately not been shown to retard progression of renal disease once it has become clinically apparent. As renal failure becomes more severe, insulin requirements may decrease, due in part to reduced insulin catabolism by the kidneys. The course from onset of proteinuria to end-stage renal failure averages about 7 years. Retinal microvascular disease is usually present by the time urinalysis first shows proteinuria.

297. The answer is A-Y, B-N, C-Y, D-Y, E-Y. *(Braunwald, ed 11, chap 221.)* Glomerular lesions may occur in 10 to 15 percent of allografts, often related to chronic rejection, but other cases are related to recurrence of the patients' primary disease. Diseases that have been known to recur include focal and segmental sclerosis, crescentic glomerulonephritis, especially of the Goodpasture's variety, IgA nephropathy, and membranoproliferative glomerulonephritis; interstitial nephritis does *not* recur. Recurrence of the primary pathologic condition does not necessarily imply loss of graft function, and the primary diagnosis is not a contraindication to transplantation, except if active glomerulonephritis is present.

298. The answer is A-Y, B-N, C-Y, D-N, E-Y. *(Braunwald, ed 11, chap 226.)* Glycosuria (with a normal blood glucose concentration) and hyperchloremic acidosis ("normal anion gap acidosis") are evidence of renal tubular dysfunction. Frequent nocturia, presumably resulting from impaired ability to concentrate urine, also suggests renal insufficiency due to a tubulointerstitial disease. Multiple myeloma may present in this manner, and similar renal abnormalities may be associated with analgesic abuse and Sjögren's syndrome. The findings presented in the case are not characteristic of primary glomerular diseases, such as diabetic nephropathy, or the membranous glomerulopathy induced by penicillamine.

299. The answer is A-Y, B-N, C-Y, D-Y, E-N. *(Braunwald, ed 11, chap 227.)* Clinical features of hypertension developing secondary to renal artery stenosis include an age of onset of under 30 years (usually fibromuscular dysplasia as a cause) or over the age of 50 years (usually of atherosclerotic etiology), poor response to medical therapy, and abdominal bruit. Routine laboratory evaluation usually discloses evidence of secondary hyperaldosteronism with hypokalemia. Captopril is particularly effective in treating renovascular hypertension, but it may cause renal failure in patients with bilateral renal artery stenosis or stenosis of the artery to a solitary kidney. Intravenous pyelography is a relatively insensitive screening procedure with only about one fourth of patients with renovascular hypertension demonstrating the classic "triad" of late appearance of contrast in a small kidney and late hyperconcentration of contrast material in the renal pelvis. If clinical suspicion of renovascular hypertension is high, the best initial study might be digital subtraction angiography.

300. The answer is A-N, B-Y, C-N, D-Y, E-N. *(Braunwald, ed 11, chap 227.)* Renal impairment, though rarely the presenting feature of scleroderma, eventually affects about half the persons with the disease. Renal involvement often is heralded by accelerated hypertension ("malignant hypertension"). Characteristic renal lesions in such cases include arterial and arteriolar narrowing and degeneration, not proliferative glomerulonephritis. Recent studies have shown that aggressive vasodilator therapy may preserve renal function. Transplantation has been performed successfully in persons with scleroderma; maintaining vascular access for hemodialysis, however, is often difficult.

301. The answer is A-N, B-Y, C-Y, D-Y, E-Y. *(Braunwald, ed 11, chaps 226, 228).* This patient with recurrent renal calculi and nephrocalcinosis has a normal serum calcium concentration. The serum electrolyte pattern is typical of distal (type 1) renal tubular acidosis with evidence of renal potassium wasting, hyperchloremic metabolic acidosis, and an alkaline urine. The nephrocalcinosis and distal RTA could be consistent with hypervitaminosis D, medullary sponge kidney, hyperparathyroidism, sarcoidosis, or multiple myeloma. However, in all of these conditions except medullary sponge kidney, an increased serum calcium concentration is responsible for the nephrocalcinosis. Intravenous pyelography would better define the defect seen in medullary sponge kidney; it shows a typical "paintbrush" pattern in the renal papillae with tiny papillary cysts containing the calcium deposits. Although medullary sponge kidney is usually not inherited, type 1 distal RTA is often hereditary and relatives should be screened.

302. The answer is A-Y, B-N, C-Y, D-N, E-Y. *(Braunwald, ed 11, chap 228.)* Clinical disease due to cystinuria, an autosomal recessive disorder, results entirely from stone formation; if stone formation is prevented, renal function will remain normal. Increasing the urine volume and raising the urine pH reduce the tendency of cystine to precipitate and are useful therapeutic measures. Restriction of methionine intake, though theoretically valuable, is impractical and unnecessary. Heterozygotes generally excrete less amino acid and usually do not form stones; thus, unless a patient's spouse carries the trait, the prevalence of which is about 1 in 7000, offspring probably will not have clinical disease.

303–305. The answers are: 303-C, 304-D, 305-C. *(Braunwald, ed 11, chap 41.)* Careful workup of a person presenting with hyponatremia may require a search for central nervous system disease, pulmonary disease, hypothyroidism, and occult malignancy, as well as a close review of medication use.

Hyponatremia in persons with meningitis is caused by inappropriate release of antidiuretic hormone (ADH). This hormone has little net effect on renal excretion of potassium and hydrogen ions; thus, serum potassium and bicarbonate concentrations remain relatively normal. Inappropriate retention of water leads to mild (nonedematous) hypervolemia. The kidneys respond with an increase in glomerular filtration rate and decrease in proximal tubular fluid reabsorption, reflected in low-normal serum creatinine and BUN concentrations; because any degree of intrinsic renal disease may obscure these subtle findings, diagnosis should not depend on their presence.

Hyponatremia due to inappropriate secretion of ADH also can occur in association with the use of a variety of medications, including vincristine. Some drugs increase ADH release, others also apparently increase distal nephron responsiveness to ADH. The electrolyte pattern is identical to that seen when inappropriate release of ADH results from CNS disease or when an ADH-like substance is released by a tumor (e.g., oat cell carcinoma). A similar degree of hyponatremia can accompany hypothyroidism, which, however, would not increase glomerular filtration rate.

Hyponatremia in association with multiple myeloma is artifactual. The concentration of sodium per unit volume of serum, as measured by a flame photometer, is reduced due to the presence of a large amount of paraprotein. Sodium concentration in extracellular fluid water would be normal, as reflected by normal serum osmolality. Severe hyponatremia is rare; reduction of serum sodium level from 140 to 122 meq/L would require approximately 12 g/100 mL of paraprotein.

Hyperkalemia and mild acidosis accompany hyponatremia (choice E) in persons with adrenal insufficiency. A syndrome including hypokalemia, alkalosis, and hyponatremia (choice B) can be caused by diuretics, often in the setting of congestive heart failure. Hypokalemia, acidosis, and hyponatremia with volume depletion (choice A) may accompany loss of fluid from the lower gastrointestinal tract.

306–308. The answers are: 306-A, 307-C, 308-D. *(Braunwald, ed 11, chap 42.)* All the sets of laboratory values presented in the question indicate renal insufficiency with metabolic acidosis. Calculation of unmeasured anions (anion gap) is helpful in determining the etiology of the acidosis. Ethylene glycol ingestion, for example, not only causes acute renal failure but leads to rapid accumulation of metabolic acids. Acidosis is disproportionate to the degree of renal insufficiency and is characterized by a high anion gap (choice A). Amphotericin B also causes renal insufficiency with disproportionate metabolic acidosis. Acidosis, however, is due to a distal tubular acidification defect (distal, or type I, renal tubular acidosis) and is characterized by hyperchloremia, a normal anion gap, and inability to lower the urine pH (choice C). Urinary potassium loss also may be excessive. With moderate renal insufficiency caused by glomerulonephritis, metabolic acidosis is usually mild and the anion gap is only slightly, if at all, elevated (choice D).

The set of laboratory data in choice E illustrates moderate renal insufficiency with disproportionate hyperkalemia and hyperchloremic acidosis, so-called type IV renal tubular acidosis. A number of causes of renal insufficiency, most notably diabetic nephropathy but usually not acute glomerulonephritis, can produce these findings. The laboratory values in choice B illustrate an apparent reduction of the anion gap, which has been reported most frequently in association with multiple myeloma. The apparent reduction in unmeasured anions is due to the presence of abnormal circulating paraprotein which bears a positive charge.

309–312. The answers are: 309-B, 310-C, 311-A, 312-D. (*Braunwald, ed 11, chap 219.*) The 23-year-old man with edema, hypoalbuminemia, and proteinuria has nephrotic syndrome (probably secondary to minimal-change disease), and the urine sediment discloses an "oval fat body" cast (under polarized lens with the typical "Maltese crosses"). The patient with lymphoma has a high tumor burden, and the tumor lysis syndrome has developed postchemotherapy; she has urate crystals in her urine. The mechanism of renal insufficiency is primarily intrarenal tubular obstruction, but frequently uric acid "sludge" is seen in the urine. The patient with the prosthetic valve most likely has endocarditis with an "immune complex" type of acute glomerulonephritis. He has red blood cell casts in the urine. The man with alcoholism has evidence of rhabdomyolysis, with pressure necrosis of muscles and secondary renal insufficiency. His urine sediment shows pigmented coarse granular casts characteristic of acute tubular necrosis.

DISORDERS OF THE ALIMENTARY TRACT AND HEPATOBILIARY SYSTEM

DIRECTIONS: Each question below contains five suggested answers. Choose the **one best** response to each question.

313. A 56-year-old woman has had profuse, watery diarrhea for 3 months. Laboratory studies of fecal water show the following:

   Sodium: 39 meq/L
   Potassium: 96 meq/L
   Chloride: 15 meq/L
   Bicarbonate: 40 meq/L
   Osmolality: 270 mosmol/kgH$_2$O (serum osmolality: 280 mosmol/kgH$_2$O)

The most likely diagnosis is

(A) villous adenoma
(B) lactose intolerance
(C) laxative abuse
(D) pancreatic insufficiency
(E) nontropical sprue

314. Evaluation of a 49-year-old man with acute epigastric pain reveals that he has lipemic serum. Serum amylase level is normal. The statement that best describes this clinical situation is

(A) if the man's pain is due to acute pancreatitis, he would be likely to have hypercalcemia
(B) if the man's pain is due to acute pancreatitis, he would be likely to have chronic pancreatitis as well
(C) if the man's pain is due to acute pancreatitis, serial dilutions of his serum may reveal elevated amylase activity
(D) if the man's pain is due to acute pancreatitis, serum lipase level would be normal
(E) the normal serum amylase level excludes a diagnosis of acute pancreatitis

315. A 57-year-old man seeks emergency-room attention for weakness and melena, which he has had for 3 days. He says he has not had significant abdominal pain and had no prior gastrointestinal bleeding. On examination he is disheveled and unshaven, appears older than his stated age, and has a 20 mmHg orthostatic drop in blood pressure. Findings include bilateral temporal wasting, anicteric and pale conjunctivas, cheilosis, spider angiomas on his upper torso, muscle wasting, hepatosplenomegaly, and hyperactive bowel sounds without abdominal tenderness to palpation. Stool is melenic. Nasogastric aspiration reveals coffee-grounds material, which quickly clears with lavage. Hematocrit is 30 percent and mean corpuscular volume is 105 fL.

The appropriate next step in the management of this man's illness would be to

(A) perform gastroscopy
(B) pass a Sengstaken-Blakemore tube and begin an intravenous infusion of pitressin
(C) order an upper gastrointestinal series
(D) order immediate visceral angiography
(E) insert a large-bore intravenous line and type and cross-match the man's blood

316. A 45-year-old man says that for the past year he occasionally has regurgitated food particles eaten several days earlier. His wife complains that his breath has been foul-smelling. He has had occasional dysphagia for solid foods. The most likely diagnosis is

(A) gastric outlet obstruction
(B) scleroderma
(C) achalasia
(D) Zenker's diverticulum
(E) diabetic gastroparesis

317. During the last year, a 55-year-old man has experienced vague postprandial epigastric fullness. For the last several months, he has been anorectic and has lost 4.5 kg (10 lb.) Physical examination is unrevealing except for faintly guaiac-positive stool. Hematocrit is 26 percent. A representative x-ray from his upper gastrointestinal series is reproduced below. The man's physician should now

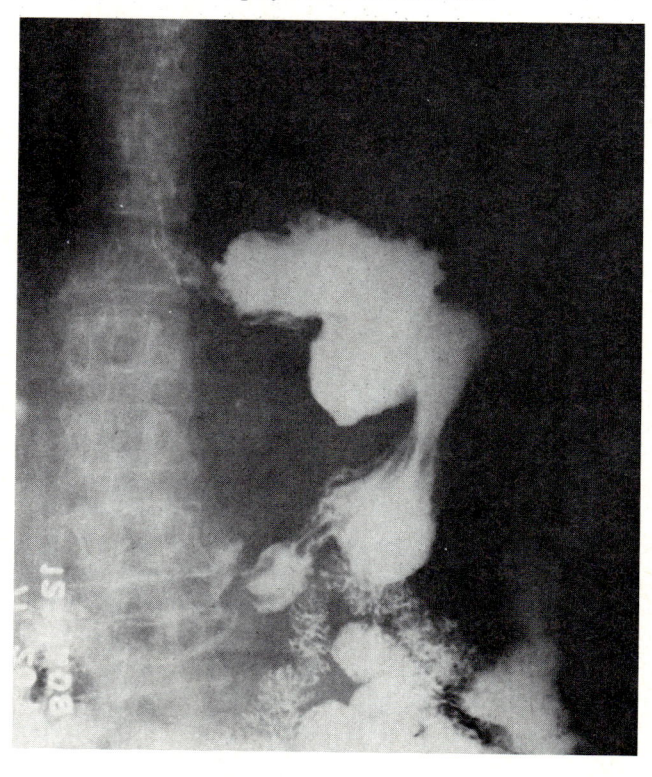

(A) prescribe cimetidine
(B) prescribe metoclopramide
(C) perform a double-contrast upper gastrointestinal series
(D) perform gastroscopy
(E) recommend total gastrectomy

318. The differential diagnosis of chylous ascites includes all of the following EXCEPT

(A) lymphoma
(B) nephrotic syndrome
(C) tuberculosis
(D) trauma
(E) congestive heart failure

319. Orally administered drugs beneficial in the treatment of persons with pseudomembranous colitis include all the following EXCEPT

(A) vancomycin
(B) bacitracin
(C) penicillin
(D) cholestyramine
(E) metronidazole

320. All of the following statements about achalasia are true EXCEPT

(A) the underlying abnormality appears to be defective innervation of the esophageal body and lower esophageal sphincter
(B) dysphagia, chest pain, and regurgitation are the predominant symptoms
(C) chest x-rays often reveal a large gastric air bubble
(D) manometry reveals a normal or elevated lower esophageal sphincter pressure
(E) nifedipine is effective in controlling symptoms in many patients

321. Conditions associated with an increased risk of squamous cell cancer of the esophagus include all of the following EXCEPT

(A) achalasia
(B) smoking
(C) Barrett's esophagus
(D) tylosis
(E) head and neck cancer

322. Four months ago, a 36-year-old man with a peptic ulcer underwent a Billroth II anastomosis: antrectomy, vagotomy, and gastrojejunostomy. He now returns for evaluation of a stomal (anastomotic) ulcer. Fasting serum gastrin level is 350 pg/mL; 5 minutes after intravenous infusion of secretin the serum gastrin level is 100 pg/mL. The man should be advised that the most appropriate treatment for his condition is

(A) total vagotomy
(B) total gastrectomy
(C) resection of the distal antrum attached to the duodenal stump
(D) laparotomy to search for a gastrin-producing tumor
(E) medical therapy with liquid antacids

323. All of the following statements regarding eosinophilic enteritis are true EXCEPT

(A) peripheral blood eosinophilia is present
(B) it may affect the stomach, small intestine, and/or colon
(C) the majority of patients have a history of food allergies or asthma
(D) treatment with corticosteroids is often effective
(E) it may be difficult to distinguish from regional enteritis

324. Which of the following diagnostic studies for malabsorption is usually normal in persons who have bacterial overgrowth syndrome?

(A) Fecal fat quantitation (24 hours)
(B) Stage II Schilling test (intrinsic factor given with vitamin B_{12})
(C) D-Xylose absorption test
(D) Lactulose breath test
(E) Quantitative cultures of jejunal aspirates

325. A 26-year-old man who has juvenile-onset diabetes complains of postprandial epigastric discomfort and bloating. An upper gastrointestinal series fails to reveal an ulcer, but the fluoroscopist notes delayed gastric emptying. Which of the following therapies would be best at this stage of the man's illness?

(A) Antacids
(B) Cimetidine
(C) Metoclopramide
(D) Probanthine
(E) Gastrojejunostomy

326. For the last 6 months, a 50-year-old man has had diarrhea and migratory arthralgias and has lost 9.1 kg (20 lb.). An upper gastrointestinal barium study shows a malabsorption pattern in the small bowel. Stool fat content is 35 g/24 h. Following oral administration of 25 g of D-xylose, a 5-hour urine collection contains 0.8 g of D-xylose. A peroral small-bowel biopsy reveals subtotal villus atrophy with infiltration of the lamina propria with macrophages that stain positively with periodic acid Schiff (PAS) stain. The man's physician should now

(A) start him on a gluten-free diet
(B) prescribe prednisone, 60 mg/day and tapered over 2 months
(C) prescribe prednisone, 60 mg/day indefinitely
(D) prescribe tetracycline, 2 g/day for 12 months
(E) recommend an exploratory laparotomy with splenectomy and biopsy of retroperitoneal nodes

327. A 70-year-old Irish consular official seeks local medical attention for diarrhea and weight loss, which have been present for 2 years. He says he has always been in good health "even though I'm the runt of the litter" (he is the smallest of eight siblings). Laboratory studies include normal complete blood cell count and serum electrolyte concentrations. Serum D-xylose concentration is 15 mg/dL 2 hours after an oral challenge, and 24-hour fecal fat determination is 12 g with the man on a 100-g fat diet. A representative biopsy specimen of his small bowel is shown below. All the following are true statements about the man's illness EXCEPT

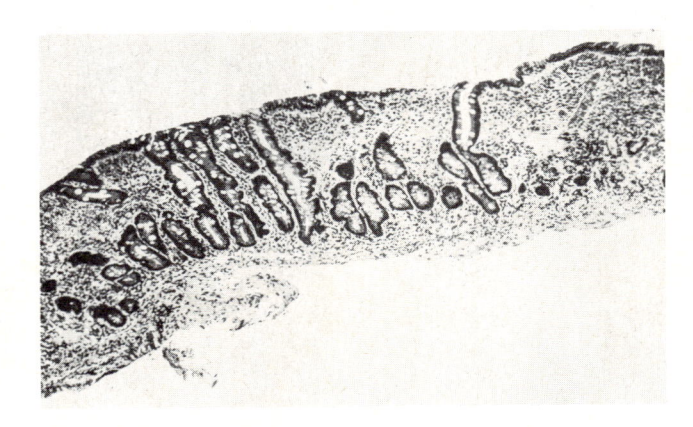

(A) this condition is associated with specific HLA genotypes
(B) abdominal pain, arthralgia, low-grade fever, and lymphadenopathy are frequently present
(C) corticosteroid therapy can reverse jejunal pathology and lessen clinical symptoms
(D) adherence to a strict gluten-free diet usually results in normalization of malabsorption tests and reversal of jejunal pathology
(E) a majority of affected persons complain of bloating after ingesting milk

328. A 62-year-old physician was well until 3 weeks ago when she developed a urinary tract infection. She was treated with ampicillin for 10 days, taking her last dose 7 days ago. Four days ago, she developed abdominal pain, fever, and bloody diarrhea. On examination, she appears acutely ill; her temperature is 38.3°C (101°F) and her abdomen is diffusely tender. Sigmoidoscopy demonstrates a hyperemic mucosa studded with plaque-like lesions. The most likely diagnosis is

(A) *Shigella* superinfection
(B) pseudomembranous colitis
(C) amebic colitis
(D) ischemic colitis
(E) toxic megacolon

329. A 28-year-old man has had diarrhea and crampy right-lower quadrant abdominal pain for the last 4 weeks. During the last 10 days, he also has had episodic low-grade fever, abdominal distention, and anorexia without vomiting but leading to a weight loss of 3.2 kg (7 lb). On examination, he is mildly uncomfortable. Vital signs are temperature, 37.8°C (100.1°F); pulse, 100/min; and blood pressure, 110/60 mmHg. His sclerae are anicteric, and there is no palpable lymphadenopathy. A tender, indistinct fullness is palpable in the right lower quadrant of the abdomen, but otherwise the abdomen is soft and without rebound tenderness or palpable hepatosplenomegaly. Rectal examination reveals no masses or focal tenderness, but the stool is guaiac-positive. Laboratory values include hematocrit, 30 percent, and white blood cell count, 11,300/mm^3 with a shift to the left. Flat-plate and upright x-rays of the abdomen show some air-filled loops of small bowel but no air-fluid levels. Sigmoidoscopy is unremarkable. On barium enema examination, barium fails to reflux into the terminal ileum, but the colon is otherwise normal. A representative film from a small-bowel barium examination is shown below.

Which of the following disorders is most consistent with the clinical picture described?

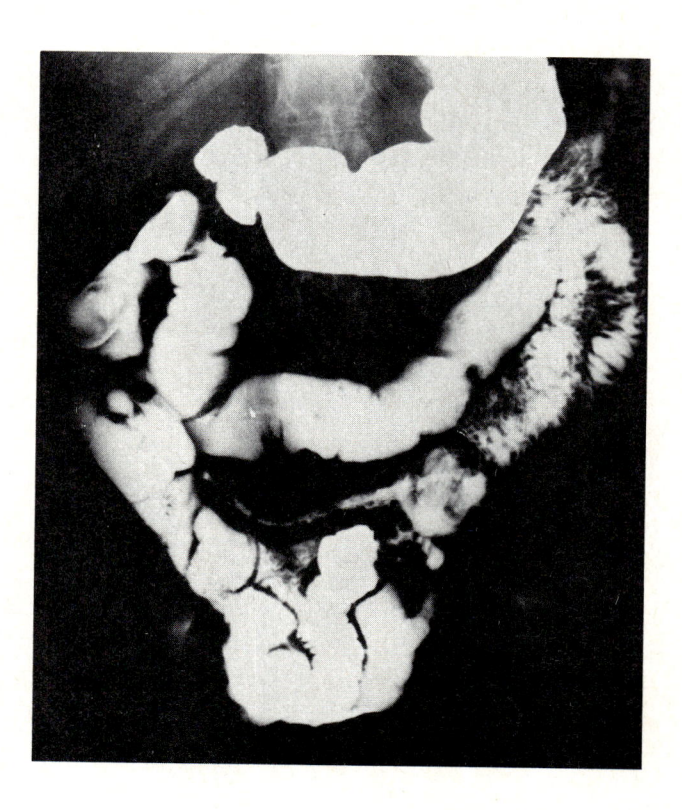

(A) Perforated appendix with appendiceal abscess
(B) Whipple's disease
(C) Regional enteritis
(D) Adenocarcinoma of the small intestine
(E) Lymphoma of the small intestine

330. A 20-year-old man was found to have ulcerative proctitis 2 years ago. Mild rectal bleeding was well controlled on daily steroid enemas, which were discontinued a year ago. For the last 3 months, he has had increasingly frequent bloody diarrhea (now 6 to 10 times a day), lower abdominal cramps, low-grade fever, anorexia, and a 5-kg (11-lb) weight loss. Physical examination of this thin, pale young man, who appears acutely ill, reveals these vital signs: temperature, 37.8°C (100°F); pulse, 110/min; and blood pressure, 120/70 mmHg. The lower abdomen is mildly and diffusely tender, but there is no rebound tenderness and bowels sounds are active. Stool is grossly bloody. Sigmoidoscopy, limited to 10 cm because of discomfort, shows marked mucosal erythema and friability; diffuse ulceration is present, and an exudate contains pus and blood.

Three hours after a barium enema, which shows ulcerations throughout the colon, the man's abdominal pain markedly worsens. Vital signs now are temperature 39.6°C (103.2°F), pulse 130/min, and blood pressure 90/60 mmHg. On examination the abdomen is distended and diffusely tender with rebound; bowel sounds are infrequent. An abdominal flat-plate x-ray is pictured below.

The most likely diagnosis for the disorder described above is

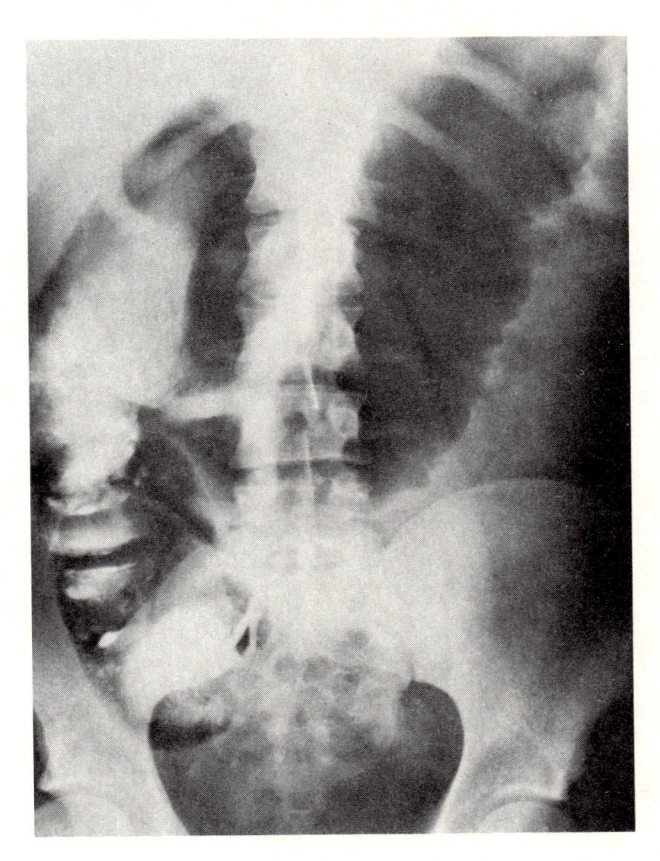

(A) acute colonic perforation
(B) inferior mesenteric artery occlusion
(C) nonthrombotic mesenteric ischemia
(D) volvulus
(E) toxic megacolon

331. All of the following are risk factors for development of cancer of the colon EXCEPT

(A) Crohn's colitis
(B) adenomatous polyps
(C) uterine cancer
(D) breast cancer
(E) juvenile polyposis

332. All of the following statements regarding primary biliary cirrhosis (PBC) are true EXCEPT

(A) a positive antimitochondrial antibody test is present in more than 90 percent of patients
(B) increased serum cryoprotein concentrations are frequently present
(C) the majority of patients are women
(D) administration of D-penicillamine appears to be an effective treatment
(E) rheumatoid arthritis, CRST syndrome, and scleroderma occur with increased frequency in patients with PBC

333. The most common organism isolated from the ascitic fluid of patients with spontaneous bacterial peritonitis is

(A) *Streptococcus pneumoniae*
(B) *Staphylococcus aureus*
(C) *Escherichia coli*
(D) *Bacteroides fragilis*
(E) *Klebsiella* sp.

334. A 27-year-old man has had ulcerative colitis for 11 years. His symptoms have been reasonably well controlled on antispasmodic medications and sulfasalazine (Azulfidine). During the last 2 months, however, he has experienced fatigability and a weight loss of 6.8 kg (15 lb). A recent barium enema x-ray is reproduced below. The most appropriate next step in the management of this man's illness would be to

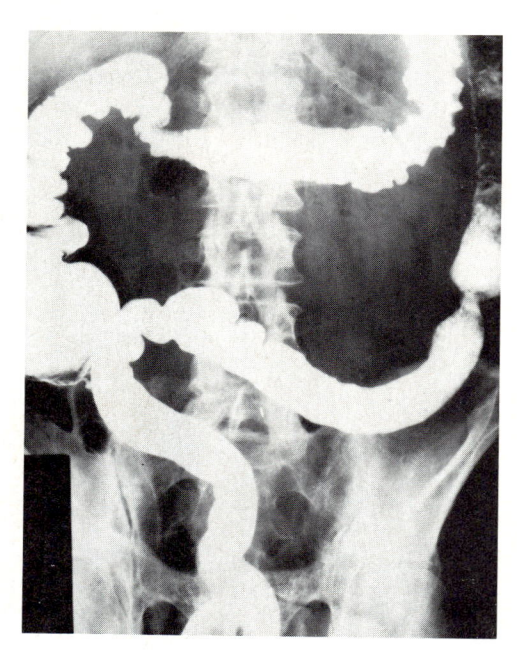

(A) order an air-contrast barium enema
(B) perform colonoscopy
(C) obtain a serum carcinoembryonic antigen level
(D) begin high-dose, intravenous steroid therapy
(E) begin azathioprine therapy

335. A 37-year-old man with chronic alcoholism is admitted to the hospital with acute pancreatitis. On the third hospital day, sudden, complete blindness develops in the left eye. The most likely explanation is

(A) alcohol withdrawal symptom
(B) transient ischemic attack (transient monocular blindness)
(C) retinal vein occlusion
(D) acute glaucoma
(E) Purtscher's retinopathy

336. Mechanical obstruction of the colon is most commonly caused by

(A) adhesions
(B) carcinoma
(C) volvulus
(D) hernia
(E) sigmoid diverticulitis

337. In which of the following causes of fatty liver is microvesicular fat seen in liver biopsy specimens?

(A) Jejunoileal bypass for morbid obesity
(B) Acute fatty liver of pregnancy
(C) Massive tetracycline therapy
(D) Prolonged intravenous hyperalimentation
(E) Carbon tetrachloride poisoning

338. The treatment of choice for Whipple's disease is administration of

(A) penicillin
(B) tetracycline
(C) trimethoprim-sulfamethoxazole
(D) metronidazole
(E) cephalexin

339. In an individual who has hepatic cirrhosis, hepatic encephalopathy can be precipitated by all the following factors EXCEPT

(A) gastrointestinal bleeding
(B) metabolic acidosis
(C) pneumonia
(D) vomiting
(E) viral hepatitis

340. One month ago, a 21-year-old woman was begun on daily isoniazid therapy because of a positive tuberculin skin test. She now feels well and her physical examination is unremarkable. Routine laboratory data include the following: serum alanine aminotransferase (ALT), 150 Karmen units/mL; total bilirubin, 1.0 mg/dL; and alkaline phosphatase, 25 units. The most appropriate intervention by the woman's physican would be to order

(A) another antituberculous drug
(B) corticosteroids
(C) a liver biopsy
(D) an ultrasound of the gallbladder
(E) continuation of isoniazid therapy

341. A 45-year-old man with Laennec's cirrhosis and a history of hepatic encephalopathy comes to the local emergency room because of alcoholic intoxication. Physical examination is remarkable for palmar erythema, spider angiomas, and bilateral gynecomastia. Liver span is 8 cm and the edge cannot be felt; a spleen tip, however, is palpable. Stool is guaiac-negative. He has no asterixis. Laboratory studies include the following:

Hematocrit: 38%
Mean corpuscular volume: 104 fL
White blood cell count: 4000/mm^3
Platelet count: 97,000/mm^3
Prothrombin time: 17.5 s
Total serum bilirubin: 0.8 mg/dL
Serum AST: 45 Karmen units/mL
Serum alkaline phosphatase: 34 units

The man is given intravenous hydration and vitamin and mineral supplements, including folic acid (1 mg), thiamine (100 mg), magnesium (2 g), and vitamin K (10 mg). After spending the night in the hospital's detoxification unit, he awakens sober and alert. Repeat prothrombin time is 12 s.
  The most likely explanation for the elevation in the man's initial prothrombin time is

(A) alcoholic hepatitis
(B) folate deficiency
(C) intestinal malabsorption
(D) disseminated intravascular coagulation
(E) laboratory error

342. A 67-year-old woman, who has previously been healthy, undergoes emergency surgery for a ruptured abdominal aortic aneurysm. Intraoperatively she requires 8 units of packed red blood cells to maintain her blood pressure and hematocrit. Following surgery she is hemodynamically stable. On the third postoperative day she appears jaundiced, but abdominal exam is unremarkable and she is afebrile. Total serum bilirubin concentration at this time is 8.3 mg/dL (direct, 6.3 mg/dL). Serum alkaline phosphatase level is 110 units, and serum AST level is 51 Karmen units/mL. The most likely explanation for the woman's jaundice is

(A) a stone in the common bile duct
(B) halothane hepatitis
(C) posttransfusion hepatitis
(D) acute hepatic infarct
(E) benign intrahepatic cholestasis

343. Clinical and laboratory findings associated with poor prognosis in persons with acute viral hepatitis include all the following EXCEPT

(A) symptoms and signs of encephalopathy
(B) prolongation of prothrombin time by more than 4 seconds
(C) plasma glucose level less than 50 mg/dL
(D) serum total bilirubin level greater than 20 mg/dL
(E) serum alanine aminotransferase level greater than 2500 Karmen units/mL

344. Chronic active hepatitis is distinguished most reliably from chronic persistent hepatitis by the presence of

(A) extrahepatic manifestations
(B) hepatitis B surface antigen in the serum
(C) antibody to hepatitis B core antigen in the serum
(D) a significant titer of anti-smooth-muscle antibody
(E) characteristic liver histology

345. A 31-year-old nephrology fellow is found to have hepatitis B surface antigen (HBsAg) in her serum during a study of hepatitis exposure in hospital personnel. She has no history of acute hepatitis or exposure to hepatitis and denies having recent episodes of fatigue, right-upper-quadrant pain, fever, or jaundice. Her physical examination is unremarkable. Liver function tests include the following:

   Total serum bilirubin: 0.8 mg/dL
   Serum AST: 44 Karmen units/mL
   Serum alkaline phosphatase: 26 units
   Serum proteins: albumin 3.9 mg/dL; globulins 2.6 mg/dL
   Prothrombin time: 11.5 s

The woman's physician should now do which of the following?

(A) Test for anti-HBs in her serum
(B) Test for other hepatitis B antigens in her serum
(C) Administer hyperimmune globulin
(D) Perform a liver biopsy
(E) None of the above

346. All the following statements regarding abdominal angiography in the evaluation and treatment of gastrointestinal hemorrhage are true EXCEPT

(A) blood loss at a rate of 0.5 to 1.0 mL/min is required to demonstrate a bleeding site
(B) intraarterial administration of vasoconstrictors often is effective in controlling bleeding from mucosal bleeding sites
(C) vasopressin injected into the superior mesenteric artery is more effective than peripheral intravenous vasopressin in controlling hemorrhage from esophageal varices
(D) hemostatic agents may be delivered through the catheter to control hemorrhage from a duodenal ulcer
(E) angiography can successfully identify actively bleeding lesions in regions of the gastrointestinal tract not accessible to endoscopy

347. A 52-year-old woman is hospitalized for medical management of severe alcoholic hepatitis. On the ninth hospital day she develops a temperature of 38.3°C (101°F) and generalized abdominal discomfort. Abdominal examination reveals significant and diffuse abdominal tenderness without guarding; hepatosplenomegaly is present but is unchanged from the admission examination. Rectal and pelvic examinations reveal no area of localized tenderness; stool guaiac testing is positive. Hematocrit is 27 percent, white blood cell count is 12,000/mm^3, and liver function tests are unchanged from admission (total serum bilirubin, 12.5 mg/dL; serum AST, 150 Karmen units/mL; and serum alkaline phosphatase, 180 units).

The procedure most likely to yield diagnosis information in this case would be

(A) serum amylase determination
(B) blood culture
(C) supine and upright x-rays of the abdomen
(D) abdominal sonography
(E) paracentesis

348. A 38-year-old woman is hospitalized for an upper gastrointestinal hemorrhage. Following an uneventful recovery, an upper gastrointestinal series (part of which is reproduced below) is obtained. The abnormality demonstrated in the x-ray suggests which of the following diagnoses?

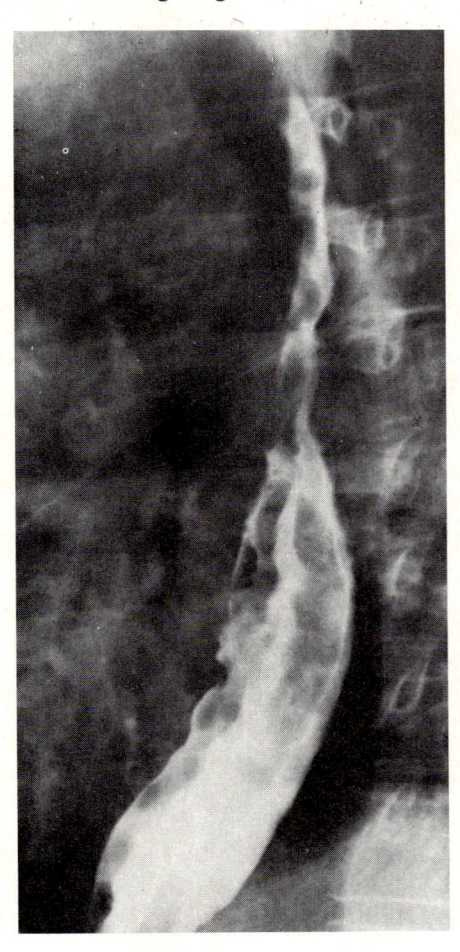

(A) Erosive gastritis
(B) Laennec's cirrhosis
(C) Hiatal hernia
(D) Gastric ulcer
(E) Reflux esophagitis

349. All the following conditions are known to predispose to the formation of cholesterol gallstones EXCEPT

(A) obesity
(B) hypercholesterolemia
(C) clofibrate therapy
(D) oral contraceptive therapy
(E) surgical resection of the ileum

350. A 58-year-old man with biopsy-proven Laennec's cirrhosis is hospitalized because of massive ascites and pedal edema. There is no evidence of respiratory compromise or hepatic encephalopahy. Initial laboratory values are as follows:

Serum electrolytes (meq/L): Na$^+$ 130; K$^+$ 3.6; Cl$^-$ 85; HCO$_3^-$ 30
Serum creatinine: 1.0 mg/dL
Blood urea nitrogen: 18 mg/dL

Bed rest and sodium and water restriction produce no significant weight change after 5 days.
Which of the following therapeutic measures would be most appropriate at this time?

(A) Intravenous furosemide, 80 mg now
(B) Oral spironolactone, 100 mg/day
(C) Oral acetazolamide, 250 mg/day
(D) Placement of a peritoneovenous (LeVeen) shunt
(E) Therapeutic paracentesis

351. A 65-year-old man with long-standing, stable, biopsy-proven postnecrotic cirrhosis develops right-upper-quadrant abdominal pain and abdominal swelling. He is afebrile. Palmar erythema, spider telangiectasias, and mild jaundice are noted on physical examination. His abdomen is distended, shifting dullness is present, a tender firm liver edge is felt 3 fingerbreadths below the right costal margin, and a spleen tip is palpable. A faint bruit is heard over the liver. Laboratory values include the following:

Hematocrit: 34%
White blood cell count: 4300/mm^3
Platelet count: 104,000/mm^3
Serum albumin: 2.6 g/dL
Serum globulins: 4.6 g/dL
Serum calcium: 11.2 mg/dL

Paracentesis reveals blood-tinged fluid.
The serum marker most specifically associated with this man's condition is

(A) antinuclear antibody
(B) α-fetoprotein
(C) antimitochondrial antibody
(D) 5'-nucleotidase
(E) chorionic gonadotropin

352. Administration of which of the following drugs or classes of drugs has been shown to prolong survival in persons with acute pancreatitis?

(A) Cimetidine
(B) Aprotinin (Trasylol)
(C) Antibiotics
(D) Anticholinergics
(E) None of the above

353. A 64-year-old man with insulin-dependent adult-onset diabetes mellitus seeks emergency medical treatment after 2 days of increasingly severe right-upper-quadrant abdominal pain, which has spread over the entire abdomen and is associated with nausea, vomiting, fever, and chills. On examination, he is alert and oriented but appears to be quite acutely distressed. Vital signs are temperature, 39.4°C (103°F); pulse, 140/min; and blood pressure, 100/60 mmHg. His sclerae are mildly icteric. His abdomen is diffusely tender with marked guarding in the right upper quadrant; there is no palpable hepatosplenomegaly, and there are no audible bowel sounds. Rectal examination reveals no focal tenderness; stool is guaiac-negative. Laboratory values are as follows:

Hematocrit: 34%
White blood cell count: 22,500/mm^3 with a marked left shift
Plasma glucose: 325 mg/dL
Blood urea nitrogen: 30 mg/dL
Serum AST: 125 Karmen units/mL
Serum alkaline phosphatase: 210 units
Serum amylase: 200 U/dL.

His abdominal flat-plate x-ray is shown below. During the first 4 hours of hospitalization, the man's condition is stabilized somewhat with the administration of intravenous fluids and insulin. A nasogastric tube is inserted, blood cultures are drawn, and he is begun on broad-spectrum antibiotics.

The most appropriate management at this point would be to order

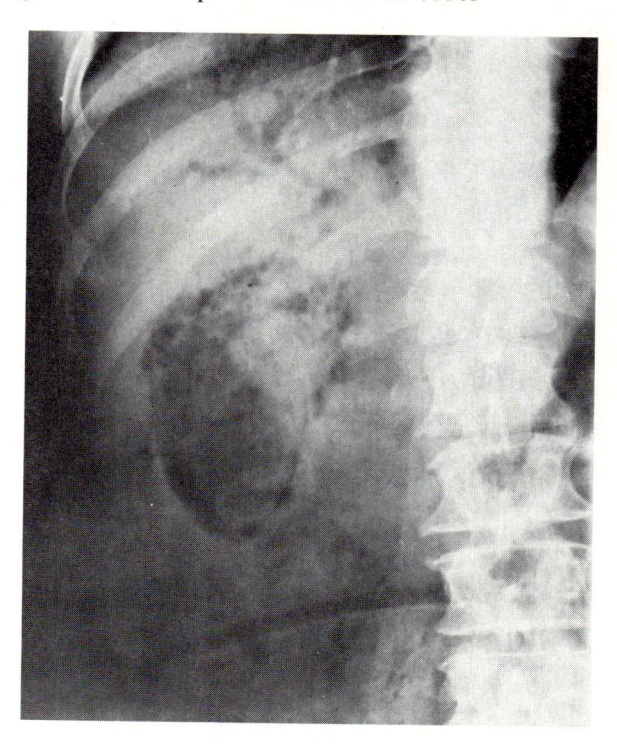

(A) conservative medical measures only for the next 48 to 72 hours
(B) an abdominal ultrasound examination
(C) an upper gastrointestinal examination with Gastrografin dye
(D) endoscopic retrograde cholangiopancreatography
(E) preparations for an emergency laparotomy

354. Complications of chronic pancreatitis include all the following EXCEPT

(A) gastric varices
(B) erythema nodosum
(C) vitamin B_{12} malabsorption
(D) pleural effusion
(E) jaundice

355. Glucagonomas can be distinguished most readily from other pancreatic endocrine tumors by their association with

(A) severe watery diarrhea
(B) refractory peptic ulcer disease
(C) necrotizing dermatitis
(D) alcohol intolerance
(E) facial flushing

DIRECTIONS: Each question below contains five suggested answers. For **each** of the five alternatives of **each** item, you are to respond either YES (Y) or NO (N). In a given item all, some, or none of the alternatives may be correct.

356. Which of the following statements regarding delta hepatitis virus (HDV) are true?

(A) HDV is a defective RNA virus
(B) HDV can infect only persons infected with HBV
(C) The HDV genome is partially homologous with HBV DNA
(D) HDV infection has been isolated only in limited areas of the world
(E) Simultaneous infection with HDV and HBV results in an increased risk of development of chronic hepatitis

357. The use of repeated phlebotomy in the treatment of persons who have symptomatic hemochromatosis may be expected to result in

(A) decreased skin pigmentation
(B) improved cardiac function
(C) return of secondary sex characteristics
(D) protection from the development of hepatocellular carcinoma
(E) longer life expectancy

358. Causes of upper gastrointestinal bleeding that usually are missed by routine upper gastrointestinal x-rays but can be diagnosed by endoscopy include

(A) Mallory-Weiss tears
(B) duodenal ulcers
(C) gastric ulcers
(D) stress gastritis
(E) Osler-Rendu-Weber syndrome

359. Which of the following statements about the management of variceal hemorrhage are true?

(A) The most accurate means of diagnosing an acute variceal hemorrhage is an upper gastrointestinal series
(B) Peripheral-vein infusion of pitressin is as effective as superior mesenteric artery infusion in controlling variceal hemorrhage
(C) The presence of preoperative jaundice and ascites increases the risk of immediate postoperative mortality in persons undergoing surgical shunting procedures for variceal hemorrhage
(D) Elective portacaval shunt surgery prevents recurrent variceal hemorrhage but does not improve life expectancy
(E) The selective, distal splenorenal shunt appears to be associated with a lower incidence than the portacaval shunt of postoperative hepatic encephalopathy

360. Chronic reflux esophagitis can lead to the development of

(A) gastrointestinal bleeding
(B) an esophageal peptic stricture
(C) a lower esophageal ring
(D) Barrett's esophagus (esophagus lined by columnar epithelium)
(E) adenocarcinoma

361. Which of the following statements regarding the prophylaxis of viral hepatitis are true?

(A) Although immune globulin (IG) is effective in preventing clinically apparent type A hepatitis, not all IG preparations have adequate anti-HAV titers to be protective
(B) If given soon enough after exposure to hepatitis B, hepatitis immune globulin (HBIG) is effective in preventing infection
(C) HBIG and hepatitis B vaccine can be effectively administered simultaneously
(D) Hepatitis B vaccine is effective in preventing delta hepatitis infection in persons who are not HBsAg carriers
(E) IG prophylaxis after needle stick, sexual, or perinatal exposure to non-A, non-B hepatitis is effective in preventing infection

362. The H-2 receptor antagonist cimetidine may increase the blood levels and/or the duration of activity of which of the following drugs?

(A) Phenytoin
(B) Warfarin
(C) Oxazepam
(D) Theophylline
(E) Lidocaine

363. Gastrointestinal manifestations of scleroderma (progressive systemic sclerosis) include

(A) reflux esophagitis
(B) pancreatitis
(C) steatorrhea
(D) gallstones
(E) pneumatosis intestinalis

364. A gastric ulcer can safely be called benign if it
(A) heals significantly after a 6-week course of antacid therapy
(B) is associated with the presence of acid in the gastric aspirate
(C) is located on the lesser gastric curvature
(D) is less than 2 cm in diameter
(E) shows no evidence of malignancy after six biopsies and brush cytology examinations

365. Which of the following statements regarding primary intestinal lymphoma are true?
(A) It may develop as a late complication of nontropical sprue
(B) Hepatosplenomegaly and peripheral adenopathy are frequently present
(C) Steatorrhea and malabsorption may be the presenting symptoms
(D) The diagnosis is best made by endoscopic biopsies
(E) Perforation and bleeding are unusual

366. The pathogenesis of duodenal ulcers can be described by which of the following statements?
(A) Relative gastric hypersecretion appears to be more important than duodenal mucosal resistance
(B) The secretion of gastrin after a protein meal is greater in persons who have duodenal ulcers than in normal controls
(C) The production of acid in response to the same dose of gastrin is greater in persons who had duodenal ulcers than in normal controls
(D) Intragastric acid is less effective in inhibiting gastrin release and gastric acid secretion in persons who have duodenal ulcers than in normal controls
(E) Gastric emptying is more rapid in persons who have duodenal ulcers than in normal controls

367. Which of the following statements about gastric cancer are true?
(A) Most gastric cancers begin as benign polyps or benign ulcers
(B) The risk of gastric cancer is increased following a Billroth II partial gastrectomy
(C) The incidence of gastric cancer is higher in persons with blood group O than in other persons
(D) Persons with atrophic gastritis have a 50 percent incidence of developing gastric cancer
(E) If achlorhydria persists despite pentagastrin stimulation in a person with a gastric ulcer, then it is likely that the ulcer is malignant

368. Which of the following statements concerning the short bowel syndrome are true?
(A) Following massive small-bowel resection, a transient syndrome of gastric hypersecretion may develop
(B) If more than 100 cm of ileum have been resected, dietary fat intake should be reduced to 40 g/day
(C) Ileal malabsorption of bile salts results in enhanced fluid and electrolyte absorption in the colon
(D) Antiperistaltic agents would aid fluid and electrolyte absorption
(E) Loss of ileal tissue is better tolerated than loss of an equal length of jejunal tissue

369. Extraintestinal complications associated with regional enteritis but **not** associated with ulcerative colitis include
(A) pericholangitis
(B) bilirubin gallstones
(C) hypocalcemia
(D) uveitis
(E) oxalate kidney stones

370. The medical therapy of Crohn's disease can be described by which of the following statements?
(A) Metronidazole may be useful if the perineal area is involved
(B) Azathioprine is ineffective as a single agent
(C) Corticosteroids are more effective in the treatment of Crohn's disease of the small intestine than in the treatment of Crohn's disease of the colon
(D) In persons in whom a remission in disease activity has been achieved, sulfasalazine decreases the frequency of relapse
(E) Sulfasalazine should never be used to treat pregnant women who have Crohn's disease

371. A 40-year-old man has a history of ulcerative colitis. Features of his illness that would contribute to an increased risk of developing colon cancer include
(A) disease duration of more than 10 years
(B) history of toxic megacolon
(C) presence of pancolitis (total colonic involvement)
(D) presence of pseudopolyps on colonoscopy
(E) high steroid requirements

372. Which of the following are true statements about carcinoembryonic antigen (CEA)?

(A) Most persons with colon cancer have elevated serum CEA levels
(B) A normal serum CEA level excludes a diagnosis of gastrointestinal malignancy
(C) A decline in serum CEA level suggests a favorable response to therapy
(D) Serum CEA level is elevated in some persons who have benign biliary disease
(E) Serum CEA level is elevated in some persons who have inflammatory bowel disease

373. Ischemic colitis can be described by which of the following statements?

(A) The usual presenting symptom is severe abdominal pain
(B) Rectal bleeding may be the presenting symptom
(C) Involvement of the rectum is uncommon
(D) Symptoms and signs of nonocclusive ischemic colitis resolve in 2 to 4 weeks
(E) Angiography is the definitive diagnostic procedure

374. Which of the following are true statements describing Meckel's diverticulum?

(A) It is the most frequent congenital anomaly of the digestive tract
(B) It accounts for approximately 50 percent of all episodes of lower gastrointestinal bleeding in children
(C) In young adults, inflammatory complications may produce a clinical syndrome indistinguishable from acute appendicitis
(D) Conventional gastrointestinal barium x-rays can demonstrate the diverticulum in more than 85 percent of cases
(E) Technetium scans are valuable in the diagnosis of those diverticula associated with gastrointestinal bleeding

375. Which of the following statements regarding acute bleeding from colonic diverticula are true?

(A) Diverticulitis usually is present
(B) The source of hemorrhage is more likely to be on the right side than on the left side of the colon
(C) Bleeding usually abates spontaneously
(D) Angiographic detection of bleeding usually is unsuccessful
(E) It is the most common cause of acute lower gastrointestinal bleeding in elderly persons

376. An 18-year-old man develops watery diarrhea shortly after returning from a vacation in Africa. Physical examination reveals a temperature of 37.8°C (100°F) and generalized abdominal tenderness. A stool sample stained with methylene blue reveals abundant mixed bacterial organisms and polymorphonuclear leukocytes. Which of the following diagnoses would be compatible with the findings described?

(A) Amebic colitis
(B) Cholera
(C) Bacillary dysentery
(D) Ulcerative colitis
(E) Giardiasis

377. Percutaneous needle liver biopsy would be indicated in a diagnostic workup for

(A) unexplained hepatosplenomegaly
(B) persistently abnormal liver function tests
(C) suspected hepatic angioma
(D) suspected miliary tuberculosis
(E) suspected obstruction of the common bile duct

378. Which of the following conditions would likely be associated with the set of serum values presented below?

Total bilirubin: 1.5 mg/dL
AST: 60 Karmen units/mL
Alkaline phosphatase: 450 units

(A) Primary biliary cirrhosis
(B) Stricture of the common bile duct
(C) Acute viral hepatitis
(D) Acetaminophen overdose
(E) Chlorpromazine therapy

379. Which of the following statements regarding adenomatous polyps of the colon are true?

(A) Most adenomatous polyps are clinically silent
(B) The majority of adenomatous polyps occur in the rectosigmoid colon
(C) The size of an adenomatous polyp correlates with the risk of malignancy
(D) Villous adenomas are more likely than tubular polyps to be malignant
(E) Colonoscopic polypectomy is adequate therapy of an adenoma that has evidence of carcinoma in situ

380. Acute viral hepatitis can be described by which of the following statements?

(A) There is a direct correlation between the concentration of HBsAg in the liver and the degree of hepatocellular damage
(B) A serum bilirubin concentration greater than 20 mg/dL, in the absence of hemolysis, is a poor prognostic sign
(C) A serum sickness-like syndrome may precede the onset of clinical jaundice caused by hepatitis B virus infection
(D) The presenting symptoms and signs are useful in predicting the specific etiologic agent responsible
(E) Steroid therapy has been shown to shorten the clinical course of the illness

381. Which of the following statements regarding non-A, non-B hepatitis are true?

(A) It accounts for approximately 90 percent of all cases of posttransfusion hepatitis
(B) Its mean incubation period is longer than that of hepatitis A but shorter than that of hepatitis B
(C) It can be spread by both percutaneous and nonpercutaneous exposure
(D) It is associated with chronic carrier states in asymptomatic individuals
(E) Treatment of exposed individuals with immune serum globulin has not provided consistent prophylaxis

382. The pathogenesis of chronic active hepatitis may be associated with

(A) hepatitis A virus infection
(B) non-A, non-B hepatitis virus infection
(C) acetaminophen overdose
(D) chlorpromazine use
(E) methyldopa use

383. Women taking oral contraceptives have a greater likelihood of developing

(A) benign hepatic adenoma
(B) peliosis hepatis
(C) focal nodular hyperplasia of the liver
(D) hepatic angiosarcoma
(E) primary hepatocellular carcinoma

384. Which of the following statements regarding Gilbert's syndrome are true?

(A) The serum total bilirubin is predominantly unconjugated and rarely exceeds 5 mg/dL
(B) Fasting increases the serum bilirubin concentration
(C) It appears to be inherited in an autosomal recessive pattern
(D) Serum bilirubin concentration increases after the administration of phenobarbital
(E) Examination by light microscopy of liver biopsy specimens discloses normal results

385. Reye's syndrome often is associated with

(A) marked hyperbilirubinemia
(B) salicylate ingestion
(C) hyperglycemia
(D) elevated serum aminotransferase levels
(E) recent viral illness

386. Which of the following statements about hepatitis B *e* antigen (HBeAg) are true?

(A) HBeAg can be detected transiently in the sera of patients ill with acute hepatitis B infection
(B) The presence of HBeAg in the serum is correlated with infectiousness
(C) The absence of HBeAg in the serum rules out chronic infection due to the hepatitis B virus
(D) The lack of detectable HBeAg in the serum rules out development of hepatocellular carcinoma
(E) The disappearance of HBeAg from the serum may be a harbinger of resolution of acute hepatitis B infection

387. Which of the following disorders are associated with an increased incidence of hepatocellular carcinoma?

(A) Hemochromatosis
(B) Alpha$_1$-antitrypsin deficiency
(C) Long-term aflatoxin ingestion
(D) Chronic hepatitis B virus infection
(E) Alcoholic liver disease

112

PRINCIPLES OF INTERNAL MEDICINE

DIRECTIONS: The groups of questions below consist of four or five lettered headings followed by several numbered items. For each numbered item choose the **one** lettered heading with which it is **most** closely associated. Each lettered heading may be used once, more than once, or not at all.

Questions 388–391

Match each of the following case histories of esophageal disease with the barium swallow x-ray with which it is most likely to be associated.

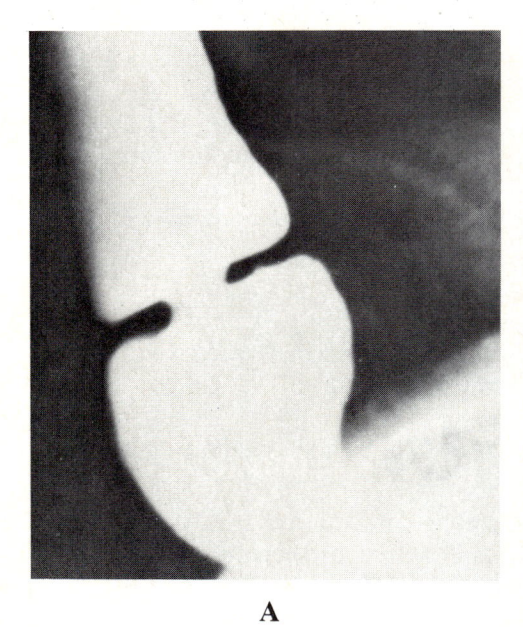

A

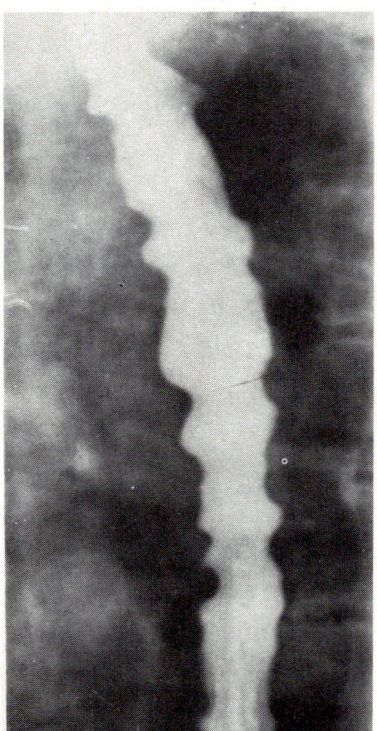

B

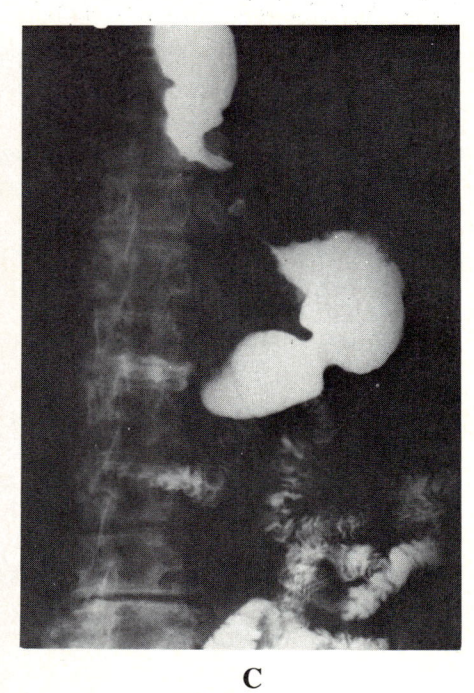

C

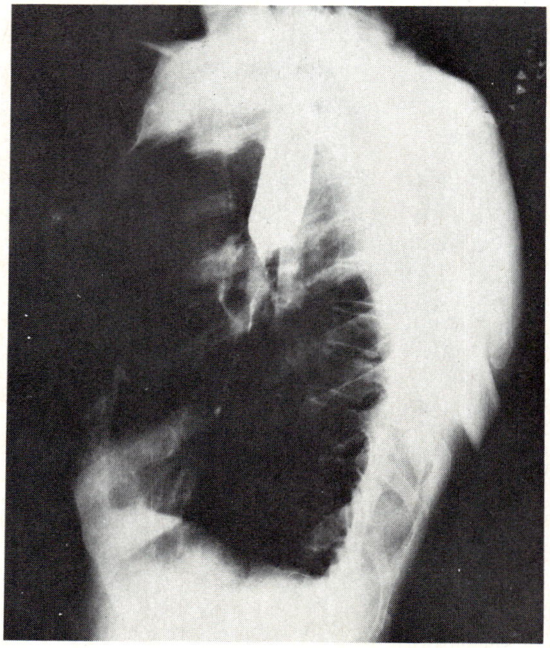

D

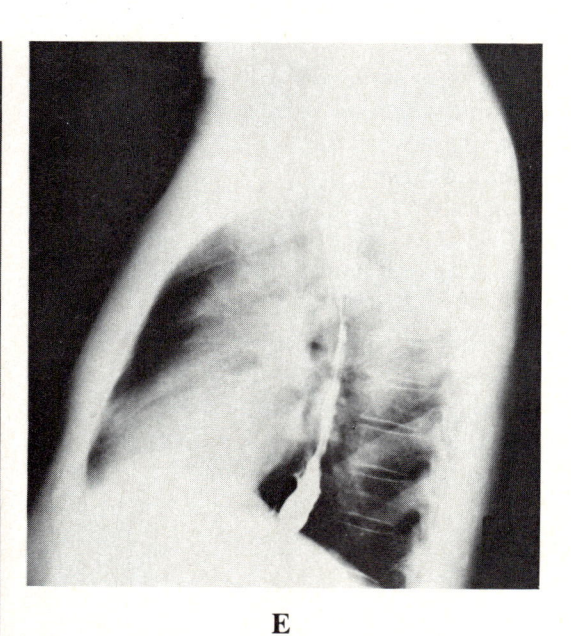

E

(A) Radiograph **A**
(B) Radiograph **B**
(C) Radiograph **C**
(D) Radiograph **D**
(E) Radiograph **E**

388. A 40-year-old truckdriver has had occasional dysphagia for solid foods for the last 5 years

389. A 61-year-old bartender has had frequent heartburn for the last 4 years and dysphagia for solid foods for the last 3 months

390. A 55-year-old alcoholic individual has had mild dysphagia for solid foods for the last month, during which time he has lost 5 kg (11 lb)

391. A 35-year-old accountant has occasional dysphagia for solid foods and frequent retrosternal chest pain that radiates to the back, occurs at rest, and lasts several minutes

---

Questions 392–396

For each clinical situation presented below, select the most likely diagnosis.

(A) Granulomatous colitis
(B) Ulcerative colitis
(C) Ischemic colitis
(D) Ulcerative proctitis
(E) Pseudomembranous colitis

392. A 28-year-old nurse with no systemic complaints reports that for the last 2 weeks he has had bright red rectal bleeding; his once-daily stools have been formed, although on occasion he has passed mucus without fecal material

393. A 79-year-old woman with a history of congestive heart failure notes the sudden onset of rectal bleeding; sigmoidoscopy is normal

394. A 22-year-old medical student has had intermittent bloody diarrhea, lower abdominal cramps, and malaise for the last 6 months

395. A 36-year-old woman suddenly develops diarrhea, lower abdominal cramps, and fever; she was treated 3 weeks ago for the development of purulent sputum following a viral upper respiratory tract infection

396. An 18-year-old student reports a 3-month history of diarrhea and fatigability; sigmoisdoscopy is normal, except for a solitary ulcer of the rectum

Questions 397–400

For each of the following serologic profiles from patients who have acute hepatitis, select the appropriate diagnostic conclusion.

(A) Acute hepatitis B
(B) Chronic hepatitis B
(C) Acute hepatitis A and B
(D) Acute hepatitis A superimposed upon chronic hepatitis B
(E) Acute hepatitis A

	HBsAg	IgM anti-HAV	IgM anti-HBc
397.	+	−	−
398.	+	+	−
399.	−	−	+
400.	−	+	−

Questions 401–404

Match each of the following patient profiles (each patient is being evaluated for chronic diarrhea) with the treatment most likely to be of benefit.

(A) Lactose-free diet
(B) Low-fat diet with medium-chain triglyceride supplementation
(C) A course (2 weeks to 1 year) of tetracycline, folate, and vitamin B_{12}
(D) Pancreatic enzyme supplementation with meals
(E) Sulfasalazine (Azulfidine)

	Serum albumin, g/dL	Serum vitamin B_{12}, pg/mL	Fecal fat on 100-g fat diet, g/day	D-Xylose in 5-h urine collection, g	Small-bowel biopsy report
401.	3.2	300	40	6	Normal
402.	4.2	700	6	10	Normal
403.	2.2	150	15	8	Dilated and telangiectatic lymphatic vessels in lamina propria and submucosa
404.	2.9	100	20	1	Shortened, thickened villi; increased crypt height; mononuclear infiltrate in lamina propria and epithelium

Questions 405–408

Match each of the following hereditary polyposis syndromes with the appropriate statement.

(A) The chance of development of colon cancer is nearly 100 percent by the age of 40 years
(B) The syndrome is associated with benign soft-tissue tumors
(C) This is the only hereditary polyposis syndrome not associated with an increased risk of development of gastrointestinal malignancy
(D) Polyps are most prominent in the small bowel
(E) The syndrome is inherited in an autosomal recessive pattern

405. Familial colonic polyposis
406. Juvenile polyposis
407. Peutz-Jeghers syndrome
408. Gardner's syndrome

Disorders of the Alimentary Tract and Hepatobiliary System

Answers

313. The answer is A. *(Braunwald, ed 11, chap 36.)* In the case described, the osmolality of fecal water is approximately equal to serum osmolality. Furthermore, there is no osmotic "gap" in the fecal water—the osmolality of the fecal water can be accounted for by the stool electrolyte composition: $[2 \times ([Na^+] + [K^+])] = [2 \times (39 + 96)] = 270$. A villous adenoma of the colon typically produces a secretory diarrhea. Lactose intolerance, non-tropical sprue, and excessive use of milk of magnesia produce osmotic diarrheas with osmotic "gaps" caused by lactose, carbohydrates, and magnesium, respectively. Pancreatic insufficiency causes steatorrhea, not watery diarrhea.

314. The answer is C. *(Braunwald, ed 11, chaps 254, 255.)* Hypertriglyceridemia (types I, IV, and V) occurs in 15 to 20 percent of persons who have acute pancreatitis. The abnormal lipid metabolism is thought to antedate the acute pancreatitis in most cases. Affected persons often have a spuriously normal serum amylase level, presumably because of the presence of uncharacterized inhibitors that interfere with measurement of amylase activity. By supposedly diluting out the inhibitor, serial dilution of the serum often unmasks elevated amylase levels. Similarly, the serum lipase level often is elevated as well. Hypercalcemia is an unrelated and uncommon cause of acute pancreatitis.

315. The answer is E. *(Braunwald, ed 11, chap 37.)* The presence of "coffee-grounds" material in a nasograstic aspirate from a person with melena indicates recent upper gastrointestinal tract bleeding. In a patient with obvious signs of cirrhosis, esophageal varices must be considered in the differential diagnosis of upper gastrointestinal bleeding; other possible diagnoses include peptic ulcer, gastroduodenitis, esophagitis, and Mallory-Weiss tear. Before diagnostic procedures, such as endoscopy or upper gastrointestinal series, are undertaken, the placement of a large-bore intravenous line and commencement of volume replacement therapy are mandatory in order to prevent hypotension. Moreover, blood should be typed and cross-matched in case of further bleeding. Diagnostic angiography is indicated only when brisk bleeding prevents diagnosis by endoscopy or barium study. Specific therapy for variceal bleeding—i.e., passage of Sengstaken-Blakemore tube and intravenous infusion of pitressin—should be considered if diagnostic studies reveal bleeding varices.

316. The answer is D. *(Braunwald, ed 11, chap 234.)* A Zenker's diverticulum typically causes halitosis and regurgitation of saliva and food particles consumed several days earlier. When a Zenker's diverticulum fills with food, it may produce dysphagia by compressing the esophagus. Gastric outlet obstruction can cause bloating and regurgitation of newly ingested food. Gastrointestinal disorders associated with scleroderma include esophageal reflux, the development of wide-mouthed colonic diverticula, and stasis and bacterial over-growth. Achalasia typically presents with dysphagia for both solids and liquids. Gastric retention caused by the autonomic neuropathy of diabetes mellitus usually results in post-prandial epigastric discomfort and bloating.

317. The answer is D. *(Braunwald, ed 11, chaps 233, 236.)* The x-ray presented shows a large malignant-appearing gastric ulcer on the lesser curvature of the stomach. Because the differentiation between benign and malignant gastric ulcer by x-ray is not infallible (there are as many as 25 percent false positives and negatives), the diagnosis of gastric cancer should be confirmed by fiberoptic gastroscopy with brush cytology and at least six biopsies from the ulcer margin. Gastroscopy is useful in diagnosing primary gastric lymphoma, which is associated with a much better 5-year survival rate than is adenocarcinoma. Double-contrast radiographic techniques help to detect small lesions by improving mucosal detail but do not generally improve accuracy in distinguishing benign from malignant ulcers.

318. The answer is E. *(Braunwald, ed 11, chaps 39, 242.)* Chylous ascites contains thoracic or intestinal lymph and has a turbid, milky appearance. There is an increased triglyceride content, and microscopic examination reveals Sudan-staining fat globules. Chylous ascites is usually the result of lymphatic obstruction. The leading causes are trauma, tumors, tuberculosis, and filariasis. Chylous ascites is also occasionally associated with the nephrotic syndrome.

319. The answer is C. *(Braunwald, ed 11, chap 238.)* Pseudomembranous colitis results from mucosal damage caused by an enterotoxin produced by the bacterium *Clostridium difficile*. Therapy can be directed against either the microorganism or the toxin. Cholestyramine and cholestipol are resins that bind the enterotoxin and are effective in the treatment of mild to moderate cases of pseudomembranous colitis. The *C. difficile* organism is exceedingly sensitive both in vitro and in vivo to several antibiotics, namely vancomycin, metronidazole, and bacitracin. Currently, vancomycin is considered the antibiotic of choice. Despite the fact that *C. difficile* has shown in vitro sensitivity to penicillin, this antibiotic has not been demonstrated to be clinically effective in the treatment of pseudomembranous colitis.

320. The answer is C. *(Braunwald, ed 11, chap 234.)* Achalasia is a motor disorder of esophageal smooth muscle in which the lower esophageal sphincter (LES) does not relax properly in response to swallowing and in which normal esophageal peristalsis is replaced by abnormal contractions. Manometry reveals a normal or elevated LES pressure and a reduced or absent swallow-induced relaxation. A decreased number of ganglion cells is seen in the esophageal body and LES of patients with achalasia, suggesting that defective innervation of these parts is the underlying abnormality. Dysphagia, chest pain, and regurgitation are the predominant symptoms. The chest x-ray often reveals absence of the gastric air bubble and the barium swallow reveals a dilated esophagus. Calcium-channel antagonists such as nifedipine relax smooth muscle and have been effective in treating some patients. However, the mainstay of therapy remains pneumatic dilation.

321. The answer is C. *(Braunwald, ed 11, chap 234.)* Squamous cell cancer of the esophagus is the fifth most common cancer in adult males. In the United States, epidemiologic studies have linked smoking and alcohol to squamous cell cancer of the esophagus and may explain the association of this tumor with head and neck carcinoma. The long-term stasis associated with achalasia leads to chronic irritation of the esophagus which is thought to predispose to cancer formation. Tylosis is a genetically acquired disease characterized by thickening of the skin of the hands and feet and is associated with squamous cell cancer of the esophagus. Barrett's esophagus is associated with adenocarcinoma but not squamous cell carcinoma of the esophagus.

322. The answer is C. *(Braunwald, ed 11, chap 235.)* The causes of stomal (anastomotic) ulceration following peptic ulcer surgery include incomplete vagotomy, retained gastric antrum, the Zollinger-Ellison syndrome (gastrinoma), poor gastric emptying, and ingestion of ulcerogenic drugs. In the case presented, if the previous antrectomy had been complete, the serum gastrin level should not be elevated. An elevated serum gastrin level that declines after intravenous administration of secretin is characteristic of a retained gastric antrum attached to the duodenal stump. Neither frequent antacid therapy nor a total vagotomy is effective in healing a stomal ulcer; thus, resection of the retained antrum is indicated. In the Zollinger-Ellison syndrome, the serum gastrin level paradoxically increases after intravenous infusion of secretin.

323. The answer is C. *(Braunwald, ed 11, chap 237.)* Eosinophilic enteritis is a disorder of the stomach, small intestine, and/or colon in which some part of the gut wall is infiltrated by eosinophils. The diagnosis also requires the presence of peripheral blood eosinophilia. Although early reports emphasized the presence of food allergies, less than half the patients have a history of food allergies or asthma. The presence of anemia, Hemoccult-positive stools, abnormalities of the ileum and cecum on barium radiographic studies, and a favorable response to administration of steroids may make eosinophilic enteritis difficult to distinguish from Crohn's disease. Although no controlled trials of corticosteroid therapy have been performed, symptoms usually respond to short-term corticosteroid therapy.

324. The answer is C. *(Braunwald, ed 11, chap 237.)* Malabsorption due to bacterial overgrowth results from bacterial utilization of ingested vitamins and the deconjugation of bile salts by bacteria in the proximal jejunum. Deconjugated bile salts do not form micelles in the jejunum, and long-chain fatty acids cannot be absorbed. The bacteria also separate ingested vitamin B_{12} from intrinsic factor, thus interfering with its absorption from the ileum. The absorption of simple carbohydrates generally is not impaired, though complex carbohydrates may be metabolized by bacteria. Thus, persons with bacterial overgrowth have steatorrhea, an abnormal Schilling test (even with administration of intrinsic factor), increased metabolism of nonabsorbable carbohydrates (e.g., lactulose), and increased bacterial concentrations in jejunal aspirates. Absorption of D-xylose, a simple carbohydrate, is often normal.

325. The answer is C. *(Braunwald, ed 11, chap 237.)* Because of autonomic neuropathy, persons who have diabetes not uncommonly display clinical symptoms and radiologic findings suggestive of gastric retention. Metoclopramide, a stimulant of gastric motility, often can help relieve symptoms of retention. Poor gastric emptying that is not due to ulceration would be unlikely to respond to antacids or cimetidine. The use of probanthine might aggravate the condition, considering that anticholinergic medications tend to retard gastric emptying. Surgical treatment is rarely necessary and should not be considered unless an adequate trial of nonsurgical therapy is unsuccessful.

326. The answer is D. *(Braunwald, ed 11, chap 237.)* The man described in the question has Whipple's disease, a bowel disorder associated with dilated lymphatics and characterized by weight loss, abdominal pain, diarrhea, malabsorption, and arthralgias. Electron microscopy has revealed the presence of bacilliform bodies in the lamina propria; these rod-shaped structures, which are located within or adjacent to macrophages that contain PAS-positive granules, resemble microorganisms, suggesting an infectious etiology of Whipple's disease. The treatment of choice is at least one year of therapy with antibiotics, such as tetracycline. Clinical recovery is accompanied by the disappearance of the bacilliform bodies.

327. The answer is B. *(Braunwald, ed 11, chap 237.)* The histologic specimen pictured in the question shows villous atrophy, crypt hyperplasia, and inflammation typical of intestinal changes in nontropical sprue (celiac disease), an illness with a high incidence in Ireland. The disease is associated with an increased incidence of histocompatibility antigens HLA-B8 and HLA-DW3. Although two-thirds of symptomatic cases present in childhood, the onset of clinical symptoms of malabsorption may occur at any age. Persons with subclinical sprue during adolescence may have mild growth retardation and may be smaller than their siblings. Because the villous absorptive surface is markedly reduced in affected persons, an acquired lactase deficiency is often present and causes symptoms of milk intolerance. A strict gluten-free diet or use of corticosteroids usually relieves symptoms and signs of malabsorption and promotes restoration of normal jejunal histology. A malabsorptive syndrome associated with abdominal pain, arthralgias, low-grade fever, and lymphadenopathy is not typical of celiac disease and should suggest another diagnosis, such as Whipple's disease or lymphoma.

328. The answer is B. *(Braunwald, ed 11, chap 238.)* Sigmoidoscopic demonstration of a hyperemic mucosa studded with plaque-like lesions is characteristic of pseudomembranous (antibiotic-associated) colitis, which is caused by the enterotoxin of *Clostridium difficile*. Although symptoms commonly develop while the offending antibiotic is still being taken, the syndrome may not become evident until several days or weeks after completion of therapy. Ischemic colitis may cause bloody diarrhea but not the mucosal lesions described. Amebic or *Shigella* infestation is associated with punched-out ulcerations of the mucosa. Toxic megacolon is a complication of active colitis.

DISORDERS OF THE ALIMENTARY TRACT AND HEPATOBILIARY SYSTEM

329. The answer is C. *(Braunwald, ed 11, chap 238.)* Radiographic demonstration of luminal narrowing, mucosal ulceration, and cobblestoning in the ileum is compatible with a diagnosis of regional enteritis. In Whipple's disease, x-rays characteristically show marked thickening of mucosal folds in the duodenum and jejunum. On barium enema, an appendiceal abscess usually presents as a mass indenting the cecal tip. Adenocarcinoma of the small bowel usually occurs as an ulcerated mass lesion in the duodenum. Infiltrating lymphomas of the distal bowel may be difficult to distinguish from regional enteritis radiographically, but stenotic bowel segments would not suggest lymphoma.

330. The answer is E. *(Braunwald, ed 11, chap 238.)* The clinical history and x-ray presented in the question are consistent with toxic megacolon in association with severe ulcerative colitis. Toxic megacolon is most likely to occur when hypomotility agents, such as diphenoxylate or loperamide, are given to persons with severe colitis, or when such persons undergo a barium-enema radiographic procedure. In the case presented, a barium enema was not only dangerous but, in fact, unnecessary, because the presence of diarrhea and signs of systemic illness indicated that the disease no longer was limited to the rectum. Colonic perforation may also be associated with severe ulcerative colitis; the presence of subdiaphragmatic air on abdominal x-rays would be suggestive.

331. The answer is E. *(Braunwald, ed 11, chap 239.)* The specific cause of colon cancer is unknown. However, certain diseases are known to increase the risk of development of cancer of the colon. Crohn's colitis is associated with an increased risk of colon cancer, although the risk is less than that for patients with ulcerative colitis. Colon cancer has been observed to occur with increased frequency in patients with uterine or breast cancer. Patients with adenomatous polyps are at higher risk for the subsequent development of colon cancer than is the general population. Therefore, such patients should have periodic follow-up examinations. Despite the importance of these risk factors, only 1 percent of persons with colon cancer have an identifiable risk factor other than age. The polyps in juvenile polyposis are hamartomatous and have no malignant potential.

332. The answer is D. *(Braunwald, ed 11, chap 249.)* Primary biliary cirrhosis (PBC) is a disease of unknown etiology, but the frequent association with autoimmune disorders such as rheumatoid arthritis, CRST syndrome, scleroderma, and sicca syndrome have suggested that an abnormal immune response plays an etiologic role. The disease typically affects middle-aged women and runs a slowly progressive course, with death resulting from hepatic insufficiency occurring within ten years of diagnosis. A positive antimitochondrial antibody test is relatively sensitive and specific for PBC, occurring in greater than 90 percent of patients. Other serum abnormalities include increased alkaline phosphatase and 5'-nucleotidase activities and the presence of cryoproteins. Treatment is entirely supportive. Neither corticosteroids nor D-penicillamine have proven to be effective.

333. The answer is C. *(Braunwald, ed 11, chap 249.)* Spontaneous bacterial peritonitis refers to the development of acute bacterial peritonitis without an obvious primary source of infection. The diagnosis can be suspected on clinical grounds and supported by an elevated ascitic fluid leukocyte count. However, confirmation of the diagnosis can be made only by bacterial culture. In the United States, *Escherichia coli* is the leading cause of spontaneous bacterial peritonitis and is isolated from approximately 30 percent of patients. *Streptococcus pneumoniae* and *Klebsiella* species are the second and third most commonly isolated organisms. Therefore, when the diagnosis is suspected, empiric therapy with ampicillin and an aminoglycoside is frequently instituted.

334. The answer is B. *(Braunwald, ed 11, chap 238.)* The x-ray presented in the question shows loss of haustrations and shortening of the colon typical of chronic ulcerative colitis. In addition, a stricture is present at the junction of the sigmoid and descending colon. The duration of the man's colitis and the presence of a stricture raise the question of colonic cancer, which necessitates colonoscopy. Air-contrast barium enema may better define mucosal detail but cannot substitute for a tissue diagnosis. The main value of serum carcinoembryonic antigen levels is to detect promptly the presence of metastases following resection of a colonic carcinoma, not to confirm the presence of a primary tumor. Therapeutic measures, such as the use of azathioprine or steroids, are not appropriate until the diagnostic workup has been completed.

335. The answer is E. *(Braunwald, ed 11, chap 255.)* Purtscher's retinopathy is a relatively rare but devastating complication of acute pancreatitis. It is characterized by sudden loss of vision and the presence of cotton-wool spots and hemorrhages in the area of the optic disc and macula. The cause is thought to be occlusion of the posterior retinal artery by aggregated granulocytes.

336. The answer is B. *(Braunwald, ed 11, chap 240.)* Carcinoma of the colon is the most common cause of mechanical obstruction of the colon and is followed in frequency by sigmoid diverticulitis and volvulus. These three causes account for 90 percent of cases of colonic obstruction. Adhesions and hernias cause about 75 percent of cases of small-intestine obstruction but are uncommon causes of colonic obstruction.

337. The answer is B. *(Braunwald, ed 11, chap 251.)* Fatty liver refers to the infiltration of hepatocytes by triglyceride. Typically, the fat accumulates in large cytoplasmic droplets. However, in acute fatty liver of pregnancy and in Reye's syndrome, the fat is contained in small vacuoles and is termed microvesicular fat. The reason for the different morphologic appearance of fat in these two disorders is unknown, but it provides a useful histologic differential point.

338. The answer is C. *(Braunwald, ed 11, chap 237.)* Whipple's disease is a rare disorder in which macrophages of the lamina propria contain large cytoplasmic granules that stain positive with the periodic acid Schiff (PAS) reaction. Electron microscopy reveals the presence of bacilliform bodies within and adjacent to macrophages; this finding has suggested that Whipple's disease is caused by a bacterial infection. This hypothesis is further supported by the observation that antibiotic therapy usually produces a clinical remission. Treatment with trimethoprim-sulfamethoxazole for at least one year is the treatment of choice. Penicillin and tetracycline are not effective as single-agent therapy.

339. The answer is B. *(Braunwald, ed 11, chaps 244, 249.)* Gastrointestinal bleeding, which causes an increase in the production of ammonia and other nitrogenous substances in the colon, is a common predisposing factor to hepatic encephalopathy in persons with cirrhosis. Hypokalemic alkalosis, caused by excessive diuresis or vomiting, may precipitate hepatic encephalopathy by increasing the ratio of ammonia to ammonium; gut and renal absorption of ammonia increases, and more ammonia enters the brain. Acidosis has the opposite effect. Acute infection, such as pneumonia, and deterioration of liver function, such as in viral hepatitis, both can precipitate encephalopathy in cirrhotic persons.

340. The answer is E. *(Braunwald, ed 11, chap 247.)* About 10 percent of persons treated with isoniazid develop mild elevations of serum aminotransferase levels during the first few weeks of therapy. These levels usually return to normal despite continued use of isoniazid. About 1 percent of persons with elevated aminotransferase levels develop symptoms of hepatitis and are at high risk for developing fatal hepatic failure. The older the patient, the higher the risk of isoniazid hepatitis; thus, because the patient described in this question is young and asymptomatic, isoniazid can safely be continued, as long as she is watched for symptoms of hepatitis. A liver biopsy would not be indicated unless isoniazid therapy had continued for a few more months and various serologies had been obtained.

341. The answer is C. *(Braunwald, ed 11, chaps 244, 249.)* Alcohol produces impairment in the absorption of many nutrients, including vitamin K. (The use of neomycin in the treatment of hepatic encephalopathy also can lead to a decrease in vitamin K.) When hypoprothrombinemia in a person with liver disease is easily corrected by parenteral vitamin K administration, decreased intestinal absorption of vitamin K should be suspected. Coagulopathy resulting from impaired hepatic function, such as in alcoholic hepatitis, is unlikely to be corrected by exogenous vitamin K. Although the patient discussed in the question is probably deficient in folate, as evidenced by the high mean corpuscular volume, folic acid administration has no effect on prothrombin time. Exogenous vitamin K would not correct the hypoprothrombinemia associated with disseminated intravascular coagulation.

342. The answer is E. *(Braunwald, ed 11, chap 246.)* Benign postoperative intrahepatic cholestasis can develop as a consequence of major surgery for a catastrophic event, in which hypotension, extensive blood loss into tissues, and massive blood replacement are notable. Factors contributing to jaundice include the pigment load from transfusions, decreased liver function due to hypotension, and decreased renal bilirubin excretion due to tubular necrosis. Jaundice becomes evident on the second or third postoperative day, with bilirubin levels (mainly levels of conjugated bilirubin) peaking by the tenth day. Serum alkaline phosphatase concentration may be elevated up to tenfold, but aspartate aminotransferase (AST) levels are only mildly elevated. Hepatitis and hepatic infarct are unlikely diagnoses in the absence of abdominal pain or tenderness or a significant rise in AST levels. The incubation period of posttransfusion hepatitis is 7 weeks, making this diagnosis unlikely.

343. The answer is E. *(Braunwald, ed 11, chap 247.)* Persons critically ill with acute viral hepatitis have evidence of highly impaired hepatic function. Availability of clotting factors, particularly those with a short half-life (e.g., factor VII), rapidly diminishes, and prothrombin time becomes prolonged. The liver's ability to metabolize such products as bilirubin, ammonia, and amino acids is impaired, and severe jaundice and encephalopathy can result. Both anorexia and depression of hepatic gluconeogenesis and glycogen formation may predispose to life-threatening hypoglycemic episodes. The serum level of alanine aminotransferase reflects leakage of cytoplasmic liver enzymes from injured and necrosing hepatocytes; however, it does not correlate with the degree of derangement in metabolic function and is thus of no prognostic significance.

344. The answer is E. *(Braunwald, ed 11, chap 248.)* Although chronic active hepatitis may be associated with extraintestinal manifestations (e.g., arthritis) and the presence in the serum of autoantibodies (e.g., anti-smooth-muscle antibody), these factors are not invariably present. The distinction between chronic active and chronic persistent hepatitis can only be established by liver biopsy. In chronic active hepatitis there is piecemeal necrosis (erosion of the limiting plate of hepatocytes surrounding the portal triads) and extension of inflammation into the liver lobule, features not seen in chronic persistent hepatitis. Both diseases may be associated with serologic evidence of hepatitis B infection.

345. The answer is E. *(Braunwald, ed 11, chaps 247, 248.)* The presence of hepatitis B surface antigen (HBsAg) in the serum of a person whose liver function is only minimally abnormal indicates either that the person is in the incubation period of an acute hepatitis B infection or that the person is a chronic carrier of hepatitis B. Testing for hepatitis B *e* antigen (HBeAg), a marker of viral infectivity, would not distinguish between these two possibilities. Similarly, a liver biopsy in either situation may be normal or show mild active hepatitis. Hepatitis B core antigen (HBcAg) is found only in the liver cell itself; on the other hand, anti-HBcAg appears in the plasma. Anti-HBs is usually absent when HBsAg is present, and hyperimmune globulin is of no value once HBsAg is present in the serum. The best approach in the case presented would be to follow serial liver function tests and HBsAg values only if the woman develops symptoms of hepatitis; if she remains asymptomatic, HBsAg could be rechecked in 6 months to assess for persistence of the carrier state.

346. The answer is C. *(Braunwald, ed 11, chaps 37, 249.)* The value of angiography as both a diagnostic and therapeutic tool is well established in cases of gastrointestinal hemorrhage. Angiography can detect actively bleeding lesions in areas not able to be reached by an endoscope, provided the rate of blood loss is at least 0.5 to 1.0 mL/min. Hemostasis by infusion of vasoconstrictor agents through the angiography catheter has been successfully achieved in cases of duodenal ulcer and other conditions. In the control of bleeding from esophageal varices, however, intraarterial vasopressin is no more effective than peripheral intravenous vasopressin.

347. The answer is E. *(Braunwald, ed 11, chap 249.)* Persons who have cirrhosis, particularly alcoholic cirrhosis and ascites, may develop acute bacterial peritonitis without a clearly definable precipitating event. The clinical presentation of spontaneous bacterial peritonitis may be subtle, such as fever of unknown origin and mild abdominal pain, and be attributed to other causes. Diagnosis is based on a careful examination of ascitic fluid obtained by paracentesis and should include cell count, Gram stain, and culture.

348. The answer is B. *(Braunwald, ed 11, chaps 37, 249.)* The x-ray presented in the question demonstrates esophageal varices, which are associated with portal hypertension. Of the diseases listed, only Laennec's cirrhosis would lead directly to portal hypertension. Although the other lesions might be associated with upper gastrointestinal bleeding, none would be expected to produce varices.

349. The answer is B. *(Braunwald, ed 11, chap 253.)* Obesity, clofibrate therapy, and oral contraceptive therapy predispose to gallstone formation by increasing biliary cholesterol excretion. Extensive ileal resection leads to malabsorption of bile salts, depletion of the bile acid pool, and a more lithogenic bile, resulting in an increased risk of gallstone formation. No correlation exists between serum cholesterol concentration and biliary cholesterol secretion; consequently, hypercholesterolemia per se does not predispose to cholelithiasis.

350. The answer is B. *(Braunwald, ed 11, chap 249.)* If fluid and sodium restriction is unsuccessful in the mobilization of ascitic fluid, cautious diuresis is indicated; spironolactone, rather than furosemide or acetazolamide, would be the drug of choice. Aggressive diuretic therapy can lead to volume depletion, azotemia, electrolyte disturbances, and hepatic encephalopathy. Therapeutic paracentesis is indicated only in the face of respiratory compromise and significant patient discomfort; repeated paracentesis may result in volume depletion and hypoproteinemia. The peritoneovenous (LeVeen) shunt should be reserved for cases of intractable ascites; its use is accompanied by significant complications, including infection and disseminated intravascular coagulation.

351. The answer is B. *(Braunwald, ed 11, chap 250.)* The clinical constellation of tender hepatomegaly, a bruit in the right upper quadrant of the abdomen, bloody ascites, and hypercalcemia occurring in an individual with previously stable cirrhosis is characteristic of primary hepatocellular carcinoma. This disease typically is associated with very high levels of α-fetoprotein, a unique and specific fetal $α_1$-globulin. Rarely, ectopic hormones, such as chorionic gonadotropin, are found in the serum of patients with hepatocellular carcinoma. The enzyme 5'-nucleotidase may be elevated in any condition associated with hepatocellular damage. Antimitochondrial antibodies are found in primary biliary cirrhosis and are not typical of primary hepatocellular carinoma.

352. The answer is E. *(Braunwald, ed 11, chap 255.)* Conventional therapy for acute pancreatitis includes analgesia, intravenous volume replacement, and abstinence from oral intake to "rest" the pancreas. Controlled trials have not demonstrated any benefit to symptomatic recovery or survival rate by administration of cimetidine, aprotinin (an inhibitor of pancreatic enzyme release), antibiotics, or glucagon. However, antibiotics are beneficial when secondary infection supervenes (e.g., abscess, phlegmon, or ascending cholangitis). Anticholinergic agents have not been shown to be beneficial and may worsen tachycardia, bowel hypomotility, and oliguria.

353. The answer is E. *(Braunwald, ed 11, chap 253.)* The radiograph reproduced in the question shows emphysematous cholecystitis, a form of acute cholecystitis in which the gallbladder, its wall, and sometimes even the bile ducts contain gas secondary to infection by gas-producing bacteria. This condition occurs most frequently in elderly men and diabetic individuals. The morbidity and mortality rates associated with emphysematous cholecystitis exceed those of acute cholecystitis. Once preoperative preparations are complete, laparotomy and cholecystectomy should be performed promptly.

354. The answer is B. *(Braunwald, ed 11, chap 255.)* Vitamin B_{12} (cobalamin) malabsorption is commonly associated with chronic pancreatitis. The mechanism of vitamin B_{12} malabsorption is thought to be excessive binding of the vitamin by nonintrinsic-factor binding proteins, which normally are destroyed by pancreatic proteases. Consequently, the condition is corrected by administration of pancreatic enzymes. Gastric varices, which may bleed, are caused by splenic vein thrombosis due to inflammation of the tail of the pancreas. Pleural effusions, most notably left-sided, can result from leaking pseudocysts or a pancreatic-pleural fistula; effusion fluid has a high amylase content. Jaundice results from compression of the common bile duct caused by edema or inflammation in the head of the pancreas. Although persons with chronic pancreatitis may develop tender red nodules on the legs, these are due to subcutaneous fat necrosis and not to erythema nodosum.

DISORDERS OF THE ALIMENTARY TRACT AND HEPATOBILIARY SYSTEM

355. The answer is C. *(Braunwald, ed 11, chap 255.)* Glucagonomas are slow-growing alpha-cell islet tumors of the pancreas that typically present with weight loss, anemia, and glucose intolerance due to hyperglucagonemia. A distinctive migratory necrotizing dermatitis also is often present. Severe watery diarrhea with hypokalemia is characteristic of pancreatic cholera caused by excessive production of vasoactive intestinal peptide. Refractory peptic ulcer disease is typical of the gastrin-producing tumor of the Zollinger-Ellison syndrome. Flushing of the face and upper chest and intolerance to alcohol are characteristic features of the carcinoid syndrome, in which excess serotonin is produced.

356. The answer is A-Y, B-Y, C-N, D-N, E-N. *(Braunwald, ed 11, chap 247.)* The delta agent hepatitis D virus (HDV) is a recently recognized defective RNA virus that coinfects with and requires the helper function of HBV for its replication and expression. Therefore, the duration of HDV infection is determined by and limited to the duration of HBV infection. Although the delta core is encapsulated by an outer coat of HBsAg, the delta antigen has no antigenic similarity to that of any of the HBV antigens, and the RNA genome is not homologous with HBV DNA. HDV infection has a worldwide distribution and exists in two epidemiologic patterns, endemic and epidemic. In endemic areas (Mediterranean countries) HDV infection is endemic among those with HBV infection and is transmitted predominantly by nonpercutaneous routes, such as close personal contact. In nonendemic areas, such as the United States or northern Europe, HDV infection is limited to persons with frequent exposure to blood products, such as intravenous drug addicts and hemophiliacs. In general, patients with simultaneous HBV and HDV infections do not have an increased risk of development of chronic hepatitis over patients with acute HBV infection alone. HDV superinfection of patients with chronic HBV infection carries an increased risk of fulminant hepatitis and death.

357. The answer is A-Y, B-Y, C-N, D-N, E-Y. *(Braunwald, ed 11, chap 310.)* In persons symptomatic from established hemochromatosis, repeated phlebotomy, by removing excessive iron stores, results in marked clinical improvement. Specifically, the liver and spleen decrease in size, liver function improves, cardiac failure is reversed, and skin pigmentation ("bronzing") diminishes. Carbohydrate intolerance may abate in up to half of all affected persons. For unknown reasons there is no improvement in the arthropathy or the hypogonadism (due to pituitary deposition of iron) associated with hemochromatosis. Five-year survival rate is increased from 33 to 90 percent with treatment; prolonged survival may actually increase the risk of hepatocellular carcinoma, which nevertheless affects one-third of persons treated for hemochromatosis.

358. The answer is A-Y, B-N, C-N, D-Y, E-Y. *(Braunwald, ed 11, chaps 233, 235.)* Although upper gastrointestinal endoscopy is superior to radiographic techniques in its ability to identify superficial lesions of the esophagus, stomach, and duodenum, barium studies are able to detect a very high percentage of lesions that breach the mucosa. For example, most gastric and duodenal ulcers can be identified on an air-contrast upper gastrointestinal series. In contrast, stress gastritis, the telangiectasias of Osler-Rendu-Weber syndrome, and small mucosal tears of the gastroesophageal junction (Mallory-Weiss tears) are missed with the best radiographic techniques but usually are found by routine endoscopy.

359. The answer is A-N, B-Y, C-Y, D-Y, E-Y. *(Braunwald, ed 11, chap 234.)* Peripheral (intravenous) and central (superior mesenteric artery) infusions of pitressin are equally effective in temporarily controlling variceal hemorrhage. For more permanent hemostasis, surgery may be required. Elective portacaval shunt surgery can prevent recurrent variceal bleeding, although the overall survival rate is not improved. The distal splenorenal shunt, when compared to the portacaval shunt, appears to have a lower incidence of postoperative encephalopathy; for either procedure, however, the presence of jaundice, ascites, or encephalopathy portends a more unfavorable operative outlook. Endoscopy, not radiography, offers the best means of diagnosing acute variceal hemorrhage.

124   PRINCIPLES OF INTERNAL MEDICINE

360. The answer is A-Y, B-Y, C-N, D-Y, E-Y. *(Braunwald, ed 11, chap 234.)* Chronic acid-induced (reflux) esophagitis may result in bleeding due to diffuse erosions or discrete ulcerations. Peptic damage to the submucosa can result in fibrosis and subsequent stricture. Barrett's esophagus is formed as destroyed squamous epithelium is replaced by columnar epithelium, usually similar to that of the adjacent gastric mucosa. Adenocarcinoma may develop in 2 to 5 percent of individuals with a Barrett's esophagus. Lower esophageal ring in a structural lesion that is not related to reflux esophagitis.

361. The answer is A-N, B-N, C-Y, D-Y, E-N *(Braunwald, ed 11, chap 247.)* The prevention of viral hepatitis is of particular importance because of the limited therapeutic options. The prophylactic approach varies with the type of hepatitis. All preparations of immune globulin (IG) contain sufficient titers of anti-HAV to prevent a clinically apparent type A hepatitis. If given early enough, infection will be prevented in approximately 80 percent of patients. For intimate contacts, 0.02 mL/kg of IG is recommended as soon as possible after exposure. The prevention of hepatitis B is based upon both passive immunoprophylaxis with hepatitis B immune globulin (HBIG) and hepatitis B vaccine. HBIG appears to be effective in reducing clinically apparent illness but does not appear to prevent infection. Hepatitis B vaccine has been shown to be highly effective in preventing HBV infection. Because only persons with HBV infection are susceptible to delta hepatitis, hepatitis B vaccine is effective in preventing delta infection in persons who are not carriers of HBsAg. There is no effective prophylaxis of HDV infection for those patients who are already HBsAg carriers. Although it has not been shown to be effective, many authorities recommend postexposure prophylaxis of non-A, non-B hepatitis with IG because it is safe and inexpensive and may be effective.

362. The answer is A-Y, B-Y, C-N, D-Y, E-Y. *(Braunwald, ed 11, chap 235.)* The H-2 receptor antagonist cimetidine is a potent inhibitor of gastric acid secretion and is widely used to promote duodenal ulcer healing. It binds to and inhibits the P_{450} cytochrome-mixed oxygenase hepatic enzyme system, and thus increases the blood levels of drugs such as phenytoin and warfarin which are metabolized by this system. Cimetidine also reduces oxidative hepatic metabolism and affects the metabolism of drugs such as lidocaine and theophylline. Drugs metabolized by glucuronidation, such as oxazepam, are not affected by cimetidine.

363. The answer is A-Y, B-N, C-Y, D-N, E-Y. *(Braunwald, ed 11, chaps 234, 237.)* Symptomatic esophageal involvement occurs in at least half of all individuals who have scleroderma. Reduced lower esophageal tone leads to reflux esophagitis, and a loss of esophageal motility may cause dysphagia. Steatorrhea results both from bacterial overgrowth in an atonic small bowel and from obliteration of lymphatics by fibrosis. Pneumatosis intestinalis, which refers to radiolucent cysts or streaks in the wall of the small bowel, occurs more often than normal in association with scleroderma. There is no known predisposition to gallstones or pancreatitis in affected individuals.

364. The answer is A-N, B-N, C-N, D-N, E-Y. *(Braunwald, ed 11, chap 235.)* The only way to differentiate conclusively between a benign and a malignant gastric ulcer is by endoscopic or surgical biopsy. If six endoscopic biopsies of the inner margin of the ulcer crater along with brush cytologies are benign, then malignancy can be ruled out (0.95 confidence). At least 4 percent of gastric ulcers with a benign radiographic appearance prove to be malignant on biopsy. Both benign and malignant gastric ulcers occur more often on the lesser than on the greater curvature. Although ulcers greater than 3 cm in diameter are more likely to be cancerous, malignant gastric ulcers may be any size. About 70 percent of persons with gastric ulcers are not achlorhydric. Nearly three-quarters of malignant ulcers undergo significant healing, at least temporarily, during medical treatment for peptic ulcer disease.

365. The answer is A-Y, B-N, C-Y, D-N, E-N. *(Braunwald, ed 11, chaps 237, 239.)* Primary intestinal lymphoma should be distinguished from secondary involvement of the intestine by lymphoma originating elsewhere in the body. Primary intestinal lymphoma originates within the lamina propria and in the lymphoid follicles of the mucosa and submucosa. Although the intestinal involvement is usually localized, it can be diffuse. In the latter case, malabsorption often occurs as a result of extensive mucosal involvement. In addition, malabsorption may be caused by lymphatic obstruction or localized narrowing of the intestinal lumen which leads to stasis of intestinal contents and bacterial overgrowth. Hepatosplenomegaly, peripheral adenopathy, and abdominal masses are unusual, but CT scans of the abdomen may reveal enlarged abdominal lymph nodes. The diagnosis is best made by laparotomy with full-thickness biopsy. Unless the duodenum or ileum is involved, the tumor is inaccessible to the endoscope. Perforation, bleeding, and intestinal obstruction are common events, especially late in the course of the disease.

366. The answer is A-Y, B-Y, C-Y, D-Y, E-Y. *(Braunwald, ed 11, chap 235.)* For reasons that are not understood, more gastric acid is delivered to the duodenum in persons with duodenal ulcers than in persons without peptic disease, as a result of more rapid gastric emptying (food is not as effective in buffering the acid), greater acid production in response to stimulation by gastrin, and less feedback inhibition of acid secretion and gastrin release by intragastric acid. Therefore, measures that decrease acid delivery to the duodenum, such as the ingestion of liquid antacids, H-2 receptor antagonists, and anticholinergic agents, are beneficial in the therapy of duodenal ulcer disease.

367. The answer is A-N, B-Y, C-N, D-N, E-Y. *(Braunwald, ed 11, chap 236.)* Although adenomatous gastric polyps may contain regions of adenocarcinoma or be associated with carcinoma elsewhere in the stomach, most gastric cancers do not begin as polyps. Atrophic gastritis may be a predisposing factor for both polyps and cancer; however, most persons who have atrophic gastritis, a common condition among the elderly, do not develop gastric cancer. Despite the fact that most persons with a malignant ulcer secrete some acid, achlorhydria after pentagastrin stimulation usually is incompatible with a diagnosis of benign peptic ulcer. Gastric cancers do not begin as benign ulcers, even if the ulcer is recurrent. Blood group A—not blood group O—is slightly increased in frequency in persons with gastric cancer. Billroth II partial gastrectomy seems to increase the risk for gastric cancer (a higher incidence of gastric cancer is being noted 10 to 20 years postoperatively).

368. The answer is A-Y, B-Y, C-N, D-Y, E-N. *(Braunwald, ed 11, chap 237.)* Surgical resection of a significant portion of small intestine can result in a variety of clinical abnormalities, which are collectively referred to as the short bowel syndrome. By a mechanism as yet unelucidated, massive small-bowel resection can lead to transient gastric hypersecretion. The loss of ileal tissue causes poor absorption of bile salts; depletion of the bile acid pool results in steatorrhea, which is best managed by a low-fat diet (40 g/day). Increased passage of bile acids into the colon stimulates a secretory diarrhea. Antiperistaltic agents, such as belladonna alkaloids and diphenoxylate, presumably enhance absorption by prolonging mucosal contact time and thus can benefit individuals who have the short bowel syndrome.

369. The answer is A-N, B-N, C-Y, D-N, E-Y. *(Braunwald, ed 11, chap 238.)* Several extraintestinal disorders are associated with both Crohn's disease and ulcerative colitis, including pericholangitis, uveitis, and a variety of skin and joint manifestations. Complications that are unique to Crohn's disease because of inflammation of the terminal ileum include hypocalcemia, which is caused by malabsorption of vitamin D, and the formation of urinary oxalate stones, which results from increased intestinal absorption of dietary oxalate. Due to bile-salt malabsorption caused by ileal disease, cholesterol gallstones tend to form in persons having regional enteritis.

370. The answer is A-Y, B-Y, C-Y, D-N, E-N. *(Braunwald, ed 11, chap 238. Summers, Gastroenterology 77:847, 1979. Ursing, Gastroenterology 83:550, 1982.)* Among the findings of the National Cooperative Crohn's Disease Study in 1979 were that corticosteroids are more efficacious in the treatment of Crohn's disease of the small intestine than in the treatment of Crohn's disease of the colon, and that azathioprine may be a useful adjunct to corticosteroid therapy but is less effective as a single agent. Sulfasalazine was found to be effective in the therapy of active colonic disease, but neither sulfasalazine nor corticosteroids decrease the frequency of recurrence once remission has been achieved. Both drugs may be used safely in treating pregnant women. In more recent studies, metronidazole has been reported to be useful in the treatment of chronic perianal fistulas associated with Crohn's disease.

371. The answer is A-Y, B-N, C-Y, D-N, E-N. *(Braunwald, ed 11, chap 238.)* Risk factors for the development of colon carcinoma in persons who have ulcerative colitis include presence of the disease for more than 10 years, extensive mucosal involvement (pancolitis), and a family history of carcinoma of the colon. The risk of cancer in persons with pancolitis is estimated to be 12 percent at 15 years, 23 percent at 20 years, and 42 percent at 24 years. Neither a history of toxic megacolon nor the prolonged use of high-dose steroids increases the risk of cancer. Pseudopolyps, although frequently associated with severe disease, are not precancerous lesions.

372. The answer is A-N, B-N, C-Y, D-Y, E-Y. *(Braunwald, ed 11, chap 239.)* Carcinoembryonic antigen (CEA) is a glycoprotein present in fetal serum and in the serum of persons who have certain malignant and inflammatory conditions. As a marker, however, it is neither sensitive nor specific for gastrointestinal malignancies in general or colonic cancer in particular. Smoking, sclerosing cholangitis, and inflammatory bowel disease are associated with mild elevations of serum CEA concentration; very high serum levels suggest malignancy. Once a diagnosis of cancer is made in a person with an elevated serum CEA level, serial CEA determinations can be used to monitor the success of treatment and warn of possible recurrence.

373. The answer is A-N, B-Y, C-Y, D-Y, E-N. *(Braunwald, ed 11, chap 239.)* Ischemic colitis most often occurs in elderly persons who have vascular disease. Areas of the colon with extensive collateral circulation, such as the rectum, usually are spared. Angiography of arteries and veins rarely is indicated for diagnosis or therapy, because vessel occlusions are almost never detected. Even though acute ischemic colitis may present with rectal bleeding and lower abdominal pain, most cases do not present with the severity of signs and symptoms suggestive of an acute abdomen. The disease usually does not recur, and symptoms tend to resolve in 2 to 4 weeks. Ischemic colitis is sometimes diagnosed retrospectively as the cause of a colonic stricture.

374. The answer is A-Y, B-Y, C-Y, D-N, E-Y. *(Braunwald, ed 11, chap 239.)* Meckel's diverticulum is the most frequently occurring congenital anomaly of the gastrointestinal tract and is found in 2 percent of autopsied adults. The diverticulum may contain ectopic gastric mucosa, and local acid secretion may produce ileal ulceration and lower gastrointestinal bleeding. In young adults, Meckel's diverticulitis can mimic acute appendicitis. Technetium, taken up by diverticular gastric mucosa, may detect the lesion. The more common gastrointestinal barium x-rays usually do not demonstrate the diverticulum.

375. The answer is A-N, B-Y, C-Y, D-N, E-Y. *(Braunwald, ed 11, chap 239.)* Acute hemorrhage from colonic diverticula is the most common cause of lower gastrointestinal bleeding among elderly persons. Although diverticula are more common in the left side of the colon, bleeding tends to originate from the ascending (right) colon. Bleeding usually stops with bed rest and transfusion; however, when conservative measures fail to curb hemorrhage, intraarterial infusion of vasoconstrictive medications, introduced during angiography, can be effective. Although acute diverticulitis may be associated with occult bleeding, gross hemorrhage rarely occurs.

376. The answer is A-Y, B-N, C-Y, D-Y, E-N. *(Braunwald, ed 11, chap 239.)* Demonstration of polymorphonuclear leukocytes in the stool indicates an invasive inflammatory process in the bowel mucosa. Both amebae and *Shigella* bacteria may cause such a response, as might idiopathic ulcerative colitis. Diarrhea caused by cholera is due to toxin production; mucosal invasion does not occur. Giardiasis may cause striking histologic abnormalities in the small bowel, but an exudative inflammatory response is not characteristic.

377. The answer is A-Y, B-Y, C-N, D-Y, E-N. *(Braunwald, ed 11, chaps 245, 249.)* Unexplained hepatosplenomegaly and unexplained persistence of elevated liver function tests are the principal indications for percutaneous needle liver biopsy. The presence of these phenomena suggests a diagnosis either of diffuse parenchymal disease of the liver, which occurs with drug reactions and metabolic liver disease, or of multiple focal lesions, which are caused by granulomatous or metastatic disease. The diagnosis of miliary tuberculosis, for example, can often be made by liver biopsy (more than 40 percent of all cases have a positive liver biopsy). A focal defect identified on liver scan also can be evaluated by percutaneous liver biopsy, often with sonographic guidance of the needle. A percutaneous liver biopsy should never be performed, however, when a vascular lesion of the liver, such as an angioma, is suspected. Although liver biopsy can confirm the presence of suspected biliary obstruction, ultrasonography, computerized tomography, and transhepatic or endoscopic cholangiography are better techniques for determining the cause of common bile duct obstruction.

378. The answer is A-Y, B-Y, C-N, D-N, E-Y. *(Braunwald, ed 11, chap 245.)* Elevated levels of serum alkaline phosphatase (of hepatic origin) generally reflect impaired hepatic excretory function. Thus, the concentration of this enzyme may be elevated in individuals with incomplete extrahepatic biliary obstruction (e.g., bile duct stricture) or intrahepatic cholestasis (e.g., chlorpromazine-induced cholestasis or early primary biliary cirrhosis); in all three of these examples, serum bilirubin concentration is only slightly elevated. Both acute viral hepatitis and acetaminophen hepatotoxicity are associated with extensive hepatocellular damage and frequently produce peak serum aspartate aminotransferase levels of above 500 Karmen units/mL.

379. The answer is A-Y, B-Y, C-Y, D-Y, E-Y. *(Braunwald, ed 11, chap 239.)* Adenomatous polyps of the colon are very common in the general population, and the incidence increases with age. They are usually detected by screening barium enemas or colonoscopy which have been performed as part of an evaluation of occult gastrointestinal blood loss. A small minority of polyps cause bleeding or obstruction. The majority of polyps occur in the rectosigmoid colon. An increasing size correlates with an increased risk of malignancy. Polyps less than 1 cm have a 1 percent chance of containing malignant cells whereas 50 percent of polyps greater than 2 cm contain malignant cells. There are three histologic types of polyps: tubular, tubulovillous, and villous. Of these, villous adenomas tend to be the largest and have the greatest risk of malignancy. Because polyps with carcinoma in situ do not metastasize, colonoscopic resection is considered curative. However, affected patients must be examined carefully for synchronous lesions and followed for recurrent disease.

380. The answer is A-N, B-Y, C-Y, D-N, E-N. *(Braunwald, ed 11, chap 247.)* Although the titer of hepatitis B surface antigen in the serum is related directly to hepatocellular necrosis, hepatic concentrations of surface antigen do not accurately reflect activity of the disease. A prolonged prothrombin time, hypoalbuminemia, hypoglycemia, and marked hyperbilirubinemia portend a poor prognosis. A serum sickness-like syndrome is associated with hepatitis B infection, occurring in 5 to 10 percent of affected individuals. The etiologic agent cannot be surmised accurately from the presenting symptoms and signs in most persons. Steroid therapy has no value in the treatment of acute viral hepatitis.

381. The answer is A-Y, B-Y, C-Y, D-Y, E-Y. *(Braunwald, ed 11, chap 247.)* Non-A, non-B hepatitis, which is thought to be caused by a variety of agents not yet identified, accounts for 90 percent of all cases of posttransfusion hepatitis. The incubation period is variable, with a mean of approximately 50 days (mean incubation period of hepatitis A is 30 days, and hepatitis B about 75 days). In humans, the disease is spread by both percutaneous and nonpercutaneous exposure; the existence of asymptomatic chronic carrier states also has been demonstrated. Although immune serum globulin may modify the illness and minimize the chance of contracting hepatitis, it cannot ensure complete immunity and its prophylactic value has been inconsistent.

382. The answer is A-N, B-Y, C-N, D-N, E-Y. *(Braunwald, ed 11, chap 248.)* The most common agents implicated as etiologic factors in chronic active hepatitis are the hepatitis B virus and the non-A, non-B agent; the latter may be responsible for cases of chronic active hepatitis following posttransfusion hepatitis. Hepatitis A virus does not cause chronic liver disease. Drugs implicated in the pathogenesis of chronic active hepatitis include oxyphenisatin (a laxative), methyldopa, isoniazid, and nitrofurantoin. Withdrawal of the offending drug results in clinical and histologic recovery, although cirrhosis, if present, is irreversible. Chlorpromazine is associated with a clinical and histologic picture resembling biliary cirrhosis. Excessive acetaminophen ingestion can produce liver cell necrosis but does not lead to chronic liver disease.

383. The answer is A-Y, B-Y, C-Y, D-N, E-N. *(Braunwald, ed 11, chap 250.)* Rare hepatic diseases that occur with increased frequency in women who use oral contraceptive agents include hepatic adenoma, which is encapsulated, and focal nodular hyperplasia, which is not. Both may regress when use of the oral contraceptive is discontinued. Peliosis hepatis (blood-filled, dilated sinusoids) has been described in users of oral contraceptives as well as in persons taking androgenic steroids. Angiosarcoma, a malignant vascular tumor, has been described in association with vinyl chloride exposure, past administration of Thorotrast (a radioactive contrast agent in wide use 30 to 40 years ago), use of androgenic steroids, but **not** use of oral contraceptives. A presumed association between oral contraceptives use and primary hepatocellular carcinoma has been refuted by recent epidemiologic evidence.

384. The answer is A-Y, B-Y, C-N, D-N, E-Y. *(Braunwald, ed 11, chap 246.)* Gilbert's syndrome is a benign disorder in which a partial deficiency of bilirubin glucuronyl transferase leads to mild unconjugated hyperbilirubinemia. The serum total bilirubin concentrations fluctuate between 1 and 3 mg/dL and rarely exceed 5 mg/dL. No clear pattern of inheritance has been identified. Fasting reliably raises the serum bilirubin concentration and is a useful diagnostic test. Phenobarbital, which enhances glucuronyl transferase activity, results in a decrease in serum bilirubin concentration. Although a liver biopsy is not required for the diagnosis, liver biopsy specimens are normal when examined by light microscopy.

385. The answer is A-N, B-Y, C-N, D-Y, E-Y. *(Braunwald, ed 11, chap 251.)* Reye's syndrome typically occurs in children recovering from a viral illness. There is often a history of aspirin ingestion during the viral illness. Marked elevations in the serum aminotransferase and ammonia levels as well as in prothrombin time are usually present, and affected children often develop hypoglycemic episodes. Despite these biochemical and physiologic signs of deranged hepatic function, jaundice is usually minimal.

386. The answer is A-Y, B-Y, C-N, D-N, E-Y. *(Braunwald, ed 11, chap 247.)* Hepatitis B e antigen (HBeAg) is a protein that is associated with the HBV core particle. Due to this close association, the presence of HBeAg in the serum is linked with infectiousness, and the antigen is present during the viremic period of acute hepatitis B. Although HBeAg correlates well with viral replication, detection of HBeAg in serum has not been found to predict the subsequent development of chronic hepatitis B infection; equally, the absence of HBeAg in serum does not preclude the development of chronic hepatitis B infection. In acute hepatitis B, the disappearance of HBeAg from serum often presages resolution of the acute infection; however, HBeAg-negative persons should be considered infectious until antibody to hepatitis B surface antigen is detected in the serum. Although persons with chronic hepatitis B infection may be at increased risk for developing hepatocellular carcinoma, this risk is not influenced by whether HBeAg is present in or absent from the serum.

387. The answer is A-Y, B-Y, C-Y, D-Y, E-Y. *(Braunwald, ed 11, chap 250.)* Chronic liver disease of any etiology is associated with an increased incidence of hepatocellular carcinoma (HCC). Thus, patients with alcoholic liver disease, hemochromatosis, and alpha$_1$-antitrypsin deficiency are all at increased risk of development of HCC. Worldwide, chronic hepatitis B virus infection is an important cause of chronic liver disease and subsequent HCC. Mycotoxins such as aflatoxin are found in foodstuffs in many parts of the world and are thought to be carcinogenic.

388–391. The answers are: 388-A, 389-E, 390-D, 391-B. *(Braunwald, ed 11, chap 32, 234.)* Dysphagia for solid foods that has been present for several years indicates a benign disease and is characteristic of a lower esophageal (Schatzki) ring (radiograph A). This lesion appears as a thin, web-like constriction near the lower esophageal sphincter. Even though the ring is congenital, dysphagia, which typically is episodic, may not occur until middle age.

DISORDERS OF THE ALIMENTARY TRACT AND HEPATOBILIARY SYSTEM

Dysphagia for solid foods following a long history of heartburn suggests the development of a peptic stricture (radiograph **E**). (However, peptic stricture can develop in persons who do not have a history of heartburn.) On barium swallow, peptic strictures usually are seen to be 1 to 3 cm long and located near the squamocolumnar junction. Longer strictures may result from persistent vomiting or prolonged nasogastric intubation.

Rapidly progressive dysphagia and weight loss are characteristic of esophageal carcinoma (radiograph **D**). Dysphagia begins with solid foods but may progress to include liquids. Alcohol and tobacco use can be important predisposing factors. Barium swallow may show an ulcerating, infiltrating, or polypoid lesion.

Dysphagia caused by diffuse esophageal spasm (radiograph **B**) may occur with or without chest pain and often involves both solids and liquids. The chest pain, which may mimic the pain of myocardial ischemia, usually occurs at rest or on swallowing. Barium swallow shows uncoordinated, simultaneous contractions that may create a "corkscrew" configuration.

The radiograph labeled **C** shows features typical of achalasia. A "beak-like" tapering of the distal esophagus and proximal dilatation are prominent features. Affected persons characteristically present with dysphagia for solids and liquids, but not with pain.

392–396. The answers are: 392-D, 393-C, 394-B, 395-E, 396-A. (*Braunwald, ed 11, chap 238.*) Because rectal bleeding is frequently associated with all the conditions listed in the question, other signs and symptoms must be relied upon to suggest a diagnosis. A long history of intermittent bloody diarrhea, lower abdominal cramps, and malaise should prompt a search for ulcerative colitis. The absence of diarrhea in a young person with bright red rectal bleeding generally reflects a lack of colonic involvement and suggests a diagnosis of ulcerative proctitis. Acute rectal bleeding in an elderly individual who has underlying vascular disease but a normal sigmoidoscopic examination should suggest ischemic disease of the colon; the use of oral contraceptive pills also can be associated with ischemic colitis. The diagnosis of pseudomembranous colitis should be considered when diarrhea develops in an individual being treated with antibiotics; it is important to note that pseudomembranous colitis may develop after discontinuation of an offending antibiotic agent. Chronic diarrhea is a non-specific symptom; if associated with a solitary rectal ulcer, however, a diagnosis of granulomatous colitis should be entertained.

397–400. The answers are: 397-B, 398-D, 399-A, 400-E. (*Braunwald, ed 11, chap 247.*) Although there is no standard serologic profile for screening patients with acute hepatitis, the three serologic markers, HBsAg, IgM anti-HAV, and IgM anti-HBc form a useful triad. When IgM anti-HBc is present, the patient has an acute HBV infection, whether or not HBsAg is detectable. If HBsAg is present, then infection with HBV is present. If IgM anti-HBc is absent, the infection is considered chronic. Patients presenting with acute hepatitis but with serologic markers suggesting chronic HBV infection should be screened for HBeAg and anti-HBe to assess infectivity. In addition, other causes of acute hepatitis such as delta superinfection should be considered. The presence of IgM anti-HAV is indicative of acute type A hepatitis. If HBsAg is also present, simultaneous infection with HAV and HBV has occurred. The presence or absence of IgM anti-HBc will determine whether the HBV infection is acute or chronic.

401–404. The answers are: 401-D, 402-A, 403-B, 404-C. *(Braunwald, ed 11, chap 237.)* All four patients described in the question demonstrate various manifestations of chronic diarrhea. Persons with pancreatic insufficiency have steatorrhea but do not have protein-losing enteropathy and usually do not develop carbohydrate malabsorption. Serum folate level may be low due to inadequate nutritional intake. Pancreatic enzyme supplementation can decrease the amount of steatorrhea.

Persons with lactase deficiency can have diarrhea if their diet is rich in dairy products. Typically, diagnostic tests of malabsorption are normal except for the lactose tolerance test. Diagnosis often can be made from the clinical history alone.

Intestinal lymphangiectasia usually presents in young adults and children, who have severe protein-losing enteropathy and steatorrhea. Because carbohydrate absorption is not dependent on lymphatic vessels, it usually is not impaired. Some persons with intestinal lymphangiectasia also show symptoms of vitamin B_{12} malabsorption. Small-bowel biopsy is diagnostic. Marked symptomatic relief may be obtained by providing dietary fat in the form of medium-chain triglycerides, which are not absorbed through lymphatics.

Biopsy findings of celiac disease and tropical sprue may be similar in many cases, although in tropical sprue the changes tend to be milder. Unlike patients with celiac disease, however, patients with tropical sprue often have folate and vitamin B_{12} malabsorption and give a history of travel to or residence in tropical regions. Tropical sprue usually responds to a course of tetracycline and vitamin replacement.

405–408. The answers are: 405-A, 406-C, 407-D, 408-B. *(Braunwald, ed 11, chap 239.)* The hereditary polyposis syndromes include familial colonic polyposis, Gardner's syndrome, juvenile polyposis, and Peutz-Jeghers syndrome. Familial colonic polyposis is an autosomal dominant disorder in which hundreds of adenomatous polyps stud the colon. Because the malignant potential is extremely high, with virtually all patients experiencing carcinomatous degeneration by the age of 40 years, prophylactic colectomy is recommended for all patients. In Gardner's syndrome there are multiple colonic and duodenal adenomatous polyps as well as benign soft-tissue and bony tumors. As with familial colonic polyposis, the risk of development of colonic malignancy is high and prophylactic colectomy is recommended. Juvenile polyposis is characterized by multiple hamartomatous polyps of the small and large intestine. The risk of development of a gastrointestinal malignancy is not increased relative to the general population. The Peutz-Jeghers syndrome is characterized by multiple hamartomatous polyps of the small and large bowel in association with mucocutaneous hyperpigmentation. The polyps are most prominent in the small bowel; and although the chance of malignant degeneration is small, duodenal carcinomas are occasionally seen. All of the familial polyposis syndromes are inherited in an autosomal dominant pattern.

IMMUNOLOGIC, ALLERGIC, AND RHEUMATIC DISORDERS

DIRECTIONS: Each question below contains five suggested answers. Choose the **one best** response to each question

409. A 14-year-old boy has a history of recurrent respiratory infections with *Staphylococcus aureus* and *Aspergillus fumigatus*. When he was 7 years old he had a hepatic abscess that was drained surgically; no organism was cultured, but the problem responded to drainage and prolonged antibiotic therapy. His parents and two younger siblings are healthy, but an older brother died in infancy of infection.

The laboratory study most likely to assist in establishing the diagnosis is

(A) determination of leukocyte myeloperoxidase level
(B) quantitative determination of serum immunoglobulin levels
(C) T-lymphocyte functional and subpopulation assessment
(D) nitroblue tetrazolium reduction test
(E) bone marrow aspiration and biopsy

410. Which of the following statements about tolerance is true?

(A) It is unique to cell-mediated immunity
(B) It is the same as anergy
(C) It is easier to induce in T cells than in B cells
(D) It is difficult to induce in neonates
(E) It is the result of T4+ cell hyperactivity

411. The least mature cells in the B cell lineage are the pre-B cells. These cells are best defined by the presence of

(A) surface immunoglobulin M
(B) surface immunoglobulin D
(C) surface immunoglobulin G
(D) cytoplasmic μ chains
(E) Fc receptors

412. The hyperviscosity syndrome is most characteristic of which of the following plasma cell disorders?

(A) Multiple myeloma
(B) Heavy chain disease
(C) Indolent myeloma
(D) Waldenström's macroglobulinemia
(E) Primary amyloidosis

413. A 35-year-old woman comes to the local health clinic because for the last 6 months she has had recurrent urticarial lesions, which occasionally leave a residual discoloration. She also has had arthralgias. Sedimentation rate obtained now is 85 mm in 1 hour. The procedure most likely to yield the correct diagnosis in this case would be

(A) a battery of wheal-and-flare allergy skin tests
(B) measurement of total serum immunoglobulin E (IgE) concentration
(C) measurement of C1 esterase inhibitor activity
(D) skin biopsy
(E) patch testing

414. A 23-year-old man seeks medical attention for perennial nasal congestion and postnasal discharge. He states he does not have asthma, eczema, conjunctivitis, or a family history of allergic disease. His nasal secretions are rich in eosinophils. The test most likely to yield to a specific diagnosis in this setting is

(A) competitive radioimmunosorbent test
(B) elimination diet test
(C) pollen skin testing
(D) dust and mold skin testing
(E) sinus x-rays

415. A 47-year-old man has had fever, weight loss, arthralgias, pleuritic chest pain, and midabdominal pain for the last 2 months. One week ago he noticed difficulty dorsiflexing his right great toe. Blood pressure is 150/95 mmHg (he has always been normotensive), and laboratory studies reveal anemia of chronic disease, high erythrocyte sedimentation rate, and polymorphonuclear leukocytosis. The most likely diagnosis is

(A) giant cell arteritis
(B) allergic granulomatosis
(C) Wegener's granulomatosis
(D) polyarteritis nodosa
(E) hypersensitivity vasculitis

416. Which of the following statements regarding the renal involvement associated with systemic lupus erythematosus is true?

(A) Clinically apparent renal disease occurs in 90 percent of affected persons
(B) Interstitial nephritis is a rare finding on renal biopsy
(C) Membranous lupus nephritis responds poorly to steroid therapy
(D) Renal disease commonly develops in persons who have drug-induced lupus
(E) Urinalysis in affected persons usually reveals proteinuria but little sediment and no red blood cells

417. Which of the following statements is NOT true of cytomegalovirus (CMV) infection?

(A) CMV is the most frequent and important viral pathogen complicating organ transplantation
(B) CMV infection in patients with acquired immunodeficiency syndrome (AIDS) may cause pneumonitis, retinitis, colitis, or adrenal insufficiency
(C) Single-sample determination of CMV-specific antibody is a useful diagnostic tool for the evaluation of acute infection
(D) Treatment of CMV infections with interferon, vidarabine, or acyclovir is largely unsuccessful
(E) A heterophile antibody-negative mononucleosis syndrome is the most common manifestation of CMV infection in normal hosts beyond the neonatal period

418. The most useful and predictive tool in evaluating the condition of a patient with an acute asthmatic attack and in assessing response to therapy is

(A) chest radiography
(B) arterial blood gas measurement
(C) measurement of pulsus paradoxus
(D) observation of accessory muscle use
(E) measurement of peak expiratory flow or FEV_1

419. A 27-year-old hiker is bitten on the wrist by a coral snake. Within minutes, he notes numbness and tingling in the vicinity of the bite. He reaches an emergency room within 60 minutes of the bite, and other than minimal local swelling and fang marks on his hand, physical examination is normal. The most important measure in the treatment of this man would be to

(A) perform cutdown and suction of the bite site
(B) put ice on the bite area to neutralize the venom
(C) give coral-snake antivenom intramuscularly
(D) perform a wide surgical debridement of the bite site
(E) reassure him that there is no significant risk with coral-snake bites and that the numbness will soon disappear

420. All of the following are immunologic abnormalities detected in patients with acquired immunodeficiency syndrome (AIDS) EXCEPT

(A) deficient T-lymphocyte response to antigenic and mitogenic stimulation
(B) decreased serum levels of immunoglobulins
(C) depletion of $T4^+$ lymphocytes
(D) normal or increased numbers of $T8^+$ lymphocytes
(E) defective natural killer cell function

421. A 32-year-old homosexual male complains of weight loss, sweats, diarrhea, and swollen glands for the past 3 to 4 months. Over the previous 1 to 2 months he has had increasing dyspnea and fever and a nonproductive cough. Infection with which of the following pathogens would NOT be an important diagnostic consideration?

(A) *Pneumocystis carinii*
(B) Cytomegalovirus
(C) *Mycoplasma pneumoniae*
(D) *Cryptococcus neoformans*
(E) *Legionella pneumophila*

422. All of the following pharmacologic agents may be useful in the treatment of the *acute* manifestations of anaphylaxis EXCEPT

(A) corticosteroids
(B) aminophylline
(C) antihistamines (e.g., diphenhydramine)
(D) epinephrine
(E) oxygen

423. A 30-year-old woman presents with acute onset of migratory arthritis involving the knee and proximal interphalangeal joints and lasting for 3 to 4 days. She had a similar episode, lasting about a week, 6 months ago. Questioning reveals that her mother developed gangrene in both lower extremities. The most likely diagnosis for this woman is

(A) rheumatoid arthritis
(B) systemic lupus erythematosus
(C) gout
(D) familial hyperbetalipoproteinemia
(E) incomplete Reiter's syndrome

424. A woman who has rheumatoid arthritis suddenly develops pain and swelling in the right calf. The most likely diagnosis is

(A) ruptured plantaris tendon
(B) pes anserinus bursitis
(C) ruptured popliteal cyst
(D) deep thrombophlebitis
(E) Achilles tendonitis

425. Which of the following statements describing the use of gold therapy in persons who have rheumatoid arthritis is true?

(A) The beneficial effects of gold usually manifest themselves within the first month of treatment
(B) Persons who previously failed to respond to a course of gold may be expected to respond to gold at a later date
(C) Persons who have had a recent onset of disease are more likely to respond to gold than are those with long-standing disease
(D) Gold therapy is indicated only when other treatments for rheumatoid arthritis have failed
(E) The side effects of gold therapy, such as skin rash, are often permanent

426. Which of the following systemic manifestations is LEAST characteristic of early adult rheumatoid arthritis?

(A) High fever
(B) Weight loss
(C) Muscle wasting
(D) Anemia
(E) Lymphadenopathy

427. Which of the following conditions is LEAST likely to occur in late extraarticular seropositive rheumatoid arthritis?

(A) Neutropenia
(B) Dry eyes
(C) Leg ulcers
(D) Sensorimotor polyneuropathy
(E) Hepatitis

428. In which of the following clinical situations would a diagnosis of ankylosing spondylitis most likely be correct?

(A) For the last 10 years, a 28-year-old man has had low back pain and stiffness, worse at night and relieved with activity
(B) For the last 5 years, a 32-year-old man has had low back pain made worse with activity but improved with bed rest
(C) For the last 10 years, a 34-year-old man has had intermittent bouts of mild low back pain; now, however, he suddenly is unable to dorsiflex his right great toe
(D) For the last 10 years, a 65-year-old man has had low back pain radiating down both posterior thighs to the knees
(E) For the last 15 years, a 72-year-old man has had progressive low back pain made worse with walking but improved with rest and leaning forward

429. Arthritis associated with psoriasis can be manifest in several different ways. Each of the following is characteristic of psoriatic arthritis EXCEPT

(A) asymmetrical oligoarticular arthritis
(B) rheumatoid factor-positive symmetrical polyarthritis
(C) arthritis of distal interphalangeal joints
(D) severe destructive polyarthritis (arthritis mutilans)
(E) spondylitis and sacroiliitis with or without peripheral arthritis

430. The arthropathy of inflammatory bowel disease can be characterized by all the following EXCEPT

(A) peripheral arthritis is more common in affected individuals who also have other extraintestinal manifestations than in affected individuals who do not
(B) the presence and activity of the peripheral arthritis is related to the extent and activity of colonic involvement
(C) the peripheral arthritis is usually a symmetrical small-joint polyarthritis
(D) the peripheral arthritis resolves without residual joint damage
(E) spondylitis is not related to the extent or activity of colonic involvement

431. For the last 2 years, a 27-year-old man has had recurrent episodes of asymmetrical inflammatory oligoarticular arthritis involving his knees, ankles, and elbows and lasting from 2 to 4 weeks. He also states he has had recurrent, painful "canker sores" in his mouth for the last 10 years. Now, he presents with fever, arthritis, mild abdominal pain, severe headache, and superficial thrombophlebitis in the left leg. The most likely diagnosis in this man is

(A) regional enteritis
(B) systemic lupus erythematosus
(C) Behçet's syndrome
(D) Whipple's disease
(E) ulcerative colitis

432. Which of the following findings is LEAST characteristic of early disseminated gonoccocal infection?

(A) Fever
(B) Skin lesions
(C) Tenosynovitis
(D) Monoarticular arthritis
(E) Negative synovial fluid cultures

433. Which of the following clinical findings would be LEAST compatible with a diagnosis of tuberculous arthritis?

(A) Normal chest x-ray
(B) Absence of fever
(C) Synovial fluid white blood cell count featuring 75 percent polymorphonuclear leukocytes
(D) Acute arthritic presentation
(E) Coexistent osteomyelitis

434. A 27-year-old woman undergoes outpatient surgical repair of her deviated nasal septum. One day later she comes to the local emergency room because of fever, the appearance of a red macular rash over her face and arms, postural fainting, and pain in several joints. The most likely diagnosis is

(A) adult Still's disease
(B) toxic shock syndrome
(C) systemic lupus erythematosus
(D) rheumatic fever
(E) gonococcal arthritis-dermatitis syndrome

435. A 67-year-old man has a 10-year history of low back pain, which radiates into both anterior thighs. During the last year the pain has become progressively worse, so that it now severely limits his activities. Walking, especially walking downhill, greatly accentuates his discomfort; while resting with the lumbar spine flexed, he feels better. He has no neurologic deficits, and sciatic tension signs are not present. The most likely diagnosis is

(A) Paget's disease of the spine
(B) herniated disk
(C) degenerative disk disease
(D) osteoporosis with recurrent lumbar compression fractures
(E) lumbar spinal stenosis

436. A 50-year-old woman has had Raynaud's phenomenon of the hands for 15 years. The condition has become worse during the last year, and she has developed arthralgias and arthritis involving the hands and wrists as well as mild sclerodactyly and difficulty swallowing solid foods. Laboratory studies reveal a positive serum antinuclear antibody assay at a dilution of 1:160 (speckled pattern). The most likely diagnosis of this woman's disorder is

(A) progressive systemic sclerosis
(B) mixed connective-tissue disease
(C) overlap syndrome
(D) dermatomyositis
(E) systemic lupus erythematosus

437. A 25-year-old man has had pain and swelling in the right knee for the last year. He is otherwise well and gives no history of trauma. X-rays show several erosions at the margin of the right knee joint. Aspiration of the joint yields 25 mL of dark-brown synovial fluid of good viscosity. The most likely diagnosis is

(A) atypical rheumatoid arthritis
(B) incomplete Reiter's syndrome
(C) hemangioma
(D) osteochondritis dissecans
(E) pigmented villonodular synovitis

DIRECTIONS: Each question below contains five suggested answers. For **each** of the five alternatives of **each** item, you are to respond either YES (Y) or NO (N). In a given item all, some, or none of the alternatives may be correct.

438. Which of the following are true statements about class II major histocompatibility complex (MHC) antigens?

(A) They are present on virtually all cell types
(B) They are important in the antigen presentation function of monocytes and macrophages
(C) They are associated on the cell surface with β-2-microglobulin
(D) They are defined serologically as HLA-A, -B, and -C antigens
(E) They consist of two noncovalently linked polypeptide chains

439. Which of the following are true statements about human B lymphocytes?

(A) They represent 75 percent of lymphocytes in bone marrow
(B) They play a necessary helper function in the synthesis of lymphokines
(C) Most carry membrane-bound immunoglobulin of the IgG class
(D) They have membrane receptors for the Fc portion of IgG
(E) They have membrane receptors for the C4 component of complement

440. Which of the following are true statements about human T cells?

(A) They are the principal cells in the cortical "germinal centers" and medullary cords of lymph nodes
(B) They carry membrane-bound IgD on their surface
(C) They constitute 70 to 80 percent of circulating blood lymphocytes
(D) They arise from stem cells in the thymus
(E) They are the main effectors of antibody-dependent, cell-mediated cytotoxicity

441. Human immunoglobulin A (IgA) can be described by which of the following statements?

(A) It is the predominant immunoglobulin in plasma
(B) It exists in four subclasses, of which IgA1 is predominant
(C) It can prevent attachment of microorganisms to epithelial cell membranes
(D) It is prominent early in the immune response and is the major class of antibody in cold agglutinins
(E) It has the shortest half-life of the five classes of immunoglobulin

442. Which of the following statements about cell-mediated immunity are true?

(A) It is effected and amplified by the action of lymphokines
(B) Cooperation between T helper cells and B cells is necessary for normal function
(C) Immune competence can be assessed by sensitization and testing with dinitrochlorobenzene (DNCB)
(D) Poison-ivy dermatitis is a pathologic expression of this form of immunity
(E) Antigens with repeating linear polymeric structures are potent stimulators of this form of immunity

443. Following the activation of complement component C5, which is a protein of molecular weight 180,000, a small fragment called C5a is released. Which of the following are true statements regarding the biologic activities of C5a?

(A) It can promote non-IgE-dependent release of histamine from mast cells
(B) It stimulates lysosomal enzyme release, oxidative metabolism, and aggregation of neutrophils
(C) It promotes phagocytosis by interacting with cells possessing C5a receptors
(D) It promotes release of neutrophils from the bone marrow
(E) It stimulates activation of the alternative complement pathway

444. Persons who are diagnosed as having Di George syndrome usually have

(A) hypocalcemic tetany
(B) hypothyroidism
(C) T-cell deficiency
(D) hypogammaglobulinemia
(E) congenital heart disease

445. Which of the following statements are true of isolated immunoglobulin A deficiency?

(A) The incidence of atopic disease is high
(B) The risk of adverse reactions to transfusions is increased
(C) The incidence of autoimmune disease is increased
(D) Serum IgA levels usually are reduced, and secretory IgA levels usually are normal
(E) IgA-bearing B cells are reduced in number

446. Which of the following statements regarding immune-complex disease are true?

(A) Normally, most immune complexes are removed by the reticuloendothelial system
(B) Signs and symptoms stem from the deposition of immune complexes in tissues other than the reticuloendothelial system
(C) Persistence of immune complexes in the circulation seems to be a requirement for the development of renal manifestations
(D) Maximal renal lesions depend on antigen-antibody systems in which antigen is in slight excess
(E) The synovitis of rheumatoid arthritis may be an example of local, or extravascular, immune-complex disease

447. Which of the following statements regarding systemic lupus erythematosus (SLE) are true?

(A) Immune-complex mechanisms are important in the pathogenesis of the disease
(B) Rash, particularly the "butterfly" facial rash, is the most common presenting complaint
(C) A lack of T-cell suppressor activity has been demonstrated in individuals who have SLE
(D) Lupus-like syndromes are associated with hereditary complement-component deficiencies
(E) Five-year survival rate for affected individuals is less than 20 percent

448. A 27-year-old woman with systemic lupus erythematosus is in remission; current treatment is azathioprine, 75 mg per day, and prednisone, 5 mg per day. Last year she had a life-threatening exacerbation of her disease. She now strongly desires to become pregnant. Her physician should

(A) advise her that the risk of spontaneous abortion is high
(B) warn her that exacerbations can occur in the third trimester and in the postpatrum period
(C) tell her that outcome is best in those women who are in remission when they become pregnant
(D) stop the azathioprine just before she attempts to become pregnant
(E) stop the prednisone just before she attempts to become pregnant

449. Which of the following mechanisms of immune evasion are exhibited by schistosomes during infection?

(A) Antigenic variation
(B) Host molecule acquisition
(C) Prevention of lysosome-phagosome fusion
(D) Loss of surface antigens
(E) Immune complex blockade

450. Which of the following statements about tobacco smoking are true?

(A) Men who smoke cigarettes have death rates 30 to 80 percent higher than nonsmokers primarily because of an increased incidence of lung cancer
(B) The risk of coronary heart disease is 60 to 70 percent greater in male smokers than in nonsmokers
(C) In female smokers, the risk of coronary artery disease is increased approximately tenfold by the combined use of cigarettes and oral contraceptives
(D) Since tobacco smoking interferes with theophylline metabolism, smokers usually require lower doses of this drug
(E) Smoking during pregnancy causes an increased risk of spontaneous abortion and reduces average infant birth weight

451. Which of the following are true statements about T-lymphocyte differentiation?

(A) Rearrangement of alpha-chain and beta-chain genes occurs and generates cell surface molecules with antigen-binding specificity
(B) Immunoglobulin gene rearrangement occurs
(C) Several different beta chains may be expressed on the surface of each T cell
(D) T4 and T8 surface markers are expressed on cells during their differentiation in the thymus
(E) Thymic hormones may play a role in regulating T-cell differentiation

452. Which of the following are true statements about sarcoidosis?

(A) Accumulation of suppressor-cytotoxic T lymphocytes occurs in sites of disease activity
(B) The ratio of black to white patients in the United States may exceed 10:1
(C) Chest radiography and pulmonary function testing are sensitive means of evaluating the intensity of pulmonary inflammation
(D) Transbronchial biopsy may reveal granulomata in a high percentage of patients and is a useful means of diagnosis
(E) Asymptomatic hilar adenopathy accounts for 10 percent to 20 percent of cases of sarcoidosis in the United States

453. Exercise-induced asthma can be described by which of the following statements?

(A) It is more common in adults than in children
(B) It is usually worse in summer than in winter
(C) It can be well treated with inhaled beclomethasone
(D) It can be well treated with inhaled cromolyn sodium
(E) Exacerbations are related to cooling of the airways

454. Which of the following statements about rheumatoid factors are true?

(A) They are antibodies to the Fc fragment of immunoglobulin G
(B) They are associated with several conditions in which there is chronic antigenic stimulation
(C) Their presence in the serum of individuals who have rheumatoid arthritis correlates with a worse prognosis than for those individuals with seronegative disease
(D) Their presence correlates with articular manifestations of rheumatoid arthritis
(E) They frequently do not appear in the serum of individuals who have rheumatoid arthritis until late in the course of the illness

455. The diagnosis of many rheumatic diseases, including rheumatoid arthritis, is based entirely on clinical grounds. Which of the following clinical characteristics are associated with rheumatoid arthritis?

(A) Prolonged morning stiffness
(B) Migratory polyarthritis
(C) Arthritis involving the distal interphalangeal joints
(D) Arthritis of the cervical spine
(E) Temporomandibular joint arthritis

456. Which of the following statements regarding the use of salicylates in treating persons who have rheumatoid arthritis are true?

(A) Daily dosage of 3 to 6 g is necessary to provide an adequate anti-inflammatory effect
(B) Maximal analgesia is reached at dosages lower than needed for maximal anti-inflammatory effect
(C) The half-life of salicylates is prolonged at higher doses
(D) Acetylated salicylate (aspirin) is generally more effective, and more toxic, than non-acetylated salicylates
(E) Salicylate therapy can lead to remission in some patients

457. Systemic corticosteroid therapy, though used sparingly in treating persons who have rheumatoid arthritis, should be prescribed in order to

(A) maintain the current level of social functioning until remission can be achieved by other pharmacologic agents
(B) spare newly diagnosed patients from more toxic agents for as long as possible
(C) treat severe extraarticular manifestations, including rheumatoid vasculitis, pleuritis, and pericarditis
(D) treat exacerbations of disease in those patients otherwise controlled between flareups
(E) treat those patients who do not respond to or who are unable to tolerate any of the remission-inducing agents

458. Development of the x-ray findings shown below is linked on occasion to the presence of which of the following disorders?

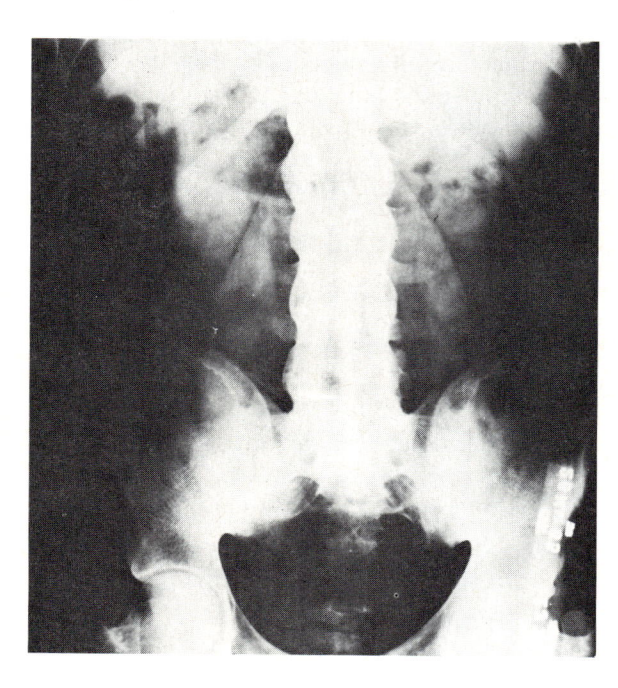

(A) Kidney stones
(B) Aortic insufficiency
(C) Peripheral neuropathy
(D) Uveitis
(E) Inflammatory bowel disease

459. A strong association exists between the HLA-B27 histocompatibility antigen and ankylosing spondylitis. Which of the following are true statements regarding this association?

(A) A positive HLA-B27 determination in a person with low back pain can verify a diagnosis of ankylosing spondylitis
(B) Half of all HLA-B27-positive individuals have sacroiliitis or spondylitis
(C) Persons who are black or of oriental heritage have a higher prevalence of both ankylosing spondylitis and HLA-B27 antigen
(D) Up to 10 percent of cases of ankylosing spondylitis are not associated with HLA-B27 antigen
(E) Women who have ankylosing spondylitis and are HLA-B27-positive have milder disease than affected HLA-B27-positive men

460. Reiter's syndrome follows certain venereal and dysenteric illnesses. Reiter's syndrome following **dysenteric** illness is associated with

(A) enteropathogenic *Escherichia coli* infection
(B) *Salmonella* infection
(C) *Shigella* infection
(D) *Yersinia* infection
(E) *Campylobacter* infection

461. Which of the following statements accurately describe the arthritis associated with the deposition of calcium pyrophosphate dihydrate crystals?

(A) Calcium pyrophosphate dihydrate crystals are thought to form from supersaturated solutions of calcium phosphate in synovial fluid
(B) Calcium pyrophosphate dihydrate crystals appear under polarized light as elongated rods with strong negative birefringence
(C) Clinical manifestations usually are limited to the knee joints
(D) Most affected individuals have radiographic evidence of chondrocalcinosis
(E) Clinical syndromes caused by deposition of calcium pyrophosphate dihydrate crystals can mimic degenerative joint disease

462. Which of the following statements describing septic arthritis are true?

(A) Hematogenous spread from a primary infection elsewhere, and not direct extension from infected bone or soft tissue, is the usual mode of joint seeding
(B) A septic joint cavity can be irrigated with sterile saline to enhance the removal of inflammatory debris
(C) Intraarticular infusion of antibiotics is a useful adjunct to intravenous antibiotic therapy
(D) To minimize the chance of joint destruction, surgical drainage is usually preferred over needle aspiration
(E) Gonococci isolated from individuals whose joint involvement is due to disseminated gonococcemia are more resistant to penicillin than those strains involved in uncomplicated genitourinary infection

IMMUNOLOGIC, ALLERGIC, AND RHEUMATIC DISORDERS

DIRECTIONS: The groups of questions below consist of four or five lettered headings followed by several numbered items. For each numbered item choose the **one** lettered heading with which it is **most** closely associated. Each lettered heading may be used once, more than once, or not at all.

Questions 463–466

For each population of cellular immune elements listed below, select the associated cell surface antigen.

(A) T4 antigen
(B) T8 antigen
(C) Major histocompatibility complex (MHC) class II antigens
(D) Interleukin 2 receptors

463. Suppressor-cytotoxic T cells

464. Activated (but not resting) T cells

465. Monocytes-macrophages and B cells

466. Subset of T cells infected by the HTLV-III/LAV AIDS virus

Questions 467–471

For each clinical situation presented, select the complement profile with which it is most likely to be associated.

(A) Deficiency of C2; other components normal
(B) Deficiency of C3; other components normal
(C) Deficiency of C8; other components normal
(D) Absence of C1 inhibitor; low C4 and C2; other components normal
(E) Reduced C3 and factor B; low CH_{50}; normal C4

467. A 29-year-old man has had episodic abdominal pain and angioedema of the lips, tongue, and larynx

468. A 20-year-old woman has had severe, recurrent bacterial infections, including streptococcal pharyngitis, pneumococcal pneumonia, and bacterial sinusitis

469. A 23-year-old woman develops proteinuria, hematuria, hypertension, and nephrotic syndrome

470. A 21-year-old man, with no current medical problems, donates blood to an immunology laboratory for complement testing

471. A 23-year-old woman presents with fever, arthralgias, and a rash; her serum lacks bactericidal activity against *Neisseria gonorrhoeae*

Questions 472–475

For each clinical setting described below, select the associated autoantibody.

(A) Antihistone
(B) Anticentromere
(C) Anti-Ro (SSA)
(D) Anticardiolipin

472. A young woman with a history of nephritis gives birth to a child with congenital heart block

473. A 37-year-old woman with a history of recurrent arterial thrombosis is found to have a prolonged partial thromboplastin time and a false-positive result on the Venereal Disease Research Laboratory (VDRL) test

474. A 60-year-old man has a rash, arthritis, and pleuritis occurring after antihypertensive therapy with hydralazine

475. A young woman has the CREST syndrome (*c*alcinosis, *R*aynaud's phenomenon, *e*sophageal hypomotility, *s*clerodactyly, and *t*elangiectasias)

Questions 476–478

Allergic asthma is a disease characterized by release of chemical mediators from mast cells and basophils following the interaction of specific antigens with cytophilic IgE antibodies on the surfaces of these cells. For each of the biologic descriptions given below, select the mediator with which it is most closely associated.

(A) Histamine
(B) Leukotriene B
(C) Leukotriene C
(D) Arylsulfatase
(E) Prostaglandin D_2

476. A secondary mediator with very potent bronchoconstrictor activity; its effect is slow in onset and exhibits a preference for peripheral airways

477. A primary mediator with bronchoconstrictor activity by direct and indirect cholinergic reflex actions; it also increases venular permeability and down-regulates mediator release

478. A secondary arachidonate-derived mediator with chemotactic activity for neutrophils

Questions 479–482

For each diagnosis that follows, select the synovial-fluid findings with which it is most likely to be associated.

(A) Fluid, clear and viscous; white blood cell count, 400/mm^3; no crystals
(B) Fluid, cloudy and watery; white blood cell count, 8000/mm^3; no crystals
(C) Fluid, dark brown and viscous; white blood cell count, 1200/mm^3; no crystals
(D) Fluid, cloudy and watery; white blood cell count, 12,000/mm^3; crystals, needlelike and strongly negatively birefringent
(E) Fluid, cloudy and watery; white blood cell count, 4800/mm^3; crystals, rhomboidal and weakly positively birefringent

479. Pigmented villonodular synovitis

480. Calcium pyrophosphate deposition disease

481. Gout

482. Degenerative joint disease

Immunologic, Allergic, and Rheumatic Disorders

Answers

409. The answer is D. *(Braunwald, ed 11, chap 56.)* This child most likely has chronic granulomatous disease, a group of inherited disorders that have in common defective oxidative metabolism of neutrophils. This defect results in a heightened susceptibility to infection with catalase-positive organisms such as staphylococci and *Aspergillus*. The diagnosis can be made by demonstrating abnormal neutrophil reduction of nitroblue tetrazolium. Most patients with isolated deficiency of myeloperoxidase are not at increased risk for infection unless another defect is present, in which case infection with *Candida albicans* may be a problem. Decreased serum levels of immunoglobulins predispose to infection with encapsulated organisms such as *Haemophilus* and streptococci, while defects in T-lymphocyte immunity are manifested as infection with viruses and protozoal pathogens such as *Pneumocystis carinii*.

410. The answer is C. *(Braunwald, ed 11, chap 62.)* Tolerance is a condition in which immune response fails to occur after administration of an antigen. In central tolerance, immune response is absent after antigenic challenge, because the responsible lymphocytes have been eliminated or inactivated. In peripheral tolerance, on the other hand, an immune response is mounted but then diminishes or ceases because of active suppressor mechanisms. Tolerance is not the same as anergy, which is an acquired, temporary loss of delayed immune responsiveness to common skin-test antigens. Tolerance does not result from $T4^+$ cell hyperactivity, because these are helper cells; in contrast, $T8^+$ cell hyperactivity can cause tolerance of the peripheral type, because $T8^+$ cells are suppressor cells. T cell tolerance can be produced with lower doses of antigen, has a briefer induction period, and persists longer than B cell tolerance. Tolerance is easier to induce in neonates than in adults.

411. The answer is D. *(Braunwald, ed 11, chap 256.)* Lymphoid cells, which are the ultimate precursors of both T and B lymphocytes, arise from hematopoietic stem cells. Those cells destined to enter the B cell lineage are first apparent in the fetal liver and shortly thereafter in the spleen and bone marrow. These pre-B cells are large lymphoid cells containing cytoplasmic μ chains, the heavy chain of immunoglobulin M (IgM), as detected by immunofluorescence. Cytoplasmic light chains are not present, and pre-B cells lack membrane-bound IgM or immunoglobulin of any other class. In the process of B cell maturation, smaller lymphoid cells appear that bear a narrow rim of cytoplasmic IgM; later, cells with membrane-bound IgM appear.

412. The answer is D. *(Braunwald, ed 11, chap 258)* Plasma cell diseases are a group of conditions in which a clone of cells capable of synthesizing and secreting immunoglobulins, or the heavy or light chain components of these molecules, proliferates abnormally. IgG immunoglobulins are the most common class produced in these diseases. Also, free light chains usually are produced in excess and are detected in urine as Bence Jones protein. Multiple myeloma is the most common of these diseases. Its classic presentation is bone pain, anemia, hypercalcemia, renal failure, and recurrent infections in an elderly person. Diagnosis is best made by looking for a homogeneous globulin peak on electrophoresis of serum, urine, or both. Waldenström's macroglobulinemia is a related condition in which the monoclonal immunoglobulin is of the IgM class. Because IgM is so large (it circulates as a pentamer), it is restricted to the bloodstream and in high concentrations tends to cause hyperviscosity of the blood. Other features differentiating Waldenström's macroglobulinemia from multiple myeloma are enlargement of lymph nodes and spleen and occasional development of chronic lymphocytic leukemia or lymphocytic lymphoma.

413. The answer is D. *(Braunwald, ed 11, chap 260.)* Urticaria and angioedema are common disorders, affecting approximately 20 percent of the population. In acute urticarial angioedema, attacks of swelling are of less than 6 weeks' duration; chronic urticarial angioedema is by definition more long-standing. Urticaria usually is pruritic and affects the trunk and proximal extremities. Angioedema is generally less pruritic and affects the hands, feet, genitalia, and face. The woman described in the question has chronic urticaria, which probably is due to a cutaneous necrotizing vasculitis. The clues to the diagnosis are the arthralgias, presence of residual skin discoloration, and elevated sedimentation rate—these would be uncharacteristic of other urticarial diseases. Diagnosis can be be confirmed by skin biopsy. Chronic urticaria is rarely allergic in etiology; hence, allergy skin tests and measurement of total immunoglobulin E levels are not helpful. Measurement of C1 esterase inhibitor activity is useful in diagnosing hereditary angioedema, a disease not associated with urticaria. Patch tests are used to diagnose contact dermatitis.

414. The answer is D. *(Braunwald, ed 11, chap 260. Jacobs, J Allergy Clin Immunol 67:253–262, 1981.)* There are three common types of rhinitis: allergic, vasomotor, and eosinophilic nonallergic (intrinsic). Allergic rhinitis can be either seasonal due to pollen exposure or perennial as a result of exposure to dust or mold spores (or both). In these IgE-mediated reactions to inhaled foreign substances, nasal eosinophilia is common. Vasomotor rhinitis is a chronic, nonallergic condition in which vasomotor control in the nasal membranes is altered. Irritating stimuli, such as odors, fumes, and changes in humidity and barometric pressure, can cause nasal obstruction and discharge in affected persons, and nasal eosinophilia is not noted. Eosinophilic nonallergic rhinitis causes perennial nasal congestion and discharge. Although it is nonallergic in etiology, it is associated with the presence of numerous eosinophils in nasal secretions. Because the man described in the question has either perennial allergic rhinitis due to dust or mold-spore allergy or eosinophilic nonallergic rhinitis, skin testing for responses to suspected allergens should be diagnostic. The competitive radioimmunosorbent test measures total serum IgE but would not be diagnostic (only 40 percent of patients with allergic rhinitis have elevated serum IgE levels). Pollen skin tests are unlikely to be helpful because of the perennial nature of the condition described. An elimination diet can be used diagnostically or therapeutically in persons with suspected food allergy; however, food allergy rarely causes rhinitis. Sinus x-rays, whether positive or negative, would not reveal the underlying cause of the rhinitis.

415. The answer is D. *(Braunwald, ed 11, chap 269.)* Polyarteritis nodosa is a vasculitis of medium-sized vessels. Early systemic features include fever, weakness, anorexia, weight loss, myalgias, and arthralgias (though severe and persistent arthritis is uncommon). Pericarditis and pleuritis also can occur. Mononeuritis multiplex develops because of involvement of the vasa nervorum; it is reflected in the man described by the sudden loss of the ability to dorsiflex his right great toe. Abdominal pain occurs in 60 to 70 percent of affected individuals and is related to disease involvement of mesenteric arteries. Hypertension develops due to arterial occlusion and occurs before renal involvement. Laboratory findings of elevated erythrocyte sedimentation rate, anemia of chronic disease, and polymorphonuclear leukocytosis all occur with polyarteritis nodosa. Pulmonary involvement is unusual and serves to distinguish this entity clinically from allergic granulomatosis and Wegener's granulomatosis. Hypersensitivity vasculitis is a term applied to small-vessel vasculitides associated with a range

IMMUNOLOGIC, ALLERGIC, AND RHEUMATIC DISORDERS

of findings—from purely cutaneous disease to minimal skin disease but life-threatening involvement of major organs. Giant cell arteritis involves the aorta and other great vessels, producing constitutional symptoms and large-vessel occlusion in young women (Takayasu's disease) and in the elderly (temporal arteritis, polymyalgia rheumatica).

416. The answer is C. *(Braunwald, ed 11, chap 262.)* Renal disease is clinically evident in about half the individuals who have systemic lupus erythematosus (SLE). However, nearly all persons with SLE have some evidence of renal disease on renal biopsy. Renal disease associated with SLE includes both glomerulonephritis and interstitial nephritis. Glomerular disease has been classified into membranous nephritis and mesangial, focal, and diffuse glomerulonephritis. Membranous nephritis is a slowly progressive disease that, like diffuse glomerulonephritis, does not respond well to steroids. Immune-complex interstitial nephritis occurs most commonly in persons who have diffuse glomerulonephritis. Urinalysis performed for persons with active renal disease usually reveals microscopic hematuria, red cell casts, and proteinuria; the exception is membranous lupus nephritis, in which proteinuria is the dominant finding. Drug-induced lupus rarely leads to renal disease.

417. The answer is C. *(Braunwald, ed 11, chap 137.)* Cytomegalovirus is a DNA virus that causes a wide spectrum of disease in normal adults, neonatal infants, and immunocompromised hosts. Latent infections are common and may be reactivated when cell-mediated immune mechanisms are compromised, such as after renal or other organ transplantation. The CMV mononucleosis syndrome resembles the disease caused by Epstein-Barr virus (EBV), with the exception that prolonged high fevers are characteristic of CMV infection, and exudative pharyngitis and cervical lymphadenopathy (common in EBV mononucleosis) rarely occur in patients with CMV mononucleosis. Most patients recover without sequelae, although CMV excretion in urine, genital secretions, and saliva may continue for months to years. Because a large segment of the population carries CMV antibody, serologic diagnosis of CMV infection should be made only when there is a four-fold or greater rise in convalescent titer. There is at present no standard treatment available for CMV disease, though promising results have been obtained with certain experimental antiviral agents including DHPG (9-[1,3-dihydroxy-2-propoxymethyl] guanine).

418. The answer is E. *(Braunwald, ed 11, chap 202.)* Several investigators have shown that the most efficient means of assessing the severity of an asthmatic attack and of following the therapeutic response is the measurement of some parameter of respiratory function such as peak flow or forced expiratory volume in one second (FEV_1). The chest radiograph will frequently show only hyperinflation in attacks of varying degrees of severity. Arterial blood gases will reflect hypoxemia and hypocapnia in all but the most severe episodes, when they may reflect respiratory fatigue and severe obstruction as rising P_{CO_2} levels. Accessory muscle use and the presence of pulsus paradoxus reflect changes in intrathoracic pressure and the work of breathing, and they may actually disappear if the patient's breathing worsens to the point of becoming shallow. Thus, these signs may be misleading.

419. The answer is C. *(Braunwald, ed 11, chap 170.)* Coral snakes rarely bite humans, but when they do their potent neurotoxin can cause death. If it is suspected that a person has been envenomed, antivenom should be given without waiting for systemic manifestations to develop. The bite of a coral snake, though it causes little pain and swelling, produces local numbness and weakness in the region of the bite; ataxia, ptosis, palatal and pharyngeal paralysis, and other neurologic symptoms may follow. If cutdown and suction are not performed promptly after a bite, a significant amount of toxin may be absorbed. Ice, no longer a recommended treatment for snake bite, does not neutralize the toxin. Wide surgical debridement would be unnecessary.

420. The answer is B. *(Braunwald, ed 11, chap 257.)* AIDS is characterized by the infection of T4+ lymphocytes by the AIDS retrovirus (HTLV-III/LAV), with subsequent deficiency in numbers and functions of this T-cell subpopulation, which includes the important helper-inducer cells necessary for production of a variety of immune responses. Thus, there is a defect in the response of T cells to soluble antigen and to mitogenic substances such as phytohemagglutinin and concanavalin A. Natural killer cell function is abnormal and may be augmented in vitro by addition of the lymphokine interleukin 2. There is polyclonal activation of B lymphocytes, with resultant increase in serum immunoglobulin levels and occasional production of autoantibodies.

421. The answer is C. *(Braunwald, ed 11, chap 257.)* The clinical situation suggests the diagnosis of the acquired immunodeficiency syndrome (AIDS). *M. pneumoniae*, while a frequent cause of mild community-acquired pneumonia in the otherwise normal host, is not commonly associated with AIDS. *P. carinii*, a protozoal pathogen, is the most frequent cause of respiratory disease in the AIDS patient, affecting some 60 percent of such patients some time during the course of their illness. Both cytomegalovirus and *C. neoformans* are less common but significant respiratory pathogens in this patient population. While *Legionella* infection is unusual in this setting, it can occur in outbreaks and may be the cause of fulminant pneumonitis with rapid deterioration in pulmonary function.

422. The answer is A. *(Braunwald, ed 11, chap 260.)* Anaphylaxis is a systemic reaction to the sudden release of mediators from sensitized mast cells triggered by interaction with specific antigen. Manifestations of anaphylaxis include: (1) cutaneous—pruritus, urticaria, and angioedema; (2) vascular collapse; (3) respiratory distress; and (4) gastrointestinal—nausea, vomiting, pain, and diarrhea. Therapeutic efforts in anaphylaxis should be directed toward preventing further mediator release and reversing the effects of mediators already released. Corticosteroids do not have any acute effect in anaphylaxis, though they may be necessary to control persistent bronchospasm or hypotension, or both. Onset of action of steroids requires several hours. Aminophylline may help ameliorate bronchospasm, while antihistamines (usually injectable diphenhydramine) will work to block histamine effects on the skin, vasculature, and airways. Epinephrine should be administered subcutaneously or intravenously, or both, in appropriate concentrations to control minor problems such as pruritus and urticaria as well as to reverse vascular instability. Oxygen should be given to combat the hypoxemia associated with bronchospasm and may be combined with inhaled bronchodilators such as isoproteronol.

423. The answer is D. *(Braunwald, ed 11, chaps 278, 315.)* Persons who have familial hyperbetalipoproteinemia may have a transient, migratory polyarthritis that affects several joints in sequence. The knees and proximal interphalangeal joints are most commonly involved. Familial hyperbetalipoproteinemia is associated with severe atherosclerotic disease. In the case described in the question, systemic lupus erythematosus would be a possible diagnosis, but less likely than a familial hyperlipidemia given the family history suggestive of atherosclerotic disease. Rheumatoid arthritis would produce a persistent arthritis, gout would be unlikely in a premenopausal woman, and Reiter's syndrome is an uncommon diagnosis in women.

424. The answer is C. *(Braunwald, ed 11, chap 263.)* Persons who have rheumatoid arthritis can develop popliteal cysts as a complication of synovitis of the knee. Popliteal cysts can expand upward into the thigh or downward into the calf. Rupture of a popliteal cyst produces sudden pain and swelling; because these symptoms resemble those of thrombophlebitis—though perhaps more dramatic in onset—an arthrogram may be needed to confirm the diagnosis. Although rupture of the plantaris tendon can occur in persons exposed to mechanical trauma, it would not be the most likely diagnosis for the woman described in the question. The anserine bursa is located on the medial aspect of the knee joint and not in the calf. Achilles tendonitis should not cause pain and swelling of the calf.

425. The answer is C. *(Braunwald, ed 11, chap 263.)* Gold salts, such as gold thioglucose (Solganol) and gold sodium thiomalate (Myochrysine), are a major element in the treatment of persons who have rheumatoid arthritis and frequently are the first drugs administered after an adequate trial of salicylates has been employed. The efficacy of gold treatment usually does not become manifest until after 8 to 10 weeks of standard therapy (a once-weekly intramuscular injection of 50 mg of gold). Gold therapy is more likely to be effective in individuals with recent onset of disease; on the other hand, it is unlikely to be of benefit for persons previously unresponsive to gold. Persons receiving gold should be monitored frequently for the appearance of a rash, leukopenia, and proteinuria; the appearance of any of these signs warrants the discontinuation of gold therapy. Fortunately, these common side effects of gold therapy, such as skin rash and mucosal ulcers, are transient, and gold can frequently be restarted after they subside.

426. The answer is A. *(Braunwald, ed 11, chap 263.)* Systemic manifestations in early rheumatoid arthritis may be severe. Weight loss and muscle wasting may be as severe as in persons who have a malignancy or primary muscle disease. Lymphadenopathy, too, may be severe, suggesting the presence of a lymphoproliferative disease; lymph node biopsy, however, would show only nonspecific reactive hyperplasia. Anemia of chronic disease is common in early rheumatoid arthritis, with hematocrit dropping to as low as 30 percent. A hematocrit less than 30 percent should alert the physician to the possibility of superimposed iron-deficiency anemia from gastrointestinal blood loss. All these systemic manifestations resolve as the disease comes under control with proper treatment.

427. The answer is E. *(Braunwald, ed 11, chap 263.)* Many of the systemic manifestations of late rheumatoid arthritis are related to the presence of rheumatoid factors in high titer in the serum. Joint disease, paradoxically, may not be active during this stage of the illness. Nail-fold thrombi, leg ulcers, and sensorimotor polyneuropathy are all manifestations of rheumatoid vasculitis and presumably are related to the effect of immune complexes containing rheumatoid factors. High levels of immune complexes are detected by immune-complex assays done at this stage of disease. Felty's syndrome, characterized by neutropenia and splenomegaly, occurs late in the course of rheumatoid arthritis and is related to the presence of high titers of rheumatoid factors. Many affected persons also have rheumatoid vasculitis. Hepatitis is not a common feature of late extraarticular, seropositive rheumatoid arthritis.

428. The answer is A. *(Braunwald, ed 11, chap 267.)* The diagnosis of ankylosing spondylitis is made on clinical grounds. Historical features suggesting inflammatory back disease include pain and prolonged stiffness that are worse at night and during rest periods and characteristically relieved with activity. In contrast, mechanical low back pain usually is eased with bed rest and made worse with activity, such as sitting, standing, walking, and lifting. Signs of nerve-root compression are not part of the clinical spectrum of ankylosing spondylitis. Ankylosing spondylitis usually presents before the age of 50 years; on the other hand, degenerative joint disease and degenerative disk disease are common causes of back pain in the elderly. Back pain made worse with walking and improved with rest and lumbar flexion is characteristic of the pseudoclaudication syndrome associated with lumbar spinal stenosis.

429. The answer is B. *(Braunwald, ed 11, chap 268.)* Five different clinical syndromes of psoriatic arthritis have been described. The most common (70 percent of cases) is an asymmetrical, oligoarticular arthritis. A second group produces arthritis mainly in distal interphalangeal joints and is associated with severe psoriatic nail changes. Severe destructive polyarthritis with lysis of joints also occurs but, fortunately, is rare. Psoriatic spondylitis is similar to the spondylitis of Reiter's syndrome. Rheumatoid factor–negative symmetrical polyarthritis also is associated with psoriasis, and this condition can look very much like rheumatoid arthritis. Persons who have psoriasis and rheumatoid factor–positive symmetrical polyarthritis are thought to have both psoriasis and rheumatoid arthritis.

430. The answer is C. *(Braunwald, ed 11, chap 268.)* Peripheral arthritis and spondyloarthropathy can be associated with inflammatory bowel disease. The characteristic peripheral arthritis involves a few joints in the lower extremities, usually in an asymmetrical fashion, and resolves in a few months without residual joint damage. The presence and activity of peripheral arthritis is related to the extent and activity of colonic involvement. In contrast, the presence and activity of spondylitis is not related to the activity of bowel disease. This form of spondylarthropathy behaves very much like ankylosing spondylitis and may even precede the emergence of bowel disease by many years.

431. The answer is C. *(Braunwald, ed 11, chap 268.)* Behçet's syndrome, a recurrent disease of unknown cause, is characterized by painful oral and genital ulcers, eye inflammation, arthritis, central nervous system symptoms, thrombophlebitis, fever, and abdominal symptoms. Some affected persons have colitis that is indistinguishable from ulcerative colitis. The combination of fever, aphthous ulcers, arthritis, and abdominal pain may mimic inflammatory bowel disease, although central nervous system involvement (e.g., severe headache) and thrombophlebitis would make this diagnosis less likely. Whipple's disease is associated with arthritis, abdominal pain, and central nervous system disease, but not with aphthous ulcers and thrombophlebitis; also, Whipple's disease usually affects middle-aged men. Fever, arthritis, abdominal pain, and headache would be compatible with a diagnosis of systemic lupus erythematosus. However, the mucosal lesions of lupus are painless and occur on the hard and soft palate, and thrombophlebitis is not a characteristic feature.

432. The answer is D. *(Braunwald, ed 11, chap 277.)* Gonococcal arthritis is the most common cause of septic arthritis in young adults. Persons with disseminated gonococcal infection usually present with fever, skin lesions, tenosynovitis, and polyarthritis. The polyarthritis may evolve in a few days to a monoarticular septic arthritis, heralding the change from the bacteremic to the septic joint phase of the disease. The clinical picture, however, may be quite variable—on occasion, affected persons present only with monoarticular arthritis and no systemic features. Cultures of synovial fluid are positive in less than half the cases of gonococcal joint infection.

433. The answer is D. *(Braunwald, ed 11, chap 277.)* Tuberculous arthritis is produced by direct hematogenous spread or extension from disease in adjacent bone. The process tends to be chronic and without significant constitutional symptoms, although low-grade fever and night sweats may be present. The synovial fluid white blood cell count is usually greater than 10,000/mm^3 with polymorphonuclear leukocytes predominating. Many persons who have skeletal tuberculosis do not have radiographic evidence of pulmonary disease.

434. The answer is B. *(Braunwald, ed 11, chap 277. Tofte, Ann Intern Med 96:843, 1982).* Toxic shock syndrome results from infection by certain toxin-producing staphylococci and has been associated not only with tampon use but also with infection of nasal packings used in conjunction with nasal surgery. Clinical features of toxic shock syndrome include fever, diffuse red macular skin rash, arthritis, and shock. Adult Still's disease is not associated with shock; the characteristic rash is evanescent and develops at the height of the fever. Rheumatic fever presenting for the first time in an adult is associated primarily with fever and arthritis and not with skin rash, carditis, or other usual manifestations of childhood rheumatic fever. The rash described in the question is not suggestive of the skin lesions of disseminated gonococcal infection. Systemic lupus erythematosus is a diagnostic possibility in the case described but is not the best choice given the surgical history and short duration of symptoms.

435. The answer is E. *(Braunwald, ed 11, chap 274.)* Lumbar spinal stenosis is defined as a reduction in the size of the lumbar spinal canal. It can be congenital or acquired. One cause of acquired lumbar spinal stenosis is encroachment on the spinal canal from bony overgrowth either of apophyseal joints affected with degenerative joint disease or of vertebral margins due to degenerative disk disease. This pathologic process can occur bilaterally and at multiple levels. The symptoms of spinal stenosis evolve insidiously, can be exacerbated by exercise or by assuming the lordotic position, and are relieved with rest and flexion of the lumbar spine; these symptoms would not accompany the low back pain of degenerative joint disease without spinal stenosis. Herniated disk would be an unlikely diagnosis in the case described, given the fact that the nucleus pulposus stiffens with age and does not tend to herniate in the elderly. In addition, herniated disk produces symptoms characteristic of nerve-root compression. Osteoporosis is generally asymptomatic until compression fractures occur. Pain then can be severe and is exacerbated by motion of the spine. Although Paget's disease can be associated with back pain made worse with ambulation, relief on lumbar flexion is not characteristic.

436. The answer is A. *(Braunwald, ed 11, chap 264. Kelly, chap 76, pp. 1211–1230.)* Progressive systemic sclerosis can be classified into two variants depending on whether scleroderma is present only in the fingers (sclerodactyly) or whether it is also present proximal to the metacarpophalangeal joints. The former disorder is associated with a constellation of findings labeled the CREST syndrome:

*c*alcinosis, *R*aynaud's phenomenon, *e*sophageal dysmotility, *s*clerodactyly, and *t*elangiectasia. Although once thought not to be associated with significant internal organ involvement, the CREST variant of systemic sclerosis has occurred in association with involvement of the lungs, heart, and kidneys, in this respect resembling systemic sclerosis associated with proximal scleroderma. The fluorescent antinuclear antibody (ANA) test is positive in 40 to 80 percent of persons with systemic sclerosis. Antibodies are produced to deoxyribonucleoprotein, nucleolar, centromere, and extractible nuclear antigens; antibodies to the latter three antigens produce speckled patterns of fluorescence.

Mixed connective-tissue disease is the overlap of three rheumatic disease syndromes: systemic lupus erythematosus (SLE), polymyositis, and the CREST variant of systemic sclerosis. It is associated with high titers of antinuclear antibodies directed against the extractible nuclear antigen ribonucleoprotein. Arthritis and a positive ANA are not sufficient to make a diagnosis of SLE. Overlap syndromes are diseases that fulfill diagnostic criteria for two rheumatic diseases. In the case described, symptoms and signs were insufficient to fulfill the diagnostic criteria for more than one rheumatic syndrome.

437. The answer is E. *(Braunwald, ed 11, chap 278.)* Pigmented villonodular synovitis, the cause of which is unknown, is a disorder of young adults that usually affects one joint only, frequently a knee. There is recurrent bleeding into the affected joint; the synovial fluid of that joint often contains blood and typically is dark brown in color, an indication of past bleeding from the synovium. The enlarged villi covering the synovium are made up of large numbers of round and polyhedral cells. Hemosiderin granules and cholesterol crystals can be identified in synovial cell cytoplasm as well as in interstitial spaces. Bone adjacent to the affected synovium can show evidence of erosion; however, invasion of other tissues does not occur. The synovial fluid findings in the case presented are incompatible with the diagnoses of atypical rheumatoid arthritis, incomplete Reiter's syndrome, and osteochondritis dissecans. Hemangioma usually presents in childhood.

438. The answer is A-N, B-Y, C-N, D-N, E-Y. *(Braunwald, ed 11, chap 63.)* The antigens of the major histocompatibility complex (MHC) in man are grouped as class I, II, or III. Class I antigens are denoted as HLA-A, -B, and -C and are present on all cells. Class II (or HLA-D) antigens are crucial to antigen recognition and presentation and are found on B-lymphocytes, monocyte-macrophages, and activated T-cells. Both class I and II antigens are composed of two linked protein chains; in the case of class I antigens, one of the chains is β-2-microglobulin. Class III MHC proteins are complement components that are encoded by genes within the MHC.

439. The answer is A-Y, B-N, C-N, D-Y, E-Y. *(Braunwald, ed 11, chap 62.)* The lymphoid system can be divided into two functionally distinct compartments: the thymus-dependent T-cell compartment, and the "bursal-equivalent" B-cell compartment. B cells are the precursors of plasma cells; their role is to produce immunoglobulins. B lymphocytes in humans and most other mammalian species are characterized by the presence of readily detectable surface immunoglobulins; the surface immunoglobulins on most B cells are of the IgM class, although some cells express both IgM and IgD (IgG and IgA are present on fewer B cells). In addition, most B cells have a receptor specific for the Fc portion of immunoglobulin, and some B cells have receptors for complement proteins. Recent evidence indicates that binding sites exist for the complement proteins C3b, C3d, C4, and C1q. B cells arise from pluripotential stem cells in the fetal yolk sac and then migrate to the fetal liver; following maturation, they comprise 75 percent of lymphocytes in bone marrow. Lymphokines, which are nonantibody mediators of cellular immunity, usually are produced by T cells, and their synthesis does not require interaction with B cells.

440. The answer is A-N, B-N, C-Y, D-N, E-N. *(Braunwald, ed 11, chap 62.)* T lymphocytes are the principal mediators of cellular immunity and also serve important helper and suppressor functions in the regulation of antibody synthesis by B lymphocytes. In humans, they have the property of forming rosettes with sheep erythrocytes (E-rosettes), and they lack readily detectable immunoglobulin of any class on their membranes. Although the maturation of T cells is thymus-dependent, the cells arise from precursors in bone marrow. T cells constitute about 70 to 80 percent of blood lymphocytes; they comprise greater than three-quarters of thymus lymphocytes but less than one-quarter of bone marrow lymphocytes. In lymph nodes, they are found in paracortical areas. Specific monoclonal antibodies have been developed to characterize various subsets of T cells—cells that carry a T4$^+$ surface antigen are helper cells, and those with a T8$^+$ antigen function as cytotoxic-suppressor cells. Antibody-dependent cell-mediated cytotoxicity is a property of a class of non-B, non-T lymphocytes called K, or killer, cells.

441. The answer is A-N, B-N, C-Y, D-N, E-N. *(Braunwald, ed 11, chap 62.)* Immunoglobulin A is the predominant immunoglobulin in body secretions (IgG is predominant in serum). Each secretory IgA molecule is a dimer consisting of a secretory component and a J chain. The secretory component, a protein of molecular weight 70,000, is synthesized by epithelial cells and facilitates IgA transport across mucosal tissues. The J chain is a small glycopeptide that aids the polymerization of immunoglobulins. IgA exists as two subclasses: IgA1 (75 percent of the total) and IgA2 (25 percent). IgA provides defense against local infections in the respiratory, gastrointestinal, and genitourinary tracts and prevents access of foreign substances to the general systemic immune system. It also can prevent attachment of microorganisms to epithelial cells. IgM, not IgA, is the principal immunoglobulin in the primary immune response and is the usual antibody in cold agglutinins. The half-life of IgA is about 6 days; IgE has the shortest half-life, approximately 2 to 2.5 days.

442. The answer is A-Y, B-N, C-Y, D-Y, E-N. *(Braunwald, ed 11, chap 62.)* Cellular immunity, also known as delayed hypersensitivity, is a nonhumoral form of immunity effected by sensitized T lymphocytes through the production of biologic mediators known as lymphokines. These factors recruit and activate phagocytes and nonsensitized lymphocytes. Cellular immunity protects the host against tumor cells and intracellular microorganisms, such as *Mycobacterium tuberculosis*, fungi, and certain viruses and protozoa. Competency of the cellular immune system is best tested by delayed hypersensitivity skin tests to a battery of recall antigens, such as tuberculin, *Candida albicans*, and mumps. If these tests are negative, a person can be sensitized with dinitrochlorobenzene (DNCB) and tested 2 weeks later with a cutaneous challenge. Contact eczema—for example, nickel allergy and poison ivy dermatitis—are pathologic expressions of cellular immunity. Antigens with repeating polymeric structures are thymus-independent, which means they stimulate B cells directly without requiring the presence of T helper cells. B cells are not required for the expression of cellular immunity.

443. The answer is A-Y, B-Y, C-N, D-N, E-N. *(Braunwald, ed 11, chap 62.)* Complement component C5a (molecular weight 11,200) is a cleavage product of C5. It possesses potent biologic activity, including the ability to stimulate non-IgE-dependent mediator release from mast cells, to increase vascular permeability, and to induce smooth muscle contraction (agents with these properties are known as anaphylatoxins). C5a is also a potent chemotactic agent for neutrophils, monocytes, and eosinophils, and it stimulates lysosomal enzyme release, oxidative metabolism, and aggregation of phagocytic cells. C3a (molecular weight 9000) is a cleavage product of C3 and, like C5a, is an anaphylatoxin. C3b, not C5a, is the complement fragment with opsonic activity; it also plays a positive feedback role in the activation of the alternative complement pathway. C3e, a degradation product of C3b, is responsible for promoting the release of neutrophils from bone marrow.

444. The answer is A-Y, B-N, C-Y, D-N, E-Y. *(Braunwald, ed 11, chap 256.)* Di George syndrome, also called congenital thymic aplasia, is caused by abnormal development of the third and fourth pharyngeal pouches during the sixth to eighth weeks of intrauterine life. The structures arising from these pharyngeal evaginations are the thymus, the tissues of the lips and central portion of the face, the ear tubercle, the aortic arch, and the parathyroid glands. Consequently, a child demonstrating the classic presentation of Di George syndrome has the following abnormalities: hypocalcemic tetany; congenital heart disease involving aortic arch structures; cellular immunodeficiency with a T lymphopenia, absence of a thymus, and failure of blood lymphocytes to respond to phytohemagglutinin and allogeneic cells; and an abnormal facies with low-set ears, "fish-shaped" mouth, and hypertelorism. Thyroid function is normal, and B-cell immunity as measured by immunoglobulin levels and antibody response to immunization usually is unimpaired. Treatment of Di George syndrome is by transplant of a fetal thymus.

445. The answer is A-Y, B-Y, C-Y, D-N, E-N. *(Braunwald, ed 11, chap 256.)* Isolated IgA deficiency is the most common immunodeficiency disorder, with an incidence between 1:600 and 1:800. Affected persons have a normal number of B cells with surface IgA, suggesting that the disorder is caused by a failure of B cells to secrete IgA. This presumption is substantiated by in vitro studies showing that lymphocytes from IgA-deficient persons can synthesize but are unable to secrete IgA. Serum IgA and secretory IgA usually are absent, although levels of secretory IgA may be normal. Although IgA deficiency need not be associated with clinical disease, it frequently is. Recurrent sinopulmonary infection is most common. Allergy occurs with an incidence of 1:200 to 1:400, compared to 1:600 to 1:800 in the general population. Approximately 30 to 40 percent of IgA-deficient persons have antibodies directed against IgA, thus predisposing them to anaphylactoid reactions following the infusion of blood products. Persons with isolated IgA deficiency are also at greater risk for developing autoimmune diseases, including lupus and rheumatoid arthritis.

446. The answer is A-Y, B-Y, C-Y, D-Y, E-Y. *(Braunwald, ed 11, chap 261.)* Most antigen-antibody complexes are cleared by cells of the reticuloendothelial system. It appears that in some conditions the reticuloendothelial system can be overwhelmed by immune complexes, thereby impeding the removal and leading to the deposition of immune complexes. Deposition of these complexes in tissues other than those of the reticuloendothelial system is responsible for the signs and symptoms of immune-complex disease. In animal models, the persistence of complexes is necessary for the development of renal disease; also, slight antigen excess has been found to predispose to the formation of antigen-antibody complexes, which persist in the circulation and lead to inflammatory illness. The synovitis of rheumatoid arthritis can be thought of as an extravascular immune-complex disease.

447. The answer is A-Y, B-N, C-Y, D-Y, E-N. *(Braunwald, ed 11, chap 262.)* Systemic lupus erythematosus (SLE) is an autoimmune disease in which autoantibodies to a wide variety of nuclear antigens are formed. Circulating and in situ immune complexes are thought to be responsible for the pathogenesis of the disease. For example, the deposition of circulating immune complexes is believed to be responsible for subendothelial glomerular deposits associated with proliferative lupus nephritis. On the other hand, in situ formation of immune complexes is thought to cause the subepithelial and intramembranous deposits characteristic of membranous lupus nephritis, and antineuronal antibodies combine with brain tissue antigens to form immune complexes thought to be related to central nervous system lupus. T-cell suppressor activity has been shown to be diminished in affected persons giving rise to enhanced humoral immunity. Lupus-like syndromes are well recognized in association with hereditary deficiencies of complement components, predominantly C1, C4, and C2. About 75 percent of persons who have SLE are still alive 5 years after the onset of disease.

448. The answer is A-Y, B-Y, C-Y, D-N, E-N. *(Braunwald, ed 11, chap 262. Fine, Ann Intern Med 94:667, 1981.)* Although most clinicians believe that women with systemic lupus erythematosus should not become pregnant if they have active disease or advanced renal or cardiac disease, the presence of SLE itself is not an absolute contraindication to pregnancy. The outcome of pregnancy is best for those women in remission at the time of conception. Even in women with quiescent disease, exacerbations may occur (usually in the last trimester and in the immediate postpartum period), and 25 to 40 percent of pregnancies end in spontaneous abortion. Flare-ups should be anticipated and vigorously treated with steroids. The experience of renal transplant recipients who conceived while on azathioprine suggests that the drug is not teratogenic and could be continued during pregnancy if the clinical situation dictates. Steroids given throughout pregnancy also usually have no adverse effects on the child. In the case presented, the fact that the woman had a life-threatening bout of disease a year ago would argue against stopping her drugs at this time.

449. The answer is A-N, B-Y, C-N, D-Y, E-Y. *(Braunwald, ed 11, chap 152.)* As our understanding of host immune responses to parasitic infection has progressed, considerable attention has been focused on the mechanisms whereby parasites evade the normal immune reaction and establish long-term infection in the host. Antigenic variation is seen most dramatically in the African trypanosomes, where a single cloned organism may produce over 100 surface-coat proteins by expressing different genes. Prevention of lysosome-phagosome fusion occurs in cellular infection by *Toxoplasma gondii*, enabling the organism to avoid the normal intracellular killing mechanisms. Schistosomes subvert host responses by acquiring host molecules on their surfaces thereby mimicking normal tissue constituents, by losing surface antigens to which immune responses have been directed, and by shedding antigens that may blockade effector cells and antibodies.

450. The answer is A-N, B-Y, C-Y, D-N, E-Y. *(Braunwald, ed 11, chap 173.)* There are 52.4 million cigarette smokers in the United States. However, the proportion of adult smokers declined between 1965 and 1980 from 53 to 37 percent of men and 33 to 27 percent of women. Tobacco smoke contains more than 4000 substances, including carcinogens such as tar, polynuclear aromatic hydrocarbons, and nitrosamines; cocarcinogens such as phenol and cresol; and numerous irritants and ciliary toxins, including formaldehyde and acrolein. Men who smoke cigarettes have 30 to 80 percent higher mortality (age-related) than nonsmokers, with coronary heart disease as the chief cause. The risk of coronary artery disease is 60 to 70 percent greater in male smokers than in nonsmokers. Sudden cardiac death is two to three times more common in male smokers between the ages of 35 and 54 years than in nonsmokers. Female smokers also have an increased risk of coronary artery disease, and this risk is magnified about tenfold by use of oral contraceptives. Cessation of smoking reduces the risk of heart disease within 1 year. In pregnant women, smoking also carries increased risk for spontaneous abortion, reduced birth weight (on average 170 g), and the possibility of adversely affecting long-term growth in the intellectual development of the child. Cigarette smoking accelerates theophylline metabolism; consequently, smokers may require higher doses of this drug.

451. The answer is A-Y, B-N, C-N, D-Y, E-Y. *(Braunwald, ed 11, chap 256.)* T-lymphocyte precursors develop from hematopoietic stem cells and migrate to the thymus where they acquire surface glycoprotein differentiation antigens during their development. Pre-T cells bear both T4 and T8 antigens, while these markers are found on separate populations in more mature T cells. Thymosin and thymopoietin, hormones secreted by thymic tissue, may regulate cellular maturation in peripheral lymphoid tissues. As T lymphocytes develop into antigen-specific cells, the genes for the alpha and beta chains of the T-cell antigen receptor undergo rearrangements, and in each clonal population of T cells, only one particular beta-chain rearrangement is expressed. Immunoglobulin gene rearrangement is a feature of B-lymphocyte differentiation.

452. The answer is A-N, B-Y, C-N, D-Y, E-Y. *(Braunwald, ed 11, chap 270.)* Sarcoidosis is a systemic granulomatous inflammatory disorder that frequently involves the lungs, where it causes a typical interstitial lung disease that may be asymptomatic, may cause transient respiratory difficulties with or without hilar adenopathy, or may progress to end-stage pulmonary fibrosis. Extrapulmonary sarcoidosis may involve the eyes, skin, liver, bones, gastrointestinal tract, kidneys, nervous system, and heart. In the United States, 10 percent to 20 percent of cases consist of asymptomatic hilar adenopathy which is detected on chest radiographs taken for other reasons; these cases may constitute a higher fraction of the total in other countries where routine pre-employment chest radiography is more widely practiced. The disease occurs more frequently among blacks than whites by a substantial margin. At sites of disease activity, such as the lung, there is an accumulation of activated helper-inducer (T4+) lymphocytes, with release of immunologic mediators such as interleukin 2 and gamma-interferon, and resultant granuloma formation. In contrast to other interstitial lung diseases, the diagnosis may frequently be made by the demonstration of the characteristic granulomatous inflammation in tissue obtained by transbronchial biopsy. Prognosis depends on the risk of progression to advanced pulmonary fibrosis, and those persons with intense pulmonary inflammation may benefit from treatment with corticosteroids. Chest radiography and pulmonary function testing cannot distinguish accurately between active inflammation and established fibrosis; hence, most clinicians familiar with the disease utilize procedures such as bronchoalveolar lavage or gallium-67 scanning, or both, to assess the

IMMUNOLOGIC, ALLERGIC, AND RHEUMATIC DISORDERS

intensity of the alveolitis present. These procedures may be performed serially during the course of the patient's illness to follow the progress of the disease and response to therapy.

453. The answer is A-N, B-N, C-N, D-Y, E-Y. *(Braunwald, ed 11, chap 202.)* Asthma is a disease characterized by hyperresponsiveness of the airways to a variety of stimuli, including inhaled antigens (e.g., pollens), irritants (e.g., sulfur dioxide), viral infections, emotional factors, and exercise. Exercise-induced bronchospasm may occur as an isolated disorder or in association with wheezing caused by other factors as well. It is more common in children than in adults and is thought to occur from inhaling large quantities of dry, cold air through the mouth. Hence, winter sports are more likely to promote exercise-induced bronchospasm than are summer activities. Inhaled beta-adrenergic agents, inhaled cromolyn sodium, or rapidly absorbed oral theophylline tablets (when used 30 to 60 minutes before exercise) can usually prevent attacks. Inhaled beclomethasone is ineffective.

454. The answer is A-Y, B-Y, C-Y, D-N, E-N. *(Braunwald, ed 11, chap 263.)* Rheumatoid factors are antibodies to the Fc fragment of immunoglobulin G. They may be of the IgG, IgA, or IgM class; the widely used latex and sheep-cell agglutination tests detect rheumatoid factors primarily of the IgM class. Chronic antigenic stimulation is one of the processes important in the production of rheumatoid factors. Rheumatoid factors are associated not only with rheumatoid arthritis and other autoimmune diseases but also with lymphoreticular malignancies and chronic infections, such as subacute bacterial endocarditis. Rheumatoid factors are usually present within the first year of onset of rheumatoid arthritis; their presence correlates with the extraarticular manifestations of the disease. Individuals with rheumatoid arthritis who have positive serologic tests for IgM rheumatoid factor have a worse prognosis than those who are seronegative.

455. The answer is A-Y, B-N, C-N, D-Y, E-Y. *(Braunwald, ed 11, chap 263.)* Joint stiffness in the morning or after periods of inactivity lasting more than 30 minutes is characteristic of inflammatory rheumatic disease. Arthritis characteristic of rheumatoid arthritis is persistent, remaining in the same joints for months. Migratory arthritis, in which short-lived arthritic symptoms in one joint subside as symptoms begin in another joint, is not characteristic of rheumatoid arthritis. Persons who have rheumatoid arthritis can have involvement of the cervical spine, the temporomandibular joints, and all the small joints of the hand except the distal interphalangeal joints.

456. The answer is A-Y, B-Y, C-Y, D-Y, E-N. *(Braunwald, ed 11, chap 263.)* Because salicylates are as effective as and less expensive than the newer nonsteroidal anti-inflammatory drugs, they should be tried first in the treatment of persons who have rheumatoid arthritis. Even though maximal analgesia is reached at a daily dosage of about 3 g, 3 to 6 g per day are needed to provide an adequate anti-inflammatory effect. The half-life of salicylates is prolonged at higher drug concentrations—for example, for a single dose (650 mg) of aspirin, the salicylate half-life is 3.5 to 4.5 hours, while at 4.5 g per day, the average half-life is 15 to 20 hours. Therefore, adjustment of high-dose regimens should be made at weekly intervals or longer, because a new steady state takes about a week to develop. Acetylated salicylate (aspirin) is both more toxic and generally more effective than nonacetylated salicylates. Salicylates do not induce remissions in persons with rheumatoid arthritis.

457. The answer is A-Y, B-N, C-Y, D-Y, E-Y. *(Braunwald, ed 11, chap 263.)* Systemic steroid therapy should be approached with great caution in the treatment of rheumatoid arthritis because of the chronicity of the disease and the toxicity inherent in the long-term use of steroids. Nevertheless, systemic steroids can be useful in helping affected persons to continue employment or home duties while waiting for the slow-acting, remission-inducing agents to take effect. In addition, they can be used occasionally to treat flare-ups of rheumatoid arthritis in those persons whose disease usually is well controlled between flare-ups. Systemic steroids also can be used to treat those persons for whom other, more potent agents have been tried and found to be either not effective or not well tolerated; however, steroids should never be used in place of these agents. Severe extraarticular manifestations of rheumatoid arthritis, such as vasculitis, pleuritis, and pericarditis, are also indications for the use of systemic steroids.

458. The answer is A-N, B-Y, C-N, D-Y, E-Y. *(Braunwald, ed 11, chap 267.)* The x-ray shown in the question is compatible with a diagnosis of ankylosing spondylitis. Early radiographic evidence of sacroiliitis includes blurring of joint margins, irregular subchondral erosions, and sclerosis affecting both sides of the sacroiliac joint. With progression of the disease, the joint is lost completely. Radiographic findings of early spondylitis include straightening of the lumbar spine and squaring of the lumbar and thoracic vertebrae. Later, syndesmophytes appear along the lateral and anterior surfaces of the intervertebral disks and bridge adjacent vertebrae, creating the so-called bamboo spine. Complications of ankylosing spondylitis include uveitis (in 30 percent of affected persons) and aortic insufficiency (3 percent). The spondylitis of inflammatory bowel disease, which may look just like that of ankylosing spondylitis, may antedate the onset of bowel disease by years.

459. The answer is A-N, B-N, C-N, D-Y, E-Y. *(Braunwald, ed 11, chap 267.)* The diagnosis of ankylosing spondylitis is based on a characteristic history and physical examination. A determination of HLA-B27 status does not help in the diagnosis of ankylosing spondylitis. Seven percent of the normal white population in the United States are positive for HLA-B27, and 5 to 10 percent of persons with bona fide ankylosing spondylitis are negative for HLA-B27. It has been shown that 20 percent of HLA-B27-positive individuals have evidence of ankylosing spondylitis. Black and oriental individuals have a lower prevalence of HLA-B27 antigenicity and a lower prevalence of ankylosing spondylitis. Women have the disease at the same frequency as men, but it is much less severe and is diagnosed less often.

460. The answer is A-N, B-Y, C-Y, D-Y, E-Y. *(Braunwald, ed 11, chap 268.)* In the United States and Great Britain, postdysenteric Reiter's syndrome occurs much less frequently than postvenereal Reiter's syndrome. *Salmonella, Shigella, Yersinia,* and, more recently, *Campylobacter* enteric infections have been associated with the development of the disorder. Urethritis occurs in both forms of the disease, though it is more common in the postvenereal type. It is interesting that Reiter's initial description of the disease was in patients who had the postdysenteric variety.

461. The answer is A-N, B-N, C-N, D-Y, E-Y. *(Braunwald, ed 11, chap 275.)* Synovial deposition of calcium pyrophosphate dihydrate crystals occurs in pseudogout, an inflammatory disorder producing arthritis in older persons. Crystals are thought to form on the surface of articular cartilage (chondrocalcinosis) and then are shed into synovial fluid; in gout, on the other hand, crystals are thought to arise from a supersaturated solution of sodium urate. Under polarized light, calcium pyrophosphate dihydrate crystals have a weak positive birefringence and can be difficult to see if not looked for carefully. Most affected individuals have radiographic evidence of chondrocalcinosis. Common sites of involvement are the menisci of the knees, articular disk of the distal radioulnar joint, the symphysis pubis, and the annulus fibrosis of the intervertebral disks. Clinical syndromes other than pseudogout, among them pseudorheumatoid arthritis and pseudodegenerative joint disease, also involve deposition of calcium pyrophosphate crystals.

462. The answer is A-Y, B-Y, C-N, D-N, E-N. *(Braunwald, ed 11, chap 277.)* Septic arthritis, which usually results from hematogenous spread of a primary infection at another site, is considered a medical emergency. Drainage of an infected joint is an important component of treatment and usually can be performed adequately by needle aspiration; open surgical drainage is necessary in only a few circumstances, such as when septic arthritis involves a hip joint. Systemic infusion of antibiotics produces sufficient intraarticular bactericidal activity; consequently, intraarticular administration of antibiotics is unwarranted, especially in view of the fact that it can cause a chemical synovitis. Irrigation of a septic joint cavity with sterile saline can be useful in removing inflammatory debris. Bacteria commonly causing septic arthritis include *Neisseria gonorrhoeae, Staphylococcus aureus,* and *Streptococcus pneumoniae;* gonococcal organisms associated with disseminated infection are usually very sensitive to penicillin.

463–466. The answers are: 463-B, 464-D, 465-C, 466-A *(Braunwald, ed 11, chap 62.)* These cell surface markers are glycoproteins that are synthesized and expressed in certain cell types in response to activation and differentiation stimuli. The T4 antigen is found on populations of helper-inducer T-lymphocytes and is characteristic of the cell type infected by the AIDS virus, with the resultant defects in T4 function and numbers associated with this immunodeficiency. Suppressor-cytotoxic T cells express the T8 antigen on their surfaces. MHC class II antigens, important in the process of antigen presentation and distinction of self from nonself, are found on B cells, activated T cells, and cells of the monocyte/macrophage line. In combination with antigen, these antigens are recognized by the T-cell antigen receptor. The interleukin 2 receptor appears on the membranes of T cells in response to activation and interacts with interleukin 2, a lymphokine with T-cell growth factor activity that is produced by other T cells.

467–471. The answers are: 467-D, 468-B, 469-E, 470-A, 471-C. *(Braunwald, ed 11, chap 62. Alper, N Engl J Med 288:601–606, 1973. Peterson, Ann Intern Med 90:917–921, 1979.)* Hereditary angioedema is characterized by recurrent attacks of angioedema of the hands, feet, perioral and periorbital regions, and upper airway. The condition causes abdominal pain as the result of small-bowel edema and may be fatal if laryngeal obstruction is severe. In hereditary angioedema, C1 inhibitor is absent, which leads to uncontrolled activation of the early complement proteins C4 and C2. This disease has an autosomal dominant pattern of inheritance. Treatment with danazol, an attenuated androgen, has been very effective.

Deficiency of complement component C3 is a rare condition that exists in two forms: in type I, C3 is deficient as a result of a C3 inactivator; and in type II, the reduced level of C3 is associated with decreased synthesis as well as increased destruction caused by the serum enzyme C3 convertase. By virtue of its central position in both the classic and alternative complement pathways, C3 is essential for normal host defense against pyogenic bacteria. Thus, C3-deficient persons suffer from recurrent and severe infections, usually involving the upper and lower respiratory tract and the genitourinary tract.

Membranoproliferative glomerulonephritis, a disease of children and young adults, often progresses to chronic renal failure. Histologically, the kidney shows mesangial proliferation and hypertrophy and thickened glomerular basement membranes. Many patients are found to have a serum substance labeled C3 nephritic factor (C3NeF), which is an autoantibody directed against the alternative pathway. Such patients would have a complement profile featuring normal levels of C1, C4, and C2 components of the classic pathway but low levels of C3 and factor B; the overall hemolytic activity (CH_{50}) of the complement system would be depressed.

C2 deficiency is the most common hereditary deficiency of complement. It is inherited as an autosomal recessive trait; both homozygous and heterozygous forms exist, with heterozygotes possessing approximately half-normal serum levels of C2. Deficiency of C2 has been associated with systemic lupus erythematosus, chronic glomerulonephritis, and polymyositis. However, it also occurs in healthy individuals. The absence of functional and immunochemically detectable C2 in affected persons is caused by an inability of macrophages to make the C2 protein.

Disseminated gonococcal infection is characterized by fever, arthralgias, and skin lesions ranging from maculopapular to pustular and hemorrhagic in appearance. Although disseminated gonococcal infection can occur in persons who have normal complement activity, it has been reported to occur with unusual frequency in association with homozygous deficiencies of C6, C7, and C8. Although sera from persons deficient in these factors possess normal opsonic activity, they lack bactericidal activity against *Neisseria* organisms, and, as a result, these persons have a greater likelihood of contracting neisserial meningitis. This phenomenon suggests that phagocytosis is insufficient to kill these organisms and that complement-mediated lysis is required.

472–475. The answers are: 472-C, 473-D, 474-A, 475-B. *(Braunwald, ed 11, chaps 262 and 264.)* Autoantibodies to nuclear antigens and other antigenic determinants are features common to systemic lupus erythematosus (SLE) and other so-called connective-tissue disorders. Screening tests for antinuclear antibodies (ANA) may utilize human cell line substrates or murine tissues to detect multiple antibodies with different specificities. Autoantibodies reacting with specific nuclear antigens have been found to characterize certain disorders and clinical situations. Antihistone antibodies, reacting with nuclear histone proteins, are found in approximtely 95 percent of patients with drug-induced lupus syndromes, while anticentromere antibodies are present in most patients with the CREST variant of progressive systemic sclerosis. Anti-Ro (SSA) antibodies recognize an RNA polymerase, are present in approximately 30 percent of patients with SLE (including a subset who may be ANA-negative), and have been associated with congenital heart block in infants born to women who carry this antibody. Antibodies that react with cardiolipin, a phospholipid, may be found in some 50 percent of patients with SLE. These antibodies also bind phospholipids in the prothrombin activator complex, prolong the partial thromboplastin time, and may be associated with a heightened tendency to thrombosis of the veins or arteries, or both. These antibodies also produce a false-positive reaction in the VDRL test for syphilis.

476–478. The answers are: 476-C, 477-A, 478-B. *(Braunwald, ed 11, chap 202.)* Basophils and mast cells contain or are capable of synthesizing approximately 20 chemicals that produce the clinical manifestations of immediate hypersensitivity disease. Some of these mediators are preformed and stored within the numerous granules of the cells, whereas others are formed secondarily by mast cells and basophils following an IgE reaction or by the activation of a second cell by one of the primary mediators.

Histamine is a primary mediator formed from the amino acid L-histidine by decarboxylation. It is a bronchial constrictor, and its effect is both direct on irritant receptors and indirect by reflex vagal action. Histamine enhances vascular permeability by acting on the endothelial cells of the postcapillary venules. There are two classes of cellular histamine receptors: H_1 receptors mediate smooth-muscle contraction and permeability effects; and H_2 receptors mediate suppression of lysosomal enzyme and histamine release. Through this function, histamine has a negative feedback effect on its own release.

Leukotriene B is derived from the same pathway as the C, D, and E leukotrienes. Its potent chemotactic activity for neutrophils is comparable to other chemotactic agents, such as C5a and f-met-leu-phe. Leukotriene B does not cause bronchial smooth-muscle contraction. Leukotriene C, on the other hand, is a secondary mediator with potent broncho-constrictor activity. It and two closely related factors, leukotrienes D and E, are oxidative metabolites of arachidonic acid. The collective activities of these three lipid mediators are identical to those previously ascribed to slow-reacting substance of anaphylaxis (SRS-A).

479–482. The answers are: 479-C, 480-E, 481-D, 482-A. *(Braunwald, ed 11, chap 273.)* The analysis of synovial fluid begins at the bedside. When fluid is withdrawn from a joint into a syringe, its clarity and color should be assessed. Cloudiness or turbidity is caused by the scattering of light as it is reflected off particles in the fluid; these particles are usually white blood cells, although crystals may also be present. The viscosity of synovial fluid is due to its hyaluronate content. In inflammatory joint disease, synovial fluid contains enzymes that break down hyaluronate and reduce fluid viscosity. In contrast, synovial fluid taken from a joint in a person with degenerative joint disease, a noninflammatory condition, would be expected to be clear and have good viscosity. The color of the fluid can indicate recent or old hemorrhage into the joint space. Pigmented villonodular synovitis is associated with noninflammatory fluid that is dark brown in color ("crankcase oil") as a result of repeated hemorrhage into the joint. Gout and calcium pyrophosphate deposition disease produce inflammatory synovial effusions, which are cloudy and watery. In addition, these disorders may be diagnosed by identification of crystals in the fluid—sodium urate crystals of gout are needlelike and strongly negatively birefringent, whereas calcium pyrophosphate crystals are rhomboidal and weakly positively birefringent.

DISORDERS OF THE HEMATOPOIETIC SYSTEM

DIRECTIONS: Each question below contains five suggested answers. Choose the **one best** response to each question.

483. Coumadin-induced skin necrosis is occasionally associated with the institution of oral anticoagulants in patients with

(A) antithrombin III deficiency
(B) protein C deficiency
(C) protein S deficiency
(D) plasminogen deficiency
(E) dysfibrinogenemias

484. A 26-year-old woman has painful mouth ulcers. Six weeks ago, she was started on propylthiouracil for hyperthyroidism. She is afebrile, and physical examination is unremarkable except for several small oral aphthous ulcers. White blood cell count is 200/mm³ (15 percent neutrophils, 80 percent lymphocytes, 5 percent monocytes); hemoglobin concentration, hematocrit, and platelet count are normal. The woman's physician should stop the propylthiouracil and

(A) schedule a follow-up outpatient appointment
(B) arrange for HLA typing of her siblings in preparation for bone marrow transplantation
(C) prescribe oral prednisone, 1 mg/kg
(D) hospitalize her for broad-spectrum antibiotic therapy
(E) hospitalize her for white blood cell transfusion

485. A 55-year-old woman is found to have seropositive rheumatoid arthritis, splenomegaly, and neutropenia. The therapeutic intervention LEAST likely to increase her white blood cell count would be

(A) splenectomy
(B) corticosteroid therapy
(C) androgen therapy
(D) lithium carbonate therapy
(E) penicillamine therapy

486. Paroxysmal nocturnal hemoglobinuria is associated with all the following conditions EXCEPT

(A) elevation of leukocyte alkaline phosphatase levels
(B) aplastic anemia
(C) iron-deficiency anemia
(D) venous thrombosis
(E) acute leukemia

487. Iron deficiency is LEAST likely to be associated with

(A) lead poisoning
(B) hemodialysis
(C) chronic heart-valve hemolysis
(D) hereditary hemorrhagic telangiectasia
(E) idiopathic pulmonary hemosiderosis

488. A 72-year-old man who has become progressively more fatigued is found to be anemic. Hematologic laboratory values are as follows:

Hemoglobin: 10.0 g/dL
Hematocrit: 27.5%
Mean corpuscular volume (MCV): 101 fL
Mean corpuscular hemoglobin (MCH): 30 pg
Mean corpuscular hemoglobin concentration (MCHC): 34 g/dL
Reticulocyte count: 0.5%
White blood cell count: 7300/mm³ (65% neutrophils)
Platelet count: 210,000/mm³

The most likely diagnosis is

(A) acute leukemia
(B) aplastic anemia
(C) autoimmune hemolytic anemia
(D) iron-deficiency anemia
(E) sideroblastic anemia

489. Which of the following procedures would be most sensitive in detecting early iron overload?

(A) Quantitative iron determination in a liver biopsy specimen
(B) Urinary iron excretion in response to a test dose of desferrioxamine
(C) Serum ferritin concentration
(D) Serum iron concentration, total iron-binding capacity, and calculated transferring saturation
(E) Iron stain of a bone marrow aspirate

490. Which of the following statements concerning the diagnosis of pernicious anemia is true?

(A) The presence of antiparietal-cell antibodies is diagnostic of pernicious anemia
(B) Hematologic response to folate therapy alone rules out pernicious anemia as the cause of megaloblastic anemia
(C) Radioisotopic measurement of serum vitamin B_{12} concentration is invariably reduced in persons with untreated pernicious anemia
(D) Bone marrow examination would be expected to reveal marked depletion of erythrocyte precursors in persons with untreated pernicious anemia
(E) Serum gastrin levels usually are elevated in persons with pernicious anemia

491. A 45-year-old woman with long-standing rheumatoid arthirtis is diagnosed as having "anemia of chronic disease." The predominant mechanism causing this type of anemia in persons with chronic inflammatory disorders is

(A) defective porphyrin synthesis
(B) impaired incorporation of iron into porphyrin
(C) intravascular hemolysis
(D) depressed erythroid maturation due to decreased erythropoietin production
(E) impaired transfer of reticuloendothelial storage iron to marrow erythroid precursors

492. Which of the following groups would be most likely to develop acute leukemia?

(A) Persons who have Wiskott-Aldrich syndrome
(B) Persons who have hereditary sideroblastic anemia
(C) Persons who have paroxysmal nocturnal hemoglobinuria
(D) Persons who have Hodgkin's disease and are treated with radiation therapy
(E) Persons receiving immunosuppressive therapy following renal transplantation

493. Which of the following statements best characterizes the hemolysis associated with glucose-6-phosphate dehydrogenase (G6PD) deficiency?

(A) It is more severe in affected blacks than in affected persons of Mediterranean ancestry
(B) It is more severe in females than in males
(C) It causes the appearance of Heinz bodies on Wright's staining of a peripheral smear
(D) It most often is precipitated by infection
(E) It primarily involves intravascular destruction of red blood cells

494. Most persons who have hemoglobin variants with high oxygen affinity will

(A) adapt poorly to hypoxic conditions
(B) demonstrate abnormal hemoglobin electrophoresis
(C) have erythrocytosis
(D) have abnormal red-cell morphology
(E) have increased red-cell 2,3-diphosphoglycerate (2,3-DPG) concentration

495. Evaluation of a person who has pure red blood cell aplasia would be expected to reveal

(A) markedly hypocellular bone marrow
(B) normochromic, normocytic red blood cells
(C) increased iron turnover on ferrokinetic studies
(D) a reticulocyte count greater than 2.0%
(E) decreased urinary erythropoietin content

496. A 21-year-old woman who has had severe menorrhagia is referred by her gynecologist for evaluation of a possible systemic coagulopathy. A younger sister has been noted to bleed excessively after trauma. She takes no medications; physical examination is unremarkable. Initial laboratory results include the following: platelet count, 252,000/mm³; prothrombin time, 23.6 seconds (control 11.6 seconds); and partial thromboplastin time, 26.9 seconds (control 33.3 seconds). Further laboratory testing should consist of

(A) determination of factor VIII level
(B) screening for inhibitors
(C) determination of bleeding time
(D) determination of factor VII level
(E) determination of alpha$_2$-antiplasmin level

497. Thrombocytosis would be LEAST likely to occur in persons who have

(A) polycythemia vera
(B) hemolytic-uremic syndrome
(C) sickle cell (SS) disease
(D) iron-deficiency anemia
(E) ulcerative colitis

498. A feature of idiopathic thrombocytopenic purpura common to both children *and* adults is

(A) occurrence after an antecedent viral illness
(B) presence of antibodies directed against target antigens on the glycoprotein IIb-IIIa complex
(C) absence of splenomegaly
(D) persistence of thrombocytopenia for more than 6 months
(E) necessity of splenectomy to ameliorate thrombocytopenia

499. A 16-year-old boy presented with deep vein thrombophlebitis and pulmonary embolism. There is no familial history of thromboembolic disease. The platelet count on admission was 325,000/mm^3; prothrombin time, 13.1 seconds (control 11.4 seconds); partial thromboplastin time, 55.0 seconds (control 27.9 seconds); and thrombin time, 14.5 seconds (control 15 seconds). The most likely reason for the thrombotic diathesis in this patient is the presence of

(A) dysfibrinogenemia
(B) congenital antithrombin III deficiency
(C) lupus anticoagulant
(D) factor XI deficiency
(E) protein C deficiency

500. A young woman presents with bleeding after a dental extraction. She is found to have a bleeding time of greater than 20 minutes along with a normal prothrombin time and partial thromboplastin time. There is a familial history of bleeding, and the patient's laboratory evaluation reveals the presence of a variant form of von Willebrand's disease (type IIa). The factor VIII coagulant activity is 54 percent of normal, von Willebrand factor (VWF) antigen is 48 percent of normal, and ristocetin cofactor is 13 percent of normal. The abnormal VWF multimer pattern of the patient's plasma on SDS-agarose electrophoresis is caused by

(A) defective release of VWF from endothelial cells
(B) inappropriate binding of VWF to platelets
(C) reduced synthesis of VWF by endothelial cells
(D) an inability to assemble high-molecular-weight multimers or premature catabolism of VWF
(E) an alteration in the platelet receptor for VWF

501. A 1-year-old boy bleeds significantly after an inguinal hernia repair. The patient has no siblings, and there is no familial history of a bleeding diathesis. Platelet count, bleeding time, prothrombin time, and partial thromboplastin time are all normal. The most likely diagnosis is

(A) prekallikrein deficiency
(B) factor XII deficiency
(C) factor XIII deficiency
(D) thrombasthenia
(E) protein S deficiency

502. A 75-year-old man presents with ischemic changes of the distal lower extremities. Physical examination reveals the presence of an abdominal mass. Laboratory evaluation discloses a hematocrit of 28 percent platelet count, 90,000/mm^3; prothrombin time, 16 seconds (control 12 seconds), and partial thromboplastin time, 55 seconds (control 30 seconds). The fibrinogen level was reduced to 100 mg/dL and the level of fibrin split products was elevated to 160 µg/mL. Appropriate therapy at this time should consist of

(A) plasma exchange transfusion
(B) administration of cryoprecipitate
(C) administration of aminocaproic acid (Amicar)
(D) platelet transfusions
(E) administration of fresh frozen plasma

503. Persons with polycythemia vera and a hematocrit greater than 45 percent generally have

(A) increased levels of urinary erythropoietin
(B) increased bone marrow iron stores
(C) decreased carotid blood flow
(D) hypocellular bone marrow
(E) myelophthisic changes in their peripheral blood smear, including teardrop-shaped red blood cells and normoblasts

DIRECTIONS: Each question below contains five suggested answers. For **each** of the five alternatives of **each** item, you are to respond either YES (Y) or NO (N). In a given item all, some, or none of the alternatives may be correct.

504. Macrocytosis of red blood cells, in the absence of megaloblastic changes in the bone marrow, may be due to

(A) hypothyroidism
(B) malabsorption
(C) acute hemolysis
(D) total gastrectomy
(E) liver disease

505. Defective neutrophil chemotaxis occurs in association with

(A) chronic granulomatous disease
(B) glucocorticosteroid therapy
(C) alcoholism
(D) hereditary neutrophil hyposegmentation (Pelger-Huët anomaly)
(E) deficiency of complement component C3

506. Which of the following findings would distinguish beta-thalassemia trait from iron deficiency?

(A) Microcytic red blood cells
(B) Absence of anemia
(C) Elevated hemoglobin A_2 level
(D) Normal transferrin saturation
(E) Normal serum ferritin concentration

507. Which of the following laboratory results would be expected in an individual who had a splenectomy for hereditary spherocytosis 6 months ago?

(A) Elevated platelet count
(B) Elevated reticulocyte count
(C) Decreased serum haptoglobin concentration
(D) Predominance of microspherocytic red blood cells on peripheral blood smear
(E) Increased osmotic fragility of red blood cells

508. Persons who have sickle-cell trait (AS hemoglobinopathy) have which of the following characteristics?

(A) Impaired growth and development in childhood
(B) Increased incidence of hematuria
(C) Impaired ability to concentrate urine
(D) Increased mortality rate in pregnant women
(E) Increased incidence of splenic infarction with high-altitude hypoxia

509. Methemoglobinemia is associated with

(A) cyanosis
(B) a shift to the left of the oxyhemoglobin dissociation curve
(C) oxidation of heme iron
(D) hemoglobinuria
(E) microcytic anemia

510. For the last 2 weeks, a 28-year-old previously healthy man has had progressive fatigue and spontaneous bruising. During the last 3 days, his temperature has risen to 38.9°C (102°F) and he has had shaking chills. Hemoglobin concentration is 7.2 g/dL; hematocrit, 18.0 percent; reticulocyte count, 0.1 percent; white blood cell count. 350/mm³; and platelet count, 8000/mm³. A bone marrow biopsy specimen is markedly hypocellular and consists primarily of nests of lymphocytes. Management at this point should include

(A) hospitalization
(B) androgen therapy
(C) empiric antibiotic therapy
(D) platelet transfusions from an HLA-compatible donor
(E) immediate preparation for bone marrow transplantation if an HLA-matched donor is identified

511. A 70-year-old woman presents with a recent history of increased bruising. Physical examination reveals the presence of numerous ecchymoses and splenomegaly. Laboratory evaluation discloses a hematocrit of 33 percent; MCV, 105 fL; white blood cell count, 8500/mm³; and platelet count, 110,000/mm³. A peripheral smear reveals the presence of metamyelocytes. Liver chemistries are normal, as are the prothrombin time and partial thromboplastin time. The bleeding time is prolonged at 15 minutes (normal less than 8 minutes). Initial laboratory evaluation should include all of the following EXCEPT

(A) fibrinogen, thrombin time, and fibrin split product determination
(B) platelet aggregometry
(C) bone marrow aspiration and biopsy
(D) serum vitamin B_{12} and folate level determinations
(E) liver-spleen scan

512. The absence of ristocetin-induced platelet aggregation is associated with which of the following clinical disorders?

(A) Glanzmann's thrombasthenia
(B) Bernard-Soulier syndrome
(C) Aspirin ingestion
(D) Storage pool disease
(E) von Willebrand's disease

513. Myeloproliferative disorders characteristically are associated with which of the following potential complications?

(A) Opportunistic infection
(B) Carcinoma
(C) Excessive bleeding
(D) Thromboembolism
(E) Acute myelogenous leukemia

DIRECTIONS: The groups of questions below consist of four or five lettered headings followed by several numbered items. For each numbered item choose the **one** lettered heading with which it is **most** closely associated. Each lettered heading may be used once, more than once, or not at all.

Questions 514–518

For each case history that follows, select the peripheral blood smear pictured in Color Plates T through X with which it is most likely to be associated.

- (A) Smear **A**
- (B) Smear **B**
- (C) Smear **C**
- (D) Smear **D**
- (E) Smear **E**

514. A 68-year-old man complains of painful and discolored fingers. Physical examination reveals acrocyanosis and mild scleral icterus. Hematocrit is 26 percent, and reticulocyte count 9 percent

515. A 48-year-old woman is found to be anemic 3 years after mastectomy for breast carcinoma

516. A 39-year-old man presents with abdominal pain and is found to have gallstones. Physical examination reveals splenomegaly. Hematocrit is 33 percent, and reticulocyte count 8 percent

517. A previously healthy 50-year-old woman is brought to the hospital after a focal motor seizure. Hematocrit is 22 percent; reticulocyte count, 11 percent; white blood cell count, 12,200/mm³; platelet count, 25,000/mm³; blood urea nitrogen, 45 mg/dL; prothrombin time, normal; and partial thromboplastin time, normal

518. A healthy 22-year-old black man is found to be slightly anemic on routine screening. Physical examination is normal. Hemoglobin is 12.2 g/dL, and MCV is 64.7 fL

Questions 519–522

For each type of anemia listed below, select the ferrokinetic profile obtained following injection of radioactive iron, with which it is most likely to be associated.

	Plasma iron clearance	Plasma iron turnover	Red-cell iron incorporation
(A)	Increased	Increased	Increased
(B)	Increased	Increased	Decreased
(C)	Normal	Normal	Normal
(D)	Decreased	Increased	Increased
(E)	Decreased	Decreased	Decreased

519. Iron-deficiency anemia

520. Thalassemia major

521. Aplastic anemia

522. Pernicious anemia

Questions 523–526

For each mechanism of pharmacologic action that follows, select the antithrombotic drug with which it is most likely to be associated.

(A) Coumadin
(B) Tissue plasminogen activator
(C) Dipyridamole
(D) Urokinase
(E) Heparin
(F) Indomethacin
(G) Aspirin

523. Unable to differentiate between free and fibrin-bound plasminogen

524. Inhibits a liver enzyme necessary for the gamma-carboxylation of several coagulation proteins

525. Reversibly inhibits platelet cyclooxygenase

526. Natural anticoagulant that is able to enhance the binding of antithrombin to thrombin

Disorders of the Hematopoietic System

Answers

483. The answer is B. *(Braunwald, ed 11, chap 281.)* Several reports have recently described the association of coumarin-induced skin necrosis in patients with congenital protein C deficiency. The skin lesions occur on the breasts, buttocks, legs, and penis. They appear to be a result of diffuse thrombosis of the venules with interstitial bleeding. This condition is presumed to result from an imbalance in hemostatic mechanism activity favoring thrombosis during the early phases of coumadin administration; a rapid drop in the effective concentration of protein C, which has a relatively short half-life within the circulation (about 14 hours) compared with that of some of the procoagulant vitamin K-dependent procoagulant clotting factors (factor X and prothrombin) which have longer half-lives, could produce such a situation.

484. The answer is A. *(Braunwald, ed 11, chap 56. Young, Clin Haematol 9:483, 1980.)* Severe neutropenia is a rare idiosyncratic reaction to certain drugs, including propylthiouracil. In addition to having sore throat and oral and anal mucosal ulcerations, affected persons are susceptible to overwhelming, life-threatening infections. However, in the absence of fever or clinical signs of infection, they should be followed as outpatients, saving them exposure to nosocomial pathogens in the hospital. Empirical use of broad-spectrum antibiotics without fever or other signs of infection is not advisable, and corticosteroid therapy is not useful. White blood cell transfusions can be accompanied by serious morbidity (particularly, pulmonary leukostasis) and should be reserved for persons with transient neutropenia and documented septicemia. Because severe drug-induced neutropenia is generally self-limited once use of the offending drug has been stopped, consideration of bone marrow transplantation is not justified.

485. The answer is E. *(Braunwald, ed 11, chap 56. Spivak, Johns Hopkins Med J 141:156, 1977).* The treatment of Felty's syndrome—rheumatoid arthritis, splenomegaly, and neutropenia—is controversial. In persons with severe neutropenia and frequent infections, splenectomy is often beneficial. Lithium carbonate and androgens may stimulate neutrophil production, and corticosteroids cause a shift of neutrophils from the marginal to the circulating pool in both normal persons and persons with Felty's syndrome. Penicillamine has been implicated as a cause of neutropenia.

486. The answer is A. *(Braunwald, ed 11, chap 243. Hartman, Ann Rev Med 28:187, 1977.)* Paroxysmal nocturnal hemoglobinuria (PNH) is an acquired disease caused by injury to or mutation in the bone marrow stem-cell pool. PNH can develop following recovery from aplastic anemia, and pancytopenia becomes evident in many affected persons sometime during the course of their illness. Iron deficiency, resulting from urinary iron loss, is a frequent complication of the chronic, intermittent, intravascular hemolysis associated with PNH. Thrombosis is a major cause of morbidity and mortality. In a minority of affected patients, PNH transforms into acute myelogenous leukemia. Functional leukocyte defects have been demonstrated in the disease, and leukocyte alkaline phosphatase level is typically reduced (as in chronic myelogenous leukemia).

DISORDERS OF THE HEMATOPOIETIC SYSTEM

487. The answer is A. *(Braunwald, ed 11, chap 284.)* Lead poisoning causes defective heme synthesis by interfering with a number of steps in the heme synthetic pathway. In severe cases, a hypochromic, microcytic anemia results. However, iron deficiency is not present, and serum iron levels may actually be increased in affected adults. Iron deficiency results from chronic, recurrent gastrointestinal bleeding in persons with hereditary hemorrhagic telangiectasia and from pulmonary bleeding in persons with idiopathic pulmonary hemosiderosis. Chronic heart-valve hemolysis leads to intravascular liberation of hemoglobin and iron depletion through hemoglobinuria and hemosiderinuria. Iron deficiency can occur due to recurrent blood loss during hemodialysis.

488. The answer is E. *(Braunwald, ed 11, chap 284. Kushner, Adv Intern Med 22:229, 1977.)* A slightly increased mean corpuscular volume and an inappropriately low reticulocyte count are characteristic of a macrocytic, hypoproliferative anemia. Iron-deficiency anemia is accompanied by microcytic red blood cell indices, and autoimmune hemolytic anemia typically is associated with reticulocytosis, unless a coexisting process, such as folate deficiency, interferes with the bone marrow erythropoietic response. Aplastic anemia and acute leukemia are unlikely diagnoses if white blood cell count and platelet count are normal. Thus, of the five disorders listed in the question, sideroblastic anemia would be the most likely diagnosis. In idiopathic refractory sideroblastic anemia, red-cell indices may be quite variable; macrocytosis may occur, even though a population of microcytic, hypochromic red blood cells often can be seen in the peripheral smear. Bone marrow aspiration, with iron staining of the sample, generally is required to make the diagnosis.

489. The answer is A. *(Braunwald, ed 11, chap 284. Fairbanks, chap 5.)* Serum iron and transferrin saturation, ferritin level, and desferrioxamine challenge are comparably sensitive, noninvasive tests of iron stores. They may all be normal in the early stages of iron overload, such as in precirrhotic affected family members of persons with idiopathic hemochromatosis. The most sensitive test for detecting early iron overload is a quantitative iron analysis, usually determined by atomic absorption spectroscopy, of a liver biopsy specimen.

490. The answer is E. *(Braunwald, ed 11, chap 285.)* Antiparietal-cell antibodies are detected in 90 percent of persons with pernicious anemia but also in persons with atrophic gastritis and 10 to 15 percent of an unselected patient population. Although folate in large doses can correct the megaloblastic anemia of pernicious anemia, it does not correct the neurologic abnormalities. Human plasma contains cobalamin analogues that can mask a vitamin B_{12} deficiency—and thus pernicious anemia—when commercial kits are used to assay serum cobalamin concentration by radioisotopic dilution; this problem does not arise with the microbiologic assay. Megaloblastic anemias are characterized by ineffective erythropoiesis and bone marrow erythroid hyperplasia. Hypergastrinemia accompanies the achlorhydria of pernicious anemia.

491. The answer is E. *(Braunwald, ed 11, chap 286. Bentley, Clin Haematol 11:465, 1982.)* A mild to moderate degree of anemia often accompanies chronic infectious, inflammatory, or neoplastic diseases. Typically, the anemia of chronic disease is normochromic and normocytic to microcytic. Bone marrow examination reveals normal erythroid maturation. Neither significant disturbance of hemoglobin synthesis nor hemolysis occurs in this type of anemia. Affected persons usually have a low serum iron concentration and a low total transferrin level (resulting in essentially normal or only slightly decreased fractional transferrin saturation). Even though storage iron is abundant, there is a decreased amount of iron in erythroblasts, reflecting a defect in the transfer of reticuloendothelial iron to developing red blood cells.

492. The answer is C. *(Braunwald, ed 11, chap 287. Linman, Blood Cells 2:11, 1976.)* Paroxysmal nocturnal hemoglobinuria, an acquired disorder of the bone marrow stem cell, affects not only red blood cells but also platelets and granulocytes. Like related myeloproliferative disorders (e.g., chronic myelogenous leukemia, essential thrombocythemia, polycythemia vera, myeloid metaplasia, and myelofibrosis), paroxysmal nocturnal hemoglobinuria may lead to acute myelogenous leukemia. Lymphoma, particularly involving the central nervous system, may develop in renal transplant recipients on immunosuppressive therapy as well as in persons with Wiskott-Aldrich syndrome. Persons who have Hodgkin's disease and have been treated with both radiation therapy and chemotherapy are at risk for developing leukemia. Acquired idiopathic refractory sideroblastic anemia leads to acute leukemia in about 10 percent of cases, but this phenomenon does not occur in hereditary forms of sideroblastic anemia.

493. The answer is D. *(Braunwald, ed 11, chap 287. Beutler, Semin Hematol 8:311, 1971.)* The gene for glucose-6-phosphate dehydrogenase (G6PD) is located on the X chromosome; thus, G6PD deficiency is a sex-linked trait. Hemolytic anemia occurs much more commonly in males than in heterozygote female carriers, who usually are asymptomatic. Of the more than 100 variants of G6PD, the most commonly encountered variant of clinical significance in the United States is the A− type, which is found in about 15 percent of black males. It generally causes less severe hemolysis than the Mediterranean variant. Hemolysis usually is precipitated by an environmental oxidant stress, most commonly viral or bacterial infection. Certain drugs, such as antimalarial agents, sulfonamides, phenacetin, and vitamin K, also can trigger hemolysis. These oxidant stresses cause precipitation of hemoglobin, because affected persons are unable to maintain adequate intracellular levels of reduced glutathione. Precipitated hemoglobin forms Heinz bodies which are visualized only with supravital stains; these inclusions cause premature destruction of the red cells, predominantly in the spleen.

494. The answer is C. *(Braunwald, ed 11, chap 288.)* Several hemoglobin variants have an increased affinity for oxygen. This abnormality causes defective oxygen unloading to tissues, leading to erythropoietin-mediated erythrocytosis. Because reduced tissue oxygen delivery usually is compensated for fully by the development of erythrocytosis, levels of red-cell 2,3-diphosphoglycerate (2,3-DPG) are normal. Routine hemoglobin electrophoresis often is normal with these variants, and red blood cell morphology is not altered. Affected persons are not at a disadvantage when exposed to hypoxic conditions.

495. The answer is B. *(Braunwald, ed 11, chap 290.)* Pure red blood cell aplasia is characterized by a normochromic, normocytic anemia and little production of reticulocytes. Erythroblasts are selectively absent from the bone marrow of affected persons; white blood cell and platelet production is preserved. In contrast to aplastic anemia, the bone marrow in persons with pure red blood cell aplasia is normocellular or even hypercellular. Iron kinetic studies reveal prolonged plasma iron clearance and reduced iron turnover. Erythropoietin levels usually are markedly elevated.

496. The answer is D. *(Braunwald, ed 11, chaps 54, 280.)* A marked prolongation of the prothrombin time with a normal partial thromboplastin time localizes the hemostatic defect to the extrinsic limb of the coagulation cascade. Congenital factor VII deficiency is a rare, autosomal recessive disorder. Factor VIII deficiency and the presence of specific inhibitors directed towards a coagulation factor (most commonly factor VIII) would be associated with a prolongation of the partial thromboplastin time. Nonspecific inhibitors (lupus anticoagulants) most commonly are associated with prolongation of the partial thromboplastin time and occasionally with prolongation of the prothrombin time (particularly when hypoprothrombinemia is present). Patients with alpha$_2$-antiplasmin deficiency have a bleeding disorder associated with accelerated clot lysis. Both the prothrombin time and the partial thromboplastin time are normal in these persons.

497. The answer is B. *(Braunwald, ed 11, chaps 279, 286.)* The hemolytic-uremic syndrome occurs predominantly in children and is related to thrombotic thrombocytopenic purpura. It is characterized by microangiopathic hemolytic anemia and thrombocytopenia. Polycythemia vera, as well as the other myeloproliferative disorders, often is associated with thrombocytosis. Thrombocytosis also is a long-term sequela of splenectomy or splenic infarction (e.g., in sickle cell disease) and chronic inflammatory states (e.g., inflammatory bowel disease). For reasons that are unclear, thrombocytosis frequently is associated with iron deficiency.

498. The answer is C. *(Braunwald, ed 11, chap 279.)* The onset of severe thrombocytopenia after an antecedent viral illness is common in children with a diagnosis of idiopathic thrombocytopenic purpura (ITP). Unlike childhood ITP, adult ITP tends to be a chronic disease in which spontaneous remissions are rare, and a majority of patients will have a fall in their platelet count after the withdrawal of corticosteroids, necessitating elective splenectomy. The presence of antibodies directed against target antigens on the glycoprotein IIb-IIIa complex has been noted in some adults with chronic ITP but not in children. Splenomegaly is not a feature of ITP; it is a common finding in patients with secondary thrombocytopenia.

499. The answer is C. *(Braunwald, ed 11, chaps 280, 281.)* The presence of nonspecific anticoagulants (lupus type) may predispose patients to thrombosis and is also associated with habitual abortions in some women. Patients with congenital dysfibrinogenemias may have variable results on screening coagulation tests. They often have slight prolongations in the prothrombin time or partial thromboplastin times, prolonged thrombin times, and a disparity between functional and immunologic assays of fibrinogen. Despite these abnormalities, patients may have either no symptoms or moderate bleeding, and a few dysfibrinogenemias have been associated with hypercoagulability. Congenital deficiencies of antithrombin III and protein C are familial thrombotic disorders and are not associated with abnormalities of the various clotting times. Factor XI deficiency is an autosomal recessive disorder often associated with bleeding following trauma or during the perioperative period.

500. The answer is D. *(Braunwald, ed 11, chap 279.)* There is no information as yet available regarding the precise molecular defects in von Willebrand's disease (VWD), but electrophoretic analysis has allowed the delineation of three major types of this disorder. The most common abnormality (type I disease) is characterized by a moderate decrease in the plasma level of von Willebrand factor (VWF antigen) resulting from defective release of the protein from endothelial cells. There are usually concordant reductions in antihemophilic factor or factor VIII coagulant activity as well as ristocetin cofactor activity.

The various forms of type II disease are characterized by normal or near normal levels of dysfunctional protein. In both types IIa and IIb, there is a loss in high-molecular-weight multimers on SDS-agarose electrophoresis. In type IIa patients, the pattern is caused by either an inability to assemble the larger multimers or by premature catabolism in the circulation. In contrast, individuals with type IIb have inappropriate binding of the abnormal larger VWF forms to platelets resulting in the formation of intravascular platelet aggregates. These are rapidly cleared from the circulation causing mild, cyclic thrombocytopenia.

A severe recessive form of VWD (type III disease) results from reduced synthesis of VWF by endothelial cells. A hyperactive platelet receptor (glycoprotein Ib) with increased affinity for larger VWF multimers is the defect in so-called platelet-type VWD or pseudo-VWD.

501. The answer is C. *(Braunwald, ed 11, chap 280.)* Factor XIII deficiency may be inherited or acquired and frequently causes severe bleeding problems. In this disorder, the bleeding time, prothrombin time, and partial thromboplastin time (PTT) are all normal. The screening test for factor XIII deficiency is a clot solubility assay. Persons with deficiencies of factor XII (Hageman factor) or prekallikrein often have dramatic prolongations of the PTT, but do not have bleeding problems even with surgery or trauma. The presence of a normal bleeding time excludes thrombasthenia, an inherited disorder in which there is defective platelet aggregation in response to agonists that require fibrinogen binding, such as adenosine diphosphate, thrombin, or epinephrine. Protein S is a vitamin K-dependent plasma protein which is a cofactor for the expression of the anticoagulant activity of activated protein C. Familial protein S deficiency is associated with a thrombotic diathesis.

502. The answer is E. *(Braunwald, ed 11, chap 280.)* This patient has chronic disseminated intravascular coagulation in association with an abdominal aortic aneurysm. The prothrombin time and partial thromboplastin time are prolonged and the fibrinogen level is decreased on the basis of consumption. Appropriate therapy would include administration of fresh frozen plasma, while cryoprecipitate, a source of only factor VIII and fibrinogen, would be inadequate. Plasma exchange transfusions are the treatment of choice for thrombotic thrombocytopenic purpura. Aminocaproic acid (Amicar) is contraindicated in this setting, because it inhibits fibrinolysis and can therefore potentially induce thrombosis. The degree of thrombocytopenia is not of sufficient severity to require platelet transfusions.

503. The answer is C. *(Braunwald, ed 11, chap 289.)* Persons with polycythemia vera and a hematocrit greater than 45 percent usually have diminished cerebral blood flow and are particularly at risk for developing thrombotic complications. Functional platelet abnormalities may cause both thrombotic and bleeding problems (the gastrointestinal tract is a common site of bleeding), and affected persons frequently are iron-deficient even at the time of presentation. Erythropoietin production is suppressed in polycythemia vera, a disease characterized by loss of normal control of erythroid stem-cell proliferation. The bone marrow is hypercellular, with hyperplasia of all marrow elements. Therapy is aimed at reducing the hematocrit below 45 percent.

504. The answer is A-Y, B-N, C-Y, D-N, E-Y. *(Braunwald, ed 11, chaps 283, 285.)* Macrocytosis of red blood cells may be caused by defective DNA synthesis (i.e., megaloblastic anemias), among other factors. Reticulocytosis due to either blood loss or hemolysis may be associated with macrocytic indices, because reticulocytes are about 20 percent larger than mature red blood cells. Increased red-cell membrane surface area due to increased membrane cholesterol incorporation occurs in liver disease and obstructive jaundice. In hypothyroidism, nonmegaloblastic macrocytic anemia develops; the cause is unclear. Vitamin B_{12} and folate deficiency states, following total gastrectomy or accompanying malabsorption syndromes, cause megaloblastic anemia.

505. The answer is A-N, B-Y, C-Y, D-N, E-Y. *(Braunwald, ed 11, chap 56.)* The stages of neutrophil defense against bacterial invasion include chemotaxis, phagocytosis, and microbicide. Accumulation of neutrophils in response to inflammation (chemotaxis) is impaired by alcohol and glucocorticosteroids. Neutrophil dysfunction may occur with various complement abnormalities; C3 deficiency, for example, results in both defective chemotaxis and defective phagocytosis. In chronic granulomatous disease, bacterial infections occur due to failure of the normal metabolic burst following phagocytosis as well as to impaired generation of bactericidal free oxygen radicals; chemotaxis and phagocytosis are normal. Hereditary neutrophil hyposegmentation (Pelger-Huët anomaly) is not associated with abnormal neutrophil function.

506. The answer is A-N, B-N, C-Y, D-Y, E-Y. *(Braunwald, ed 11, chaps 284, 288. Cook, Semin Hematol 19:6, 1982.)* Iron deficiency frequently is confused with thalassemia trait, both alpha and beta, in that all three of these conditions are characterized by a microcytic anemia. Iron stores, as reflected by transferrin saturation, serum ferritin level, and bone marrow iron staining, are depleted in iron deficiency but normal in both types of thalassemia trait. Hemoglobin electrophoresis reveals an increased hemoglobin A_2 level in beta-thalassemia trait but subnormal levels in iron deficiency and alpha-thalassemia trait. (In the presence of concomitant iron deficiency, hemoglobin A_2 levels may be normal in persons with beta-thalassemia, but levels rise once iron stores are replenished.)

507. The answer is A-Y, B-N, C-N, D-Y, E-Y. *(Braunwald, ed 11, chap 287.)* Because the spleen is the primary site of destruction of abnormal red blood cells in persons with hereditary spherocytosis, splenectomy generally restores hematologic laboratory indices to normal. Reticulocyte count decreases, and serum haptoglobin concentration, which may be low as a result of extravascular as well as intravascular hemolysis, also returns to normal following splenectomy. Although hemolysis is ameliorated by splenectomy, the intrinsic erythrocyte membrane defect is unaffected, as reflected by the persistence of increased osmotic fragility and the presence of microspherocytes on peripheral blood smear. Postsplenectomy thrombocytosis may persist for years.

508. The answer is A-N, B-Y, C-Y, D-N, E-Y. *(Braunwald, ed 11, chap 228.)* Hematuria and hyposthenuria both are increased in incidence in sickle-cell trait; the mechanism of both abnormalities probably is related to the relatively hypertonic, acidotic, and hypoxic conditions of the renal medulla, which predispose to local sickling. Splenic infarction may develop at altitudes above approximately 3000 meters (10,000 feet) during flights in unpressurized airplanes. A prospective study of matched pairs of individuals has shown no deficits in standard measurements of growth and development in children with sickle cell trait when compared to other children. Mortality rates during pregnancy are not affected appreciably by sickle cell trait.

509. The answer is A-Y, B-Y, C-Y, D-N, E-N. *(Braunwald, ed 11, chap 228.)* Methemoglobin is the type of hemoglobin in which iron has been oxidized to the ferric form. It accumulates in excess when red blood cells are exposed to oxidant stress and when they are deficient in enzymatic reduction mechanisms. Methemoglobin cannot bind oxygen, and excessive concentrations of methemoglobin lead to a progressive increase in oxygen affinity of the remaining functioning heme residues on the hemoglobin tetramer (i.e., shift to the left of the oxyhemoglobin dissociation curve). A methemoglobin level greater than 1.5 g/dL causes visible cyanosis. Methemoglobinemia is not associated with hemolysis or red-cell morphologic changes.

510. The answer is A-Y, B-N, C-Y, D-N, E-Y. *(Braunwald, ed 11, chaps 290, 291.)* Severe aplastic anemia is defined as marked pancytopenia: neutrophil count less than 500/mm^3; platelet count less than 20,000/mm^3; and anemia accompanied by a reticulocyte count less than 1 percent. Affected persons have a poor prognosis for spontaneous recovery, with bleeding and infection being the major causes of morbidity and mortality. A febrile, neutropenic patient should be hospitalized; potential sources of infection should be sought promptly by culture, and empiric broad-spectrum antibiotic therapy should begin immediately, to be modified subsequently according to culture results. Androgens do not appear to be beneficial in treating severe aplastic anemia but may stimulate the marrow in milder cases. In severe aplastic anemia occurring in younger persons having an HLA-matched donor, prompt bone marrow transplantation is the treatment of choice. If a bone marrow transplant is considered, HLA-compatible family members should not be used as blood donors, to avoid sensitization of the potential recipient to minor transplantation antigens.

511. The answer is A-Y, B-N, C-N, D-N, E-N. *(Braunwald, ed 11, chap 279.)* There are no clinical findings to suggest the presence of disseminated intravascular coagulation or a fibrinogen abnormality, so that ordering fibrinogen, thrombin time, and fibrin split product determinations would be inappropriate. The clinical and laboratory picture in this patient is consistent with the presence of a myeloproliferative disorder. Further evaluation might include bone marrow aspiration and biopsy and liver-spleen scan, as well as serum vitamin B$_{12}$ and folate level determinations which are often elevated in such a setting. In patients with these disorders, an acquired platelet functional defect occasionally develops, with abnormalities demonstrable on platelet aggregometry. The most frequent abnormality is a lack of platelet responsiveness to administration of epinephrine.

512. The answer is A-N, B-Y, C-N, D-N, E-Y. *(Braunwald, ed 11, chap 279.)* The interaction of von Willebrand's factor (VWF) with the platelet is most readily studied in vitro by measuring the effect of the antibiotic ristocetin on platelet aggregation. Patients whose platelets are not aggregated by ristocetin either lack VWF activity (most persons with von Willebrand's disease except those with the type IIb variant) or the platelet receptor for VWF (glycoprotein Ib). The latter situation is found in the Bernard-Soulier syndrome, a rare clinical condition also characterized by reduced levels of several other platelet membrane proteins, mild thrombocytopenia, and large, lymphocytoid platelets. Platelets from patients with Glanzmann's thrombasthenia are deficient in the glycoprotein IIb-IIIa complex. This receptor serves as the binding site for fibrinogen in platelet-platelet interactions. Hence, thrombasthenic platelets adhere normally and will agglutinate with ristocetin but will not aggregate with any of the agonists that require fibrinogen binding, such as adenosine diphosphate (ADP), thrombin, or epinephrine. Aspirin specifically acetylates the platelet cyclooxygenase enzyme decreasing the production of thromboxane A$_2$. This results in a defect in secondary platelet aggregation in response to agonists such as ADP and epinephrine. A similar situation is found in persons with storage pool disease whose platelet granules lack releasable stores of ADP and serotonin.

168   PRINCIPLES OF INTERNAL MEDICINE

513. The answer is A-N, B-N, C-Y, D-Y, E-Y. *(Braunwald, ed 11, chap 289. Laszlo, Semin Hematol 12:409, 1975.)* The myeloproliferative disorders (polycythemia vera, essential thrombocythemia, chronic myelogenous leukemia, myeloid metaplasia, and myelofibrosis) are a group of related diseases of the bone marrow stem cell. All cell lines—erythroid, myeloid, and megakaryocytic—are affected. Several functional platelet defects have been identified in these disorders and result paradoxically in both bleeding and thromboembolic complications, which are the major causes of morbidity and mortality. All myeloproliferative disorders may develop into acute leukemia, especially if alkylating agents are used in treatment. Although abnormal white blood cell function also may be associated with these disorders, opportunistic infections generally are not encountered.

514–518. The answers are: 514-D, 515-E, 516-B, 517-A, 518-C. *(Braunwald, ed 11, chap 53.)* In cold agglutinin disease (illustration D), cold-active IgM antibodies react against red blood cell antigens. Cold agglutinins may arise secondary to infections (particularly viral and *Mycoplasma* infections), in association with lymphoproliferative disorders (e.g., lymphoma), or due to idiopathic cold agglutinin disease. Symptoms are due to vasoocclusion in cold-exposed regions of the circulation; fresh blood specimens may dramatically agglutinate during withdrawal into a cooler syringe.

Myelophthisic anemia occurs in situations in which bone marrow has been invaded by nonmarrow elements, such as granulomas, fibrous tissue (myelofibrosis), or metastatic tumor. The peripheral smear (illustration E) typically shows marked anisocytosis and poikilocytosis of the red blood cells, with "teardrop" forms, nucleated red cells, and sometimes a "leukoerythroblastic reaction," which is characterized by leukocytosis and immature white blood cells. The diagnosis is made by bone marrow biopsy.

Hereditary spherocytosis is a relatively common hemolytic anemia, in which intrinsically defective red blood cells are prematurely destroyed in a normally functioning spleen. Adults frequently develop gallstones due to increased bilirubin production. Peripheral smears (illustration B) typically show a predominance of microspherocytes and variable polychromatophilia (reticulocytosis).

Thrombotic thrombocytopenic purpura is characterized by microangiopathic hemolytic anemia (with marked red-cell fragmentation in the peripheral smear—illustration A), thrombocytopenia, and widely variable and fluctuating neurologic abnormalities. Disseminated intravascular coagulation is not present, and prothrombin and partial thromboplastin times usually are normal. The typical pathologic lesion responsible for these changes is hyaline occlusion of small vessels.

Alpha-thalassemia trait and beta-thalassemia trait usually are asymptomatic conditions, characterized by mild anemia and markedly microcytic red-cell indices. The blood smear (illustration C) typically reveals variable degrees of anisocytosis and poikilocytosis, target cells, cell fragments, misshapen cells, and basophilic stippling.

519–522. The answers are: 519-A, 520-B, 521-E, 522-B. *(Braunwald, ed 11, chap 284. Finch, Medicine 49:17, 1970.)* Ferrokinetic studies, using an injected radioactive iron (^{59}Fe) tracer, provide valuable dynamic information about marrow iron supply and erythropoiesis. In iron-deficiency anemia, ^{59}Fe is removed avidly from plasma by the "iron-starved" marrow, leading to increased plasma iron clearance and increased plasma iron turnover. Because erythropoiesis proceeds effectively, red-cell incorporation of iron also is increased.

In thalassemia major, ineffective erythropoiesis takes place in the bone marrow; intramedullary red-cell destruction also occurs. Erythropoiesis, even though it is largely ineffective, is increased in the marrow, and erythroid hyperplasia typically is seen on examination of bone marrow aspirates. Ferrokinetic studies usually show increased plasma iron clearance and plasma iron turnover, but impaired red-cell utilization of iron.

In aplastic anemia, plasma iron clearance is slow, and plasma iron turnover is decreased because of the absence of normal erythropoiesis. Furthermore, because production of red blood cells is suppressed, red-cell iron incorporation also is decreased. Erythropoiesis is ineffective in untreated megaloblastic anemias (e.g., pernicious anemia or folate deficiency); therefore, the ferrokinetic profile is similar to that seen in thalassemia.

523–526. The answers are: 523-D, 524-A, 525-F, 526-E. *(Braunwald, ed 11, chaps 280, 281.)* Urokinase is able to accelerate the lysis of blood clots by directly converting plasminogen to plasmin. It cannot discriminate between free and fibrin-bound plasminogen, and therefore can produce profound hypofibrinogenemia and a systemic lytic state. On the other hand, tissue plasminogen activator is a fibrin-specific activator of plasminogen and should be able to lyse clots without producing severe systemic fibrinolysis and bleeding.

Vitamin K is a fat-soluble vitamin that supports the gamma-carboxylation of a group of glutamic acid residues on factors II, VII, IX, and X, and proteins C and S. This reaction allows these factors to be fully functional by providing carboxyl groups, which can bind calcium; calcium, in turn, provides a link to phospholipid surfaces. Coumadin blocks the activity of a liver microsomal epoxide reductase; this enzyme is able to convert the vitamin K epoxide generated by the carboxylation reaction back into an active form of the vitamin.

Indomethacin is a competitive and hence reversible inhibitor of platelet cyclooxygenase activity. This enzyme results in the conversion of arachidonic acid to endoperoxide intermediates and ultimately thromboxane A_2, a potent inducer of platelet aggregation. Aspirin irreversibly acetylates platelet cyclooxygenase.

Antithrombin III is the major naturally occurring inhibitor of thrombin. It is also able to inactivate several other activated coagulation factors (factors IX_a, X_a, XI_a, and XII_a). Heparin binds to antithrombin III and markedly accelerates the rate of hemostatic enzyme-inhibitor complex formation. Once the inactive complex has formed, heparin is released and is again available for binding to free inhibitor. Heparin-like molecules with anticoagulant activity have been identified on the surface of vascular endothelial cells.

Dipyridamole is a widely used antiplatelet agent. While the mechanism of action of this drug is not completely understood, it is able to prolong platelet survival in individuals with increased platelet turnover. It does not impair platelet aggregation in vitro at doses that produce the in vivo effects on platelet survival.

NEOPLASIA

DIRECTIONS: Each question below contains five suggested answers. Choose the **one best** response to each question.

527. All of the following hereditary syndromes are associated with the development of malignancies EXCEPT

(A) the Chédiak-Higashi syndrome
(B) chronic granulomatous disease of childhood
(C) ataxia-telangiectasia
(D) familial polyposis coli
(E) Fanconi's anemia

528. Metabolic derangements associated with neoplastic diseases and their treatment can best be described by which of the following statements?

(A) Secondary gout is a common concomitant of lymphoproliferative neoplasms
(B) Acidification of the urine may help promote renal excretion of uric acid and prevent urate nephrolithiasis
(C) Cytotoxic therapy of highly drug-sensitive tumors may result in serious hyperphosphatemia, hypocalcemia, and hyperkalemia
(D) Lactic acidosis may be a complication of treatment of leukemia and Burkitt's lymphoma
(E) The excessive toxicity of mithramycin makes it an undesirable agent for the treatment of tumor-associated hypercalcemia

529. All of the following statements describe characteristics of the superior vena cava (SVC) syndrome EXCEPT

(A) clinical features of the syndrome include conjunctival suffusion, lower extremity edema, and pulsus paradoxus
(B) administration of corticosteroids and diuretics may be useful as temporizing measures until a diagnosis is established
(C) diffuse histiocytic lymphomas and small cell carcinomas of the lung are the most common neoplasms associated with the syndrome
(D) the SVC syndrome is rarely a cause of death in patients in whom it develops
(E) definitive therapy should include local irradiation and, if possible, systemic chemotherapy for the neoplasm in question

530. Which of the following characteristics is more apt to be associated with Hodgkin's disease than with non-Hodgkin's lymphoma?

(A) "B" symptoms
(B) Involvement of Waldeyer's ring
(C) Extralymphatic presentation
(D) Dissemination at the time of diagnosis
(E) Most common type (60 percent) of lymphoma

531. In persons who have chronic myelogenous leukemia, the Philadelphia chromosome most commonly is found in

(A) all cells of the body
(B) all three hematopoietic cell lines but not in nonhematopoietic cells
(C) all cells of the granulocytic cell line but not in nongranulocytic cells
(D) all morphologically abnormal (malignant-appearing) granulocytes
(E) occasional malignant-appearing granulocytes

532. Which of the following statements describes the relationship between testicular tumors and serum markers?

(A) Pure seminomas produce α-fetoprotein (AFP) or β-human chorionic gonadotropin (β-HCG) in more than 90 percent of cases
(B) More than 40 percent of nonseminomatous germ cell tumors produce no cell markers
(C) Both β-HCG and AFP should be measured in following the progress of a tumor
(D) Measurement of tumor markers the day following surgery for localized disease is useful in determining completeness of the resection
(E) β-HCG is limited in its usefulness as a marker, because it is identical to human luteinizing hormone

533. The cytotoxic action of anticancer agents is thought to be defined by first-order kinetics, which means that these agents

(A) kill a constant fraction of tumor cells
(B) kill a constant number of tumor cells
(C) kill a number of tumor cells directly proportional to the time of exposure to the agent
(D) kill a number of tumor cells directly proportional to the molar concentration of the agent
(E) act directly on cells and do not require metabolism to an intermediate

534. The use of tamoxifen, an antiestrogen agent, in treating women with metastatic breast cancer is LEAST likely to cause

(A) hot flashes
(B) nausea
(C) virilization
(D) fluid retention
(E) acute hypercalcemia

535. A 59-year-old postmenopausal woman underwent radical mastectomy 3 years ago for carcinoma of the breast. All nodes biopsied were negative, and the estrogen receptor status of the tumor was positive at 150 fmol/mg of cytosol protein. No further therapy was ordered. Now the woman presents with right upper leg pain. Plain films reveal a 3-cm lytic lesion in the right upper femur, and a bone scan shows not only the femoral lesion but also three separate lesions in her ribs, two in her skull, and one in her pelvis. Chest x-ray is unremarkable, and liver function tests are normal.

The most appropriate therapeutic option now would be

(A) tamoxifen, 10 mg twice daily
(B) tamoxifen, 10 mg twice daily, plus CMF combination chemotherapy (cyclophosphamide, methotrexate, and 5-fluorouracil)
(C) tamoxifen, 10 mg twice daily, plus external-beam radiation to the femoral lesion
(D) tamoxifen, 10 mg twice daily, plus prophylactic internal fixation of the right femur followed by external-beam radiation
(E) tamoxifen, 10 mg twice daily, plus both CMF and external-beam radiation to the femoral lesion

536. A 27-year-old man has a testicular mass. Chest x-ray reveals six discrete tumor nodules, and an abdominal CT scan shows enlarged paraaortic nodes. Serum α-fetoprotein level is elevated. He undergoes transinguinal orchiectomy, which reveals teratocarcinoma. Treatment is started with three cycles of combination chemotherapy consisting of bleomycin, vinblastine, and *cis*-platinum; he tolerates the chemotherapy well. Four of the six lung nodules resolve completely, the paraaortic nodes disappear, and α-fetoprotein levels return to normal. The two remaining pulmonary nodules, one in each lung, have diminished in size to about 2 cm. The man receives a fourth cycle of the same drugs with no change in his clinical status.

At this stage, his physician should

(A) continue the same chemotherapy for one more cycle but increase the dosage of drugs by 50 percent
(B) switch to a new drug regimen
(C) perform thoracotomy in order to biopsy and remove the nodule on one side
(D) administer low-dose, whole-lung radiation
(E) administer high-dose spot radiation to the individual lung nodules

537. A 60-year-old man with known lung cancer has recently developed lower back pain. Physical examination, including careful neurologic examination, is normal. Plain films of the back reveal several blastic lesions around T12 and L1. The next step in the man's management should be

(A) careful observation and frequent neurologic examinations
(B) electromyography with nerve conduction studies
(C) lumbar puncture
(D) CT scan of the spine
(E) corticosteroid therapy

538. The Health Insurance Plan of New York evaluated mammography as a screening tool for breast cancer in 62,000 individuals. After a 9-year follow-up period, it was found that the screened population

(A) showed a 30 percent reduction in mortality from breast cancer, compared to a control group, for women 50 years of age or older
(B) showed a 30 percent reduction in mortality from breast cancer, compared to a control group, for women 35 to 50 years of age
(C) showed a 30 percent reduction in mortality from breast cancer for women at high risk for the development of breast cancer (i.e., women having prior breast cancer or an affected first-degree relative)
(D) demonstrated no change in mortality from breast cancer for women of any age group, despite having an earlier stage of cancer at diagnosis
(E) had an increased mortality from breast cancer probably due to the carcinogenic effects of radiation delivered during mammography

539. All the following statements concerning risk factors for breast cancer are true EXCEPT

(A) irregularity of the menstrual cycle increases a woman's chance of developing breast cancer
(B) late menopause (after 55 years of age) increases a woman's chance of developing breast cancer
(C) artificial menopause before 35 years of age diminishes a woman's chance of developing breast cancer
(D) bearing a first child before 18 years of age diminishes a woman's chance of developing breast cancer
(E) the effects of childbearing and menstruation are unimportant in determining the risk of breast cancer in women past the age of 75 years

540. A 38-year-old premenopausal woman has a 3-cm mass in her left breast. Breast biopsy reveals infiltrating ductal carcinoma, and a left modified radical mastectomy is performed. Pathology reports that the primary tumor is estrogen-receptor positive and that 4 of 28 lymph nodes identified are involved with tumor. Chest x-ray, bone scan, liver scan, and blood chemistries are all normal.

The most appropriate next step in the management of this case would be

(A) antiestrogen therapy (e.g., tamoxifen)
(B) appropriate combination chemotherapy
(C) postoperative radiation therapy to the left chest wall and axilla
(D) bilateral oophorectomy
(E) follow-up in 2 months

541. Bone marrow transplantation for persons who have acute nonlymphocytic leukemia and are in first remission can best be described by which of the following statements?

(A) It leads to cure in approximately 30 percent of cases
(B) It generally should be restricted to adults, because younger persons do not tolerate the procedure well
(C) It is unwarranted, given the excellent results of chemotherapy for this disease
(D) The major causes of death have been graft-versus-host disease and infection
(E) The best donor usually is a histocompatible parent

542. A 76-year-old man complains of fatigue. His physical examination is normal except for pallor and resting tachycardia. His complete blood cell count reveals a hematocrit of 24 percent, a platelet count of 224,000/mm^3, and a white blood cell count of 18,000/mm^3 of which 60 percent are granulocytes, 10 percent are lymphocytes, and 30 percent are myeloblasts. Bone marrow examination reveals generalized myeloid hyperplasia with approximately 35 percent myeloblasts. After transfusion with packed red blood cells, the man is asymptomatic.

The most appropriate step at this time would be to

(A) begin therapy with vincristine and prednisone
(B) begin therapy with daunomycin and cytosine arabinoside
(C) begin hydroxyurea therapy
(D) begin busulfan therapy
(E) discharge the man and check his blood counts in a week

543. A 28-year-old man with newly diagnosed acute myelogenous leukemia spikes a temperature of 38.7°C (101.7°F) on the sixth day of induction therapy. He feels well and has no physical complaints. His only medicine is intravenous cytosine arabinoside, 140 mg every 12 hours. Physical examination is unrevealing. His white blood cell count is 900/mm^3, of which 10 percent are granulocytes and the rest mostly lymphocytes; platelet count is 24,000/mm^3. Chest x-ray and urinalysis are normal.

After obtaining appropriate cultures, the man's physician should

(A) observe closely for the development of a clinically evident source of fever
(B) begin antibiotic therapy with gentamicin, carbenicillin, and a cephalosporin
(C) begin granulocyte transfusion and antibiotic therapy with gentamicin, carbenicillin, and a cephalosporin
(D) begin gammaglobulin treatment and antibiotic therapy with gentamicin, carbenicillin, and a cephalosporin
(E) begin antibiotic therapy with amphotericin, gentamicin, carbenicillin, and a cephalosporin

544. Which of the following statements concerning the immunologic abnormalities associated with Hodgkin's disease is NOT true?

(A) Antibody production is normal in most affected persons
(B) The ability of untreated persons to respond to a battery of skin-test antigens is usually abnormal if they have stage III or stage IV disease
(C) A lymphocyte count of less than 1000/mm^3 is associated significantly with cutaneous anergy
(D) The major immunologic defect in affected persons appears to reside in the T lymphocyte
(E) Following successful drug or radiation therapy, affected persons regain full immunologic competence within 12 to 24 months

545. It is important to recognize Bowen's disease (squamous cell carcinoma of the skin in situ), because

(A) the lesions are difficult to treat by surgical excision and require aggressive radiotherapy
(B) the lesions usually become invasive and metastasize early if not appropriately treated
(C) affected persons are at significant risk for development of carcinomas of the respiratory, genitourinary, and gastrointestinal tracts
(D) affected persons are at increased risk for the development of leukemia
(E) the disease is associated with developing incompetence of the immune system

546. All of the following statements about the acute leukemias are true EXCEPT

(A) the majority of cases of acute lymphocytic leukemia (ALL) express both T-cell antigens and surface immunoglobulin
(B) leukemic cells in most cases of ALL contain terminal deoxynucleotidyl transferase (TdT), an enzyme only rarely present in acute myelogenous leukemia (AML) cells
(C) the T-cell form of ALL occurs typically in adolescent males; it is frequently associated with an increased leukocyte count and an anterior mediastinal mass
(D) the cells of B-cell ALL frequently contain the t(8;14) chromosomal abnormality characteristic of Burkitt's lymphoma
(E) patients with the acute promyelocytic (M3) subtype of AML frequently present with disseminated intravascular coagulation (DIC)

547. Which of the following statements best describes the human T-lymphotropic viruses (HTLV)?

(A) A viral etiology has been established for the majority of cases of acute lymphocytic leukemia (ALL)
(B) Common features among different variants of HTLV include tropism for the T4$^+$ lymphocyte and the presence of genes encoding for an RNA-directed DNA polymerase (reverse transcriptase)
(C) Leukemias/lymphomas caused by HTLV-I are usually characterized by an indolent course
(D) There is little genetic variation among different isolates of HTLV-III/LAV
(E) HTLV-II infection has been implicated in the usual B-cell type of hairy-cell leukemia

548. All of the following are neoplasms of B-lymphocyte lineage EXCEPT

(A) chronic lymphocytic leukemia
(B) follicular lymphomas
(C) Burkitt's lymphoma
(D) mycosis fungoides
(E) small lymphocytic (well-differentiated) lymphomas

549. All of the following statements about the carcinoid syndrome are true EXCEPT

(A) elevated urinary excretion of 5-hydroxyindoleacetic acid (5HIAA) may also be associated with acute intestinal obstruction, nontropical sprue, or dietary ingestion of bananas or walnuts
(B) the full-blown syndrome is a frequent accompaniment of primary nonmetastatic tumors in the gastrointestinal tract
(C) pharmacologic therapy directed toward blocking the effects of the humoral mediators with antihistamines, serotonin antagonists, corticosteroids, and phenothiazines may be clinically useful
(D) supplemental niacin may be necessary to prevent pellagra in patients with markedly increased urinary excretion of 5HIAA
(E) flushing attacks associated with bronchial carcinoid tend to be prolonged and severe and may be associated with excessive lacrimation and salivation, bronchoconstriction, and periorbital edema

550. Which of the following clinical scenarios is NOT likely to be a paraneoplastic syndrome resulting from oat cell tumors of the lung?

(A) Weakness and fatigability, primarily of proximal muscles; electromyographic results show increasing amplitude of contraction with repetitive stimulation
(B) Cerebellar ataxia, dysarthria, deafness, pleocytosis of cerebrospinal fluid, and cerebellar atrophy on CT scan of the brain
(C) Moon facies, truncal striae, hypertension, hypokalemia, and hyperglycemia
(D) Hypercalcemia, polydipsia, polyuria, and mental status changes in the absence of bony metastases
(E) Mental status changes, muscle weakness, hyponatremia, and decreased serum osmolality with inappropriately elevated urine osmolality

DIRECTIONS: Each question below contains five suggested answers. For **each** of the five alternatives of **each** item, you are to respond either YES (Y) or NO (N). In a given item all, some, or none of the alternatives may be correct.

551. Which of the following statements concerning the relationship between cigarette smoking and cancer are true?

(A) Approximately 40 percent of all cancers are related directly or in part to cigarette smoking
(B) Bladder cancer has been associated with cigarette smoking
(C) Heavy smokers should have a yearly chest x-ray to screen for early signs of lung cancer
(D) Alcohol, asbestos, and uranium exposure act synergistically with cigarette smoking to increase the risk of cancer
(E) Women who are heavy smokers are three times as likely to develop breast cancer as are other women

552. Which of the following statements about doxorubicin (Adriamycin) cardiotoxicity are true?

(A) Acute cardiotoxicity, which is characterized by arrhythmias and other abnormal electrocardiographic changes, is brief and rarely serious
(B) Chronic cardiotoxicity occurs in fewer than 3 percent of individuals whose lifetime dose of doxorubicin is below 500 mg/m^2
(C) The congestive heart failure associated with doxorubicin therapy usually responds to digitalis therapy
(D) Congestive heart failure frequently develops 6 months or more after the last dose of doxorubicin
(E) Previous cardiac irradiation and exposure to cyclophosphamide or anthracycline antibiotics other than doxorubicin increase the risk of cardiotoxicity

553. Which of the following statements concerning the relationship between radiation exposure and the development of neoplasia are true?

(A) An unlimited linear dose-response relationship exists between radiation exposure and the development of leukemia
(B) Infants and pregnant women are at greatest risk for developing radiation-induced neoplasia
(C) Exposure to radiation below the established minimum threshold dose is considered safe
(D) The incidence of leukemia reaches a peak approximately 7 years after radiation exposure
(E) An increase in the frequency of breast cancer in women undergoing repeated chest x-ray has been shown with as low a dose as 17 rads

554. For a given clinical stage of Hodgkin's disease, which of the following would affect prognosis **adversely**?

(A) Presence of anergy
(B) Presence of fever
(C) Pruritus
(D) Abnormal absolute lymphocyte count
(E) Abnormal in vitro lymphocyte phytohemagglutinin response

555. The use in combination of nitrogen mustard, vincristine (Oncovin), prednisone, and procarbazine (MOPP) in the treatment of persons who have advanced-stage Hodgkin's disease can be described by which of the following statements?

(A) Persons for whom radiotherapy has failed respond more poorly to MOPP than do previously untreated persons whose disease is of the same stage and histologic subtype
(B) Up to 80 percent of previously untreated persons achieve a complete remission with MOPP
(C) More than two-thirds of persons who achieve a complete remission with MOPP remain free of disease for up to 12 years
(D) Most persons who relapse do so within the first 2 years following treatment
(E) Two years of MOPP maintenance therapy, after an initial induction of remission, improves disease-free survival rate

556. Which of the following statements concerning staging laparotomy for Hodgkin's disease are true?

(A) The mortality rate is 1.5 percent and the complication rate is approximately 12 percent
(B) The majority of persons with Hodgkin's disease require this operation in order to be appropriately staged
(C) Laparotomy should nearly always be performed if positive findings would advance the stage of the disease
(D) The spleen should nearly always be removed during staging laparotomy
(E) Removal of the spleen at laparotomy is associated with better tolerance of chemotherapy

557. Which of the following statements about hairy-cell leukemia are true?

(A) Palpable splenomegaly is present in only a minority of cases
(B) In approximately 30 percent of patients, an associated vasculitic disorder will develop, with erythema nodosum, other cutaneous nodules, or visceral involvement similar to polyarteritis nodosa
(C) Virtually all treated patients have exhibited a positive response to administration of alpha-interferon
(D) Infectious complications are unusual
(E) The disorder results from expansion of neoplastic B-lymphocytes which sometimes produce a monoclonal immunoglobulin

558. Which of the following factors influence the frequency of dissemination of cutaneous malignant melanoma?

(A) Primary tumor site
(B) Dermatologic level of invasion
(C) Thickness of the primary lesion
(D) Geographic area of residence
(E) Presence or absence of lymphocytic infiltrate of the lesion

DIRECTIONS: The groups of questions below consist of four or five lettered headings followed by several numbered items. For each numbered item choose the **one** lettered heading with which it is **most** closely associated. Each lettered heading may be used once, more than once, or not at all.

Questions 559–562

Match each of the following chemotherapeutic agents to their appropriate mechanism of action

(A) Inhibits DNA synthesis and reacts with DNA to cause strand scission
(B) Binds with DNA, causing untwisting of the double helix
(C) Blocks thymidylate synthetase
(D) Produces metaphase arrest by direct binding to tubulin
(E) Causes depurination and miscoding errors by its alkylating action

559. Bleomycin

560. Doxorubicin

561. Vinblastine

562. 5-Fluorouracil

Questions 563–567

Match the histologic subtype of lung cancer with the clinicopathologic description.

(A) Small cell carcinoma
(B) Large cell carcinoma
(C) Epidermoid carcinoma
(D) Adenocarcinoma
(E) Bronchoalveolar carcinoma

563. Hypercalcemia common

564. Initial presentation in the peripheral part of the lung

565. Extrathoracic involvement at the time of presentation in the majority of cases

566. Frequent association with prior fibrotic lung disease

567. Frequent association with ACTH production

Questions 568–570

For each toxic reaction that follows, select the chemotherapeutic agent with which it is most likely to be associated.

(A) Procarbazine
(B) L-Asparaginase
(C) Cyclophosphamide
(D) 6-Thioguanine
(E) 6-Mercaptopurine

568. Simultaneous ingestion of ethanol can produce a disulfiram (Antabuse)-like reaction

569. Simultaneous administration of allopurinol can greatly enhance toxicity if the dose of this agent is not appropriately lowered

570. Simultaneous administration of barbiturates may increase the toxicity of this agent

Neoplasia

Answers

527. The answer is B. *(Braunwald, ed 11, chap 78.)* Certain familial and genetic syndromes are associated with an increased propensity to development of malignant neoplasms. Most patients with the Chédiak-Higashi syndrome, a disorder associated with abnormal cellular function and neurologic dysfunction, succumb to infections in childhood or young adulthood; those who survive the infections are prone to the development of lymphoproliferative disorders. Chronic granulomatous disease of childhood, in contrast, is a disorder of oxidative metabolism in phagocytes and is not associated with neoplasia. Ataxia-telangiectasia, an autosomal condition in which there is abnormal cellular immunity, conjunctival telangiectasias, and progressive spinocerebellar atrophy, is also associated with lymphoma. Carcinoma of the colon develops in almost all persons with familial polyposis coli and is found at the time of initial diagnosis of the polyps in about 40 percent of cases. Fanconi's anemia is one of a group of familial disorders associated with cytogenetic abnormalities and an increased risk of development of cancer.

528. The answer is C. *(Braunwald, ed 11, chap 79.)* Hyperuricemia occurs frequently in patients with acute leukemia, but it may also be associated with other malignant conditions. Secondary gout, however, is quite unusual, except in patients with polycythemia vera. The solubility of urate in the urine is increased at *alkaline* pH, and thus administration of bicarbonate may prevent the precipitation of urate crystals in the renal tubules and parenchyma. Cytotoxic therapy of highly drug-sensitive tumors may cause massive release of intracellular phosphate and potassium, leading to sudden alteration of blood electrolytes which may result in fatal cardiac rhythm disturbances. Lactic acidosis occasionally occurs in untreated patients with leukemia and Burkitt's lymphoma, because of the excessive production of lactate by these metabolically active tumors, and it may be reversed by appropriate chemotherapy. The treatment of choice for tumor-associated hypercalcemia is therapy of the underlying malignancy, but mithramycin is a useful ancillary agent, with toxicity that is limited if the drug is used in careful and recommended fashion.

529. The answer is A. *(Braunwald, ed 11, chap 79.)* Obstruction of the superior vena cava, the SVC syndrome, is a complication of malignancies involving the mediastinum and upper lung fields, most commonly caused by diffuse histiocytic lymphomas and small cell carcinomas of the lung. The syndrome is characterized clinically by headache, conjunctival injection and suffusion, plethoric facies, distention of veins in the neck and upper extremities, loss of venous pulsations, and (in severe cases) convulsions. Lower extremity swelling and pulsus paradoxus suggest the presence of pericardial tamponade, another complication of chest malignancies. While the SVC syndrome is a serious medical problem, it is rarely a cause of death, and time is usually available to allow pursuit of a specific histologic diagnosis. During this interval, therapy with corticosteroids and diuretics may be useful, pending a diagnosis and the institution of more specific therapy, which should include local irradiation and systemic treatment of the tumor.

530. The answer is A. *(Braunwald, ed 11, chap 294.)* Hodgkin's disease can be distinguished from non-Hodgkin's lymphomas (NHL) by a variety of characteristics. The "B" (or constitutional) symptoms described for Hodgkin's disease are less common in patients with NHL, although the presence of these symptoms is thought to influence the prognosis negatively. Involvement of Waldeyer's ring occurs more commonly in NHL than in Hodgkin's disease. Extralymphatic presentation is more frequent with NHL than with Hodgkin's disease, and NHL is more often disseminated at the time of diagnosis. Approximately 60 percent of all lymphomas are NHL.

531. The answer is B. *(Braunwald, ed 11, chap 78.)* In about 85 percent of persons who have chronic myelogenous leukemia, the material comprising approximately one-half of the long arm of the G22 chromosome is translocated to the end of the C9 chromosome. This abnormality, called the Philadelphia chromosome, involves all three hematopoietic cell lines. It is thought to represent an acquired somatic cell mutation in the bone marrow, with preferential survival and proliferation of the affected cell clone.

532. The answer is C. *(Braunwald, ed 11, chap 78.)* Ninety percent of persons with nonseminomatous germ cell tumors produce either α-fetoprotein (AFP) or β-HCG; in contrast, persons with pure seminomas usually produce neither. These tumor markers are present for some time after surgery—if the presurgical levels are high, 30 days or more may be required before meaningful postsurgical levels can be obtained. After treatment, unequal reduction of β-HCG and AFP may occur, suggesting that the two markers are synthesized by heterogeneous clones of cells within the tumor; thus, both markers should be followed. Beta-HCG is similar to luteinizing hormone except for its distinctive beta subunit.

533. The answer is A. *(Braunwald, ed 11, chap 79.)* By following first-order kinetics, anticancer agents kill a constant fraction, rather than a constant number, of tumor cells. A course of therapy that has been shown to be capable of killing three orders of magnitude of cells (i.e., 3 logs) will do so regardless of total number of tumor cells. Because most chemotherapeutic agents have been found to reduce the number of tumor cells by only 1 to 3 logs, their effectiveness in treating cancers with a trillion cells (10^{12}) has been limited, unless the tumor burden is reduced first.

534. The answer is C. *(Braunwald, ed 11, chap 79.)* Tamoxifen is a useful antiestrogen agent in the treatment of metastatic breast cancer and usually is very well tolerated. However, it can be associated with hot flashes, nausea, mild fluid retention, and acute hypercalcemia. Virilization is uncommon with tamoxifen.

535. The answer is D. *(Braunwald, ed 11, chap 79.)* The appropriate systemic therapy for postmenopausal women with ER-positive breast cancer metastic to bone is either tamoxifen, 10 mg twice daily, or diethylstilbestrol. Radiation therapy can relieve bone pain and may prevent fractures if used prophylactically to treat lesions of weight-bearing bones. For lytic lesions greater than 2.5 cm in diameter in weight-bearing bones, prophylactic internal fixation followed by radiation therapy is the treatment of choice, especially if the lesions involve the cortex.

536. The answer is C. *(Braunwald, ed 11, chap 79.)* Persons with disseminated teratocarcinoma treated with combination chemotherapy achieve complete remission in more than 70 percent of cases. Occasionally, residual masses remain after chemotherapy and on biopsy prove to be benign mature teratomas rather than residual malignant disease. In these cases, partial responders can be converted to complete responders—and even cured—by surgical removal of residual masses.

537. The answer is D. *(Braunwald, ed 11, chap 79.)* Epidural spinal cord compression is an important complication of metastatic cancer. Local or radicular pain is the most frequent and earliest clinical symptom; subsequently, weakness and bladder and bowel dysfunction can develop. The diagnosis, which should always be considered even if neurologic exam is normal, is confirmed by demonstrating a lesion on myelography or CT scan. Lumbar spinal taps should be avoided because herniation of the cord into a decompressed region can occur after withdrawal of fluid. Surgery usually is recommended for persons with rapidly progressive neurologic signs; radiation is useful in treating persons who have slowly progressive deficits due to radiosensitive tumors. Neither systemic chemotherapy nor corticosteroids should be employed in place of surgery or radiotherapy.

NEOPLASIA

538. The answer is A. *(Braunwald, ed 11, chap 295.)* The Health Insurance Plan of New York evaluated mammography as a screening tool in 62,000 persons. Their screening procedure included physical examination as well. A 9-year follow-up assessment showed a 30 percent reduction in mortality, when compared to a control group, for women 50 years of age or older who had been screened.

539. The answer is E. *(Braunwald, ed 11, chap 295.)* Early menarche, late menopause, and irregularity of the menstrual cycle all increase a woman's risk of developing breast cancer. Women who have undergone artificial menopause before the age of 35 years and women who bear their first child before the age of 18 years have a lower risk overall. These risk factors hold true throughout the woman's life.

540. The answer is B. *(Braunwald, ed 11, chap 295.)* For premenopausal women who have stage II carcinoma of the breast (axillary metastases only), the drug regimen combining cyclophosphamide, methotrexate, and 5-fluorouracil (CMF), when employed as an adjuvant therapy, leads to a statistically significant reduction in recurrence rate. It is the treatment of choice following mastectomy in this group of women. Mortality rate after 4 years is decreased 20 percent in women treated with CMF.

541. The answer is D. *(Braunwald, ed 11, chap 292.)* Approximately 60 percent of persons who have acute nonlymphocytic leukemia (ANL) and receive bone marrow transplants while in first remission are still without evidence of recurrent leukemia more than 4 years after transplantation. The donor is usually a histocompatible sibling. Younger persons seem to tolerate the transplant procedure better than do older persons. The major causes of death are graft-versus-host disease and infection, not recurrent leukemia.

542. The answer is E. *(Braunwald, ed 11, chap 292.)* Remission rates with appropriate chemotherapy generally are poorer for acute nonlymphoblastic leukemia (e.g., acute myelocytic leukemia, as in the case presented) than for acute lymphoblastic leukemia. Furthermore, induction of remission is much more dangerous to attempt in elderly persons than in younger persons. Thus, for an elderly person with acute nonlymphoblastic leukemia whose disease is slowly progressive ("smoldering leukemia"), supportive treatment alone may suffice, at least temporarily. Only when the disease shows evidence of progression should such an individual be treated with antileukemic therapy.

543. The answer is B. *(Braunwald, ed 11, chap 292.)* If not attacked promptly, infection in neutropenic individuals can be quickly fatal. Often, these individuals display neither the signs nor the symptoms of infection. Fever should be regarded as an indication of infection, and antibiotic therapy should begin immediately after appropriate cultures are obtained. An effective initial antibiotic regimen would consist of a cephalosporin, carbenicillin, and gentamicin. Gammaglobulin is of little benefit in the treatment of cancer patients. Granulocyte transfusions and amphotericin administration may be of benefit in selected cases.

544. The answer is E. *(Braunwald, ed 11, chap 294.)* T lymphocytes are reduced in number and in function in all persons with Hodgkin's disease, even those who have been treated successfully with chemotherapy or radiation therapy. Cutaneous anergy becomes significant when the lymphocyte count drops below 1000/mm^3. Individuals with advanced-stage Hodgkin's disease respond abnormally to skin testing with such recall antigens as histoplasmin and intermediate-strength PPD. Antibody production is normal in most persons who have Hodgkin's disease.

545. The answer is C. *(Braunwald, ed 11, chap 300.)* Bowen's disease—squamous cell carcinoma of the skin in situ—is easily treated by surgical excision. Metastasis occurs in less than 2 percent of cases. Affected persons are at significant risk for development of respiratory, genitourinary, and gastrointestinal carcinomas. The risk is especially high in persons whose Bowen's disease is on a region of skin not usually exposed to sunlight.

546. The answer is A. *(Braunwald, ed 11, chap 292.)* The most common type of ALL (approximately 60 percent of cases) is termed common ALL. The cells are positive for terminal deoxynucleotidyl transferase (TdT), express the common ALL antigen, and express neither T-cell antigens nor surface immunoglobulin. About 20 percent of cases of ALL are of the T-cell type and occur typically as described above. Less than 5 percent of cases of ALL are of the B-cell type. The cells in this form of the illness frequently express a monoclonal surface immunoglobulin, are TdT-negative, and have the cytogenetic abnormalities also associated with Burkitt's lymphoma, another B-cell neoplasm. While there are only subtle clinical differences among the subtypes of AML, the DIC associated with the M3 (promyelocytic) variant may be profound, is typically present at the time of diagnosis, and may be exacerbated markedly during chemotherapy.

547. The answer is B. *(Braunwald, ed 11, chap 293.)* While nearly all cases of adult T-cell leukemia/ lymphoma (ATL) are caused by HTLV-I, these cases represent a minority of T-cell neoplasms in the United States. ATL is usually characterized by an aggressive course, frequent hypercalcemia, opportunistic infections, and leukemic skin infiltrates. HTLV-II was originally isolated from a T-cell variant of hairy-cell leukemia but has not been implicated in the more usual B-cell form of the disease. A considerable amount of information has been learned about the molecular biology of the HTLV family. These viruses are human retroviruses, characterized by an RNA genome and the presence of the virally encoded enzyme reverse transcriptase, which makes a DNA copy of the viral RNA template. All the HTLV exhibit a striking tropism for the $T4^+$ lymphocyte. Restriction enzyme analysis of the genomes of various HTLV-III isolates reveals considerable variation in their nucleotide sequences, especially in the envelope gene. This variation appears to arise during transcription of the viral RNA genome to the DNA form or during integration of the DNA copy into the host cell DNA.

548. The answer is D. *(Braunwald, ed 11, chap 294.)* Neoplasms may be classified as to their cell of origin by the use of antisera and monoclonal antibodies against certain cell surface phenotypic markers and, more recently, by the use of DNA probes for immunoglobulin genes and genes for the beta chain of the T-cell receptor. The malignant cell in chronic lymphocytic leukemia is a morphologically normal but functionally abnormal B lymphocyte. Follicular lymphomas arise from the proliferative part of the B-cell system, the lymphoid follicle, while the diffuse, small lymphocytic lymphomas are derived from the secretory compartment of the medullary cords. The Burkitt's lymphoma cell is a malignant cell of B-lymphocyte lineage, in many cases bearing a characteristic chromosomal translocation. In contrast to these B-cell neoplasms, mycosis fungoides is a peripheral T-cell lymphoma in which helper-cell function and phenotype have been identified.

549. The answer is B. *(Braunwald, ed 11, chap 299.)* The carcinoid syndrome is caused by the production of serotonin and other vasoactive amines by carcinoid tumors in the bronchus, gastrointestinal tract, pancreas, and thyroid and in ovarian or testicular teratomas. The most useful test for diagnosing the syndrome is the quantitation of 5HIAA, the chief urinary metabolite of serotonin, in a 24-hour collection of urine. If increases related to excessive dietary consumption of foods such as bananas and walnuts can be excluded, marked increases in 5HIAA excretion are diagnostic of the syndrome. Minor increases, however, can also be associated with acute intestinal obstruction and nontropical sprue. Mediators released from tumors draining into the portal venous system are rapidly cleared by the liver; thus the syndrome usually results from the presence of hepatic metastases or tumors in other locations, such as the lung or in ovarian or testicular teratomas. The manifestations of the syndrome associated with bronchial carcinoids may be dramatic and include excessive lacrimation and salivation, bronchoconstriction, periorbital edema, hypotension, tachycardia, anxiety and tremulousness, nausea, vomiting, and explosive diarrhea. Pharmacologic blockade of the mediator effect may be a useful adjunct to more definitive therapy of the tumor. If large amounts of dietary tryptophan are shunted into the production of hydroxylated metabolites by the tumor, niacin deficiency and a pellagra-like condition may result, requiring the administration of supplemental niacin.

550. The answer is D. *(Braunwald, ed 11, chaps 303 and 304.)* Oat cell neoplasms of the lung are associated with a wide variety of paraneoplastic syndromes, some of which are humorally mediated, while others are of unknown pathophysiology. The Eaton-Lambert syndrome, characterized by proximal muscle weakness and the characteristic electromyographic findings, is associated almost exclusively with oat cell tumors. Subacute cortical cerebellar degeneration is associated with the findings outlined in scenario B and also with oat cell tumors and some cases of ovarian cancer, carcinoma of the breast, and Hodgkin's disease. Cushing's syndrome, with all the effects of hypersecretion of glucocorticoids, and the syndrome of inappropriate secretion of antidiuretic hormone, are also associated with oat cell lung tumors, in addition to other cancers. Hypercalcemia is infrequently associated with oat cell neoplasms, but it is not an infrequent manifestation of squamous and large cell lung tumors, in which cases it may be a result of secretion of substances with parathyroid hormone-like activity or of another factor associated with the humoral hypercalcemia of malignancy.

551. The answer is A-Y, B-Y, C-N, D-Y, E-N. *(Braunwald, ed 11, chap 79.)* More than 15 carcinogens have been isolated from tobacco smoke. Approximately 40 percent of all cancers have been related to cigarette smoking. The incidence not only of lung cancer but also of head and neck, esophageal, and bladder cancer is increased in smokers. In addition, use of alcohol and exposure to asbestos and uranium act synergistically to increase the risk. Yearly chest x-rays are not helpful in increasing the cure rate of lung cancer. The incidence of breast cancer does not seem to be affected by smoking.

552. The answer is A-Y, B-Y, C-N, D-Y, E-Y. *(Braunwald, ed 11, chap 79.)* Two types of cardiotoxicity are associated with doxorubicin (Adriamycin) therapy. Acute cardiotoxicity produces electrocardiographic abnormalities, such as arrhythmias, but rarely is serious. Chronic cardiotoxicity, which rarely develops with total doxorubicin doses less than 500 mg/m^2, leads to a congestive heart failure that is unresponsive to digitalis therapy; it occurs with increased frequency in individuals who also have received cardiac irradiation, cyclophosphamide, or anthracycline compounds other than doxorubicin. Up to half of all cases of cardiotoxicity occur 6 months or more after completion of therapy.

553. The answer is A-N, B-Y, C-N, D-Y, E-Y. *(Braunwald, ed 11, chap 79.)* A minimum acceptable safe dose of radiation does not seem to exist. Doses of radiation as low as 17 rads have been shown to increase the frequency of breast cancer in women undergoing repeated fluoroscopic examination of the chest. Increasing doses of radiation increase the risk of developing leukemia, until a plateau is reached beyond which the chance of developing malignancy is not increased. Leukemia resulting from radiation exposure peaks in incidence 7 years after exposure. Infants and pregnant women are most susceptible to radiation-induced neoplasia.

554. The answer is A-N, B-Y, C-N, D-N, E-N. *(Braunwald, ed 11, chap 294.)* Within a given clinical stage of Hodgkin's disease, recent history of fever, night sweats, and weight loss adversely influences prognosis. Persons who have these symptoms have substage "B" disease; persons who do not, have substage "A" disease. Given modern therapeutic techniques, pruritus, anergy, absolute lymphocyte count, and in vitro lymphocyte phytohemagglutinin response all have no bearing on the outcome of Hodgkin's disease.

555. The answer is A-N, B-Y, C-Y, D-Y, E-N. *(Braunwald, ed 11, chap 294.)* Combination chemotherapy with nitrogen mustard, vincristine (Oncovin), prednisone, and procarbazine—MOPP—currently is the treatment of choice for most persons with advanced-stage Hodgkin's disease. Use of the MOPP regimen has led to remission in as many as 80 percent of affected individuals, two-thirds of whom stay disease-free for up to 12 years. Those individuals who relapse usually do so within 2 years. Maintenance chemotherapy with MOPP has not been shown to prolong the disease-free state. Persons who did not respond to radiotherapy are no less likely than other affected individuals to respond to MOPP.

556. The answer is A-Y, B-N, C-N, D-Y, E-N. *(Braunwald, ed 11, chap 294.)* Staging laparotomy for persons who have Hodgkin's disease carries a mortality rate of 1.5 percent and a complication rate of 12 percent. It should not be considered a routine procedure but should be performed if the result would change the treatment plan, not just the stage of the disease. Staging laparotomy should include careful needle and wedge biopsies of the liver lobes and edge, biopsy of retroperitoneal lymph nodes identified by preoperative lymphangiography, and biopsies of any suspicious area. The spleen should be removed to reduce the radiation port; however, splenectomy does not improve tolerance to chemotherapy.

557. The answer is A-N, B-Y, C-Y, D-N, E-Y. *(Braunwald, ed 11, chap 292.)* More than 75 percent of patients with hairy-cell leukemia (HCL) will have clinically apparent splenomegaly, which in some cases may be massive. The cornerstone of therapy is splenectomy, which may ameliorate the disease in most patients. Associated vasculitis is relatively common in patients with HCL, in contrast to other leukemias. Therapy with alpha-interferon has been shown to be effective in a large fraction of patients and is generally quite well tolerated. Infection is the most common cause of death in patients with HCL, and common infecting organisms include *Legionella,* atypical mycobacteria, *Nocardia, Toxoplasma,* and the more usual pyogenic organisms. The malignant cell is a B lymphocyte with the characteristic cytoplasmic projections from which the disorder derives its name. The cells stain positively for tartrate-resistant acid phosphatase (TRAP) and frequently produce a monoclonal immunoglobulin.

558. The answer is A-Y, B-Y, C-Y, D-N, E-Y. *(Braunwald, ed 11, chap 302.)* Primary malignant melanoma of the skin is the leading cause of death from all diseases arising in the skin. A number of factors have been identified that correlate with increased or decreased likelihood of dissemination. The most common site for melanoma in males is the torso, and lesions occurring on the torso offer a worse prognosis than do those occurring on a lower extremity. Both dermatologic level of invasion and thickness of the primary lesion are predictive of dissemination and, hence, of survival. There appears to be a favorable effect on prognosis of a lymphocytic response identified on histologic examination of the lesion. While geographic area of residence is an important determinant of risk of development of melanoma, with incidence of disease being higher in latitudes with greater sun exposure, it does not appear to affect risk of dissemination in those with diagnosed clinically localized disease.

559–562. The answers are: 559A, 560-B, 561-D, 562-C. *(Braunwald, ed 11, chap 79.)* Bleomycin is an antibiotic complex consisting of seven structurally related polypeptides. It both inhibits DNA synthesis and reacts with DNA to cause strand scission. Indications for the use of bleomycin include lymphomas and tumors of the head and neck, skin, testes, and penis. Doxorubicin (Adriamycin), another antitumor antibiotic, inhibits DNA synthesis and DNA-dependent RNA synthesis. It acts by binding with DNA and causing untwisting of the helix, which facilitates intercalation. Doxorubicin is useful in treating a wide variety of tumors.

A pyrimidine analogue, 5-fluorouracil blocks thymidylate synthetase, an enzyme important in the synthesis of thymidylate and DNA. Its active form is the metabolite 5-fluorodeoxyuridine monophosphate. Used topically, 5-fluorouracil is effective in treating certain neoplastic skin disorders, including superficial basal cell carcinoma.

Vinblastine and vincristine are plant alkaloids. They cause metaphase arrest in dividing cells by binding directly to tubulin; in addition, they interfere with the assembly of spindle proteins. Vinblastine is used in the treatment of persons who have Hodgkin's disease.

563–567. The answers are: 563-C, 564-D, 565-A, 566-E, 567-A. *(Braunwald, ed 11, chaps 78, 213.)* Approximately 12 percent of lung cancers may present with or develop an endocrine paraneoplastic syndrome. Ectopic parathyroid hormone production leading to hypercalcemia is seen most frequently with epidermoid carcinoma, while ectopic production of ACTH leading to Cushing's syndrome is most commonly seen in small cell cancer. Adenocarcinomas generally arise in a peripheral location unrelated to the bronchi except by contiguous growth or lymph node metastases. Although all lung cancers may be metastatic at the time of presentation, this phenomenon is most common with small cell cancer in which pretreatment staging reveals metastases to bone 40 percent of the time, to liver 30 percent of the time, and to bone marrow 15 to 25 percent of the time. Bronchoalveolar carcinoma presents either as a single nodule or in a multinodular pattern. It is usually associated with prior fibrotic lung disease, including repeated pneumonias, granulomas, and idiopathic pulmonary fibrosis. It is not strongly correlated with smoking.

568–570. The answers are: 568-A, 569-E, 570-C. *(Braunwald, ed 11, chap 79.)* Many of the anticancer chemotherapeutic drugs are associated with toxic reactions relatively unique to their use. If procarbazine, a methyl hydrazine derivative, is taken together with ethyl alcohol, a reaction may develop that resembles the acetaldehyde syndrome produced by disulfiram (Antabuse). This reaction occurs because of procarbazine's weak monoamine oxidase inhibitor activity. Because allopurinol is a xanthine oxidase inhibitor, it is capable of blocking the metabolism of 6-mercaptopurine. As a result, the likelihood of toxicity is increased if the dose of 6-mercaptopurine is not reduced accordingly. No reduction in dose of 6-thioguanine is necessary when used together with allopurinol. Barbiturates stimulate hepatic enzymes and therefore increase the activation and, consequently, the toxicity of cyclophosphamide.

ENDOCRINE, METABOLIC, AND GENETIC DISORDERS

DIRECTIONS: Each question below contains five suggested answers. Choose the **one best** response to each question.

571. A 23-year-old woman with chronic sinusitis is noted to have an enlarged sella turcica on an x-ray series of the paranasal sinuses. She has no other recognized medical problems. The next step in the evaluation of this woman should be

(A) magnetic resonance imaging
(B) CT scanning of the head
(C) measurement of plasma gonadotropins
(D) visual field testing by Goldmann perimetry
(E) repeat sella x-rays in 6 months

572. A 26-year-old diabetic man is evaluated for poor control of diabetes. He had taken 30 units of NPH insulin each morning for several years and had consistently negative or trace urine sugars before meals. However, during the last few weeks he increased the dosage to 38 units each morning because of increasing glycosuria, detected in the bedtime urine sample. He has gained 2.2 kg (5 lb) during the last month. He has noted increasingly severe hunger pangs and headaches before dinner for the last week, but bedtime urine sugars have not diminished.

The most appropriate management at this point would be to

(A) begin the man on regular insulin at 5 P.M., according to the plasma glucose level at bedtime
(B) increase the dosage of NPH insulin, according to the plasma glucose level at bedtime
(C) decrease the dosage of NPH insulin gradually (initially by 10 percent)
(D) continue the same dosage of insulin but decrease the caloric intake at dinner
(E) switch from ordinary NPH to pork NPH insulin

573. Evidence of continuing ovarian estrogen production in a 29-year-old woman being evaluated for secondary amenorrhea is

(A) normal plasma estrone and luteinizing hormone (LH) levels
(B) normal plasma prolactin level
(C) an increase in plasma estradiol level following administration of human chorionic gonadotropin (hCG)
(D) appearance of menses following a short course of progestogen therapy
(E) normal bone density

574. A 7-year-old girl is referred for evaluation of vaginal bleeding for 2 months. Her mother says that she has not been exposed to exogenous estrogens. Physical examination reveals height at the 98th percentile, Tanner stage III breast development, and no axillary or pubic hair. No abdominal or pelvic masses are palpated. Neurologic examination is normal. Radiographic and laboratory evaluation reveals the following results:

Skull films: normal sella; no intracerebral calcifications
Bone age: 10 years
Urinary 17-ketosteroids: 0.5 mg/g creatinine/24 h
Urinary gonadotropins: undetectable

The appropriate next step in the management of this girl would be

(A) exploratory laparotomy
(B) treatment with medroxyprogesterone acetate
(C) measurement of plasma androstenedione level
(D) abdominal CT scanning and pelvic sonography
(E) karyotype analysis

575. A 42-year-old man (indicated by the star in the family history below) has renal failure due to Alport's syndrome, which is hereditary nephritis associated with sensorineural deafness and is inherited as an autosomal dominant defect. He is being evaluated for a renal transplant from a living related donor. The best candidate for evaluation as a potential kidney donor for this man would be his

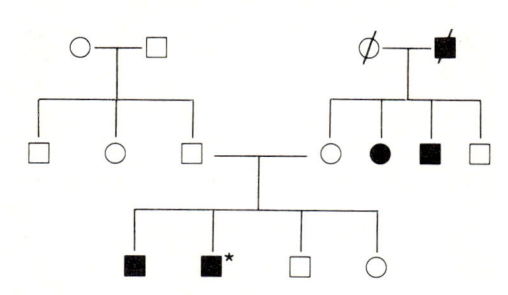

■ Renal failure
/ Deceased

(A) mother
(B) father
(C) unaffected brother
(D) sister
(E) none of the above

576. Which of the following pairs of chromosomal trisomies is most likely to allow survival of a patient into adult life?

(A) 47,XXY or trisomy 18
(B) Trisomies 21 or 13
(C) Any autosomal trisomy
(D) 47,XXX or trisomy 21
(E) Trisomy 16 or 13

577. A 42-year-old alcoholic man has eaten poorly for the last 10 days but has continued to drink. His family brings him to the emergency room. On neurologic examination he is confused but otherwise normal. Blood glucose concentration is 50 mg/dL. Intravenous infusion of a bolus of 50% glucose solution is given. His confusion worsens, and he develops horizontal nystagmus, ataxia, and a heart rate of 130/min.

At this point, the man's physician should

(A) order an immediate CT scan of the head
(B) perform a lumbar puncture
(C) administer another bolus of 50% glucose solution
(D) administer intravenous folic acid, 5 mg
(E) administer intramuscular thiamine, 50 mg

578. A 32-year-old alcoholic man is admitted to the hospital because of acute abdominal pain. Hemorrhagic necrosis of the pancreas is found during emergency laparotomy. Postoperatively, he becomes septic and hyperglycemic. Mechanical ventilation for respiratory failure is required, and attempts to wean him from the ventilator are begun 3 days later. Which of the following daily regimens would provide the most appropriate form of nutrition for this man (assuming that each regimen would include the required amounts of calories, vitamins, and minerals and that the hyperglycemia can be controlled with insulin)?

(A) A defined-formula liquid diet given through a small-bore nasogastric tube
(B) Peripheral intravenous infusion of 3 L of a 25% dextrose solution containing 2% amino acids
(C) Central intravenous infusion of 3 L of a 25% dextrose solution containing 2% amino acids
(D) Peripheral intravenous infusion of 1.5 L of a 25% dextrose solution containing 4% amino acids and mixed with 1 L of a 10% lipid solution
(E) Peripheral intravenous infusion of 1 L of a 12% dextrose solution containing 6% amino acids and mixed with 2 L of a 10% lipid solution

579. After apical scars are found on chest x-ray in a 48-year-old postmenopausal woman, chemoprophylaxis with isoniazid is begun. Two months later the woman complains of weakness, nausea, and tingling in the feet. Physical examination is unremarkable, and routine blood and urine tests are normal. Four weeks later she has a grand-mal seizure and is admitted to the hospital. Findings on the admission physical include seborrheic dermatitis, glossitis, and absent ankle and knee tendon reflexes; hematologic testing reveals microcytic anemia.

At this point, the woman's physician should

(A) order immediate electroencephalography
(B) order CT scan of the brain
(C) discontinue isoniazid and begin treatment with rifampin
(D) administer intramuscular pyridoxine, 100 mg, then give 50 mg orally daily
(E) administer intramuscular cyanocobalamin, 100 μg, then give 100 μg daily for 1 week

580. The condition LEAST likely to result in the formation of calcium-containing kidney stones is

(A) idiopathic hypercalciuria
(B) hyperuricosuria
(C) primary hyperparathyroidism
(D) cancer of the breast metastatic to bone
(E) renal tubular acidosis, distal type

581. A person with hypercalcemia due to sarcoidosis would likely have all but which one of the following?

(A) An abnormal chest x-ray
(B) Increased absorption of calcium from the gastrointestinal tract
(C) Hypercalciuria
(D) Increased serum parathyroid hormone level
(E) Hypergammaglobulinemia

582. A 67-year-old man with chronic arthritis is found to have passed a uric acid stone after an episode of renal colic. On workup he is found to have multiple radiolucent stones in the left renal pelvis, uric acid excretion of 900 mg per day, a serum uric acid concentration of 9.8 mg/dL, a serum creatinine concentration of 1.8 mg/dL, and monosodium urate crystals in an effusion in the left knee. The drug of choice for long-term therapy in this patient is

(A) probenecid alone
(B) probenecid and sodium bicarbonate
(C) allopurinol
(D) colchicine
(E) sulfinpyrazone

583. Decreased levels of high-density lipoprotein (HDL) have been found to be associated with all the following EXCEPT

(A) diabetes mellitus
(B) hypertriglyceridemia
(C) obesity
(D) Tangier disease
(E) alcoholism

584. A patient has a serum triglyceride concentration of 4000 mg/dL, a serum cholesterol concentration of 600 mg/dL, eruptive xanthomas, and lipemia retinalis. The serum shows a creamy upper layer with a turbid infranatant after overnight refrigeration. These findings are most consistent with which of the following plasma lipoprotein patterns?

(A) Type 1
(B) Type 2
(C) Type 3
(D) Type 4
(E) Type 5

585. An obese woman has hypertriglyceridemia without hypercholesterolemia. The most appropriate first step in the treatment of this woman would be

(A) abstinence from alcohol
(B) weight reduction
(C) avoidance of oral contraceptives
(D) clofibrate therapy
(E) bile acid-binding resin therapy

586. Among the following hereditary hyperlipidemias, which is NOT associated with increased evidence of premature atherosclerosis?

(A) Familial hypercholesterolemia, heterozygous form
(B) Familial hypertriglyceridemia
(C) Familial lipoprotein lipase deficiency
(D) Familial combined hyperlipidemia
(E) Familial type III hyperlipoproteinemia

587. Cholestyramine and colestipol are binding resins that are used to treat patients with hypercholesterolemia. Their serum-cholesterol-lowering effects are thought to be mediated by

(A) causing mild diarrhea and a mild degree of fat malabsorption
(B) binding of intestinal cholesterol, thus decreasing its net absorption
(C) decreasing the intestinal synthesis of very low density lipoproteins
(D) interrupting the enterophepatic circulation of cholesterol by sequestering bile acids in the intestine
(E) none of the above

588. A 28-year-old woman who is 15 kg (33 lb) over ideal body weight wants to begin dieting. The best initial regimen for weight loss would be

(A) a low-calorie balanced diet
(B) a low-calorie, liquid protein diet ("protein-sparing modified fast")
(C) total starvation
(D) use of amphetamines to curb appetite
(E) an increase in exercise but no dietary changes

589. Obese persons are at an increased risk for all the following disorders EXCEPT

(A) hypothyroidism
(B) cholelithiasis
(C) diabetes mellitus
(D) hypertension
(E) hypertriglyceridemia

590. In persons who have untreated diabetes mellitus, insulin resistance most often is caused by

(A) the production of antibodies to insulin
(B) the production of antibodies to insulin receptors
(C) prolonged insulin deficiency
(D) obesity
(E) acanthosis nigricans

591. A 30-year-old woman who has had oligomenorrhea and galactorrhea for the last 2 years is found to have a serum prolactin level of 85 ng/mL. Contrast-enhanced CT scan of the sella turcica is normal. The next stage of her evaluation should be

(A) referral for formal visual field testing
(B) assessment of thyroid function
(C) measurement of plasma FSH and LH levels
(D) measurement of serum prolactin level following administration of thyrotropin-releasing hormone (TRH)
(E) assessment of galactorrhea during a 1-week trial of bromocriptine, 2.5 mg/day

592. A person with Cushing's disease undergoes transsphenoidal removal of an ACTH-secreting microadenoma. Routine endocrinologic management after recovery from surgery should include administration of

(A) hydrocortisone, 30 mg/day
(B) hydrocortisone, 100 mg/day
(C) hydrocortisone, 30 mg/day, and levothyroxine, 0.1 mg/day
(D) hydrocortisone, 100 mg/day, and desmopressin, 0.2 µg/day
(E) none of the above

593. Which of the following statements is true regarding Cushing's disease caused by bilateral adrenal hyperplasia?

(A) Cortisol production may increase during administration of metyrapone
(B) Urinary 17-ketosteroid excretion is usually normal
(C) Plasma cortisol concentration may be maintained at a level less than 20 µg/dL
(D) Administration of dexamethasone, 8 mg/day for 2 days, reduces cortisol production only minimally
(E) Administration of dexamethasone, 2 mg/day for 2 days, is not followed by a reduction in urinary free cortisol excretion

594. A 34-year-old woman, who has had insulin-dependent diabetes mellitus since 19 years of age, has developed during the preceding 8 months increasing fatigability, paresthesias and edema in the legs and feet, a 6.8-kg (15-lb.) weight gain, and oligomenorrhea. Laboratory evaluation reveals the following:

Fasting plasma glucose: 170 mg/dL
Blood urea nitrogen: 95 mg/dL
Serum creatinine: 8.8 mg/dL
Serum calcium: 6.2 mg/dL
Serum phosphorus: 7.9 mg/dL
Serum cholesterol: 350 mg/dL
Serum thyroxine: 1.5 µg/dL; resin tri-iodothyronine uptake: 85%
Plasma cortisol (following 25 units of cosyntropin): 11 µg/dL
Urine protein: 14 g/24 h

The most likely explanation for the findings presented above would be

(A) panhypopituitarism secondary to development of a chromophobe adenoma
(B) polyglandular endocrine failure involving the thyroid, adrenal, and parathyroid glands, the pancreatic islets, and the ovaries
(C) panhypopituitarism secondary to pituitary infarction
(D) inadequate adherence to prescribed diet and insulin regimen
(E) development of renal failure and secondary hyperparathyroidism

595. The most common finding in the endocrine evaluation of patients with the empty sella syndrome is

(A) hypogonadotropic hypogonadism and hyposmia
(B) hyperprolactinemia
(C) ACTH deficiency
(D) recurrent episodes of hypoglycemia
(E) none of the above

596. A 42-year-old woman has obesity, weakness, and mild hypertension. She complains of menstrual irregularity for the last few months. Physical examination discloses some pink abdominal striae. Fasting blood glucose level is 189 mg/dL. The most appropriate means to rule out Cushing's syndrome in this woman would be

(A) CT of the pituitary gland
(B) measurement of 24-hour urinary free cortisol excretion
(C) measurement of 24-hour urinary 17-hydroxycorticosteroid excretion
(D) overnight dexamethasone suppresion test
(E) measurement of the morning plasma ACTH level

597. A 28-year-old woman is referred because of failure to menstruate during the 7 months since the delivery of an infant. She is still nursing the baby. Measurement of a random serum prolactin level obtained elsewhere was 310 ng/mL. After obtaining a pertinent history and physical examination, your next step in the evaluation of this patient's condition would be which of the following?

(A) Trial of low-dose bromocriptine to assess suppressibility of the hyperprolactinemic state
(B) Computed tomography of the head and pituitary gland with contrast
(C) Magnetic resonance imaging of the head and pituitary gland with contrast
(D) Measurement of serum prolactin levels before and after nursing
(E) Delay in any further evaluation until she stops nursing

598. In the assessment of a 10-year-old girl with short stature and an abnormal growth rate, all of the following studies are of value in the initial workup EXCEPT

(A) serum thyroxine concentration
(B) measurement of random insulin-like growth factor I/somatomedin C (IGF-I/SM-C) concentration
(C) measurement of random plasma growth hormone concentration
(D) radiographic assessment of bone age
(E) chromosomal karyotype

599. A 64-year-old man seeks medical attention because of annoying cough. Physical examination is remarkable only for supraclavicular lymphadenopathy. Chest x-ray shows a parahilar mass and paratracheal lymph node enlargement. Serum and urine chemistries are as follows:

Sodium: 120 meq/L
Potassium: 4 meq/L
Bicarbonate: 23 meq/L
Serum osmolality: 250 mosmol/kg H_2O
Urine osmolality: 600 mosmol/kg H_2O
Urine sodium: 80 meq/L

The most likely pathophysiologic basis for this man's hyponatremia is

(A) production of a vasopressin-like molecule by tumor tissue
(B) production of authentic vasopressin by tumor tissue
(C) potentiation of vasopressin action on the renal tubule by a tumor product
(D) stimulation of neurohypophyseal vasopressin secretion by a tumor product
(E) central nervous system metastases resulting in loss of vasopressin regulation

600. In a person who has chronic inappropriate AVP (vasopressin) secretion due to bronchogenic carcinoma, the agent most likely to be effective in supplementing the benefit of a water restriction regimen would be

(A) ethanol
(B) phenytoin
(C) lithium
(D) desmopressin
(E) demeclocycline

601. A 27-year-old man is involved in a motor vehicle accident and sustains trauma. He is brought to the hospital unconscious. Within 24 hours he has polyuria (250 mL urine output per hour). Urine osmolality is 120 mosmol/kg H_2O. Plasma osmolality is 340 mosmol/kg H_2O, and plasma sodium concentration is 160 meq/L. In addition to volume and free water replacement as necessary, treatment of this patient should include the use of

(A) vasopressin tannate in oil
(B) lypressin nasal spray
(C) carbamazepine
(D) desmopressin
(E) chlorpropamide

602. Impaired peripheral conversion of thyroxine (T_4) to tri-iodothyronine (T_3) is associated with the administration of all the following agents EXCEPT

(A) propylthiouracil
(B) dexamethasone
(C) methimazole
(D) propranolol
(E) oral cholecystography dye

603. Eight years after surgical resection of a benign nodule in the left lobe of her thyroid gland, a 35-year-old woman presents with a right-sided neck mass. Her thyroid scan is shown below. She is asymptomatic and takes no medication. Which of the following should her physician advise?

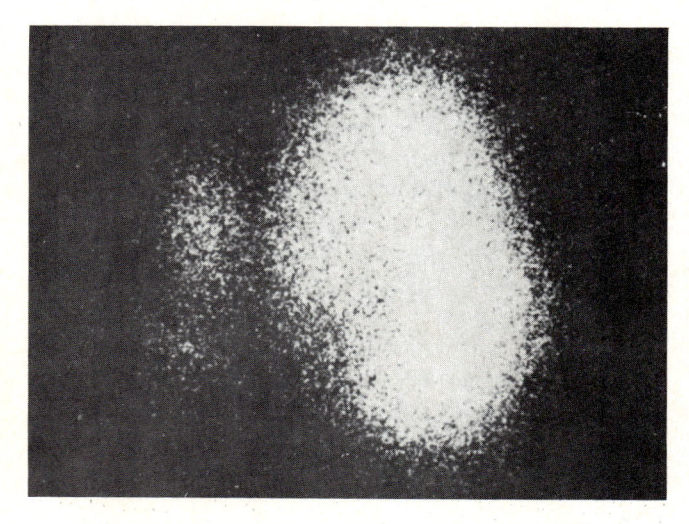

(A) Diagnostic ultrasonography
(B) Surgical exploration of the right side of the neck
(C) Measurement of plasma calcitonin concentration
(D) Reevaluation in 1 year
(E) Exogenous thyroid hormone therapy

604. A 26-year-old pregnant woman has a goiter but is clinically euthyroid. Thyroid function tests reveal a free thyroxine index that is slightly elevated. The test that would be most appropriate in determining whether the woman is euthyroid or hyperthyroid is

(A) radioactive iodine uptake
(B) technetium thyroid scan
(C) T_3 suppression test
(D) thyrotropin-releasing hormone (TRH) stimulation test
(E) thyroid-stimulating hormone (TSH) stimulation test

605. A 24-year-old woman develops Graves' disease during the third trimester of pregnancy. The most appropriate treatment would be

(A) subtotal thyroidectomy
(B) propylthiouracil
(C) propylthiouracil and levothyroxine
(D) radioactive iodine
(E) propranolol

606. In treating a 25-year-old man who has both hypothyroidism and adrenal insufficiency, his physician should

(A) prescribe an initial replacement dosage of hydrocortisone that would be higher than usual
(B) begin treatment with levothyroxine at a low dosage (less than 50 μg/day), then gradually increase it
(C) begin treatment with hydrocortisone, 30 mg/day, and levothyroxine, 100 μg/day, simultaneously
(D) check serum cortisol and thyroxine levels every 3 to 4 weeks during the first several months of hormonal replacement
(E) none of the above

607. In a 44-year-old woman with a subnormal serum thyroxine level and a history of treatment at the age of 29 years with radioactive iodine for Graves' disease, the best confirmatory test for suspected primary hypothyroidism is measurement of which of the following?

(A) Serum tri-iodothyronine (T_3) concentration
(B) Serum reverse tri-iodothyronine (rT_3) concentration
(C) Serum thyroid-stimulating hormone (TSH) concentration
(D) 24-hour radioactive iodine uptake
(E) Thyrotropin-releasing hormone (TRH) stimulation test to measure TSH reserve

608. A 20-year-old man who has been treated with high-dose daily steroids for 3 weeks during an exacerbation of asthma is switched to alternate-day prednisone therapy. Four days later, he complains of muscle weakness, arthralgias, and fatigue; in addition, his temperature is 37.8°C (100°F). His physician should

(A) order a blood sample for antinuclear antibody determination
(B) order a blood sample for creatine phosphokinase determination
(C) search for an occult infection
(D) immediately switch back to daily steroid administration
(E) reassure the man that this problem is common and self-limited

609. In persons with congenital adrenal hyperplasia due to inherited defects of adrenal steroid C-21 hydroxylase, excessive androgen production is the result of

(A) autonomous adrenal production of steroids
(B) autonomous pituitary production of ACTH
(C) extraglandular formation from large amounts of nonandrogenic adrenal steroids
(D) failure of production of an adrenal product necessary for negative feedback on pituitary ACTH secretion
(E) positive feedback on pituitary ACTH secretion by abnormal adrenal products

610. A 38-year-old woman with obesity, dermal striae, and hypertension is referred for endocrinologic evaluation of possible cortisol excess. The woman receives a midnight dose of 1 mg of dexamethasone; a plasma cortisol level drawn at 8 A.M. the next day is 14 µg/dL. At this point in the evaluation, the most appropriate diagnostic maneuver would be

(A) CT scanning of the pituitary gland
(B) abdominal CT scanning
(C) measurement of 24-h 17-hydroxycorticosteroid excretion in urine
(D) two-day low-dose dexamethasone suppression test (0.5 mg every 6 h for 48 h)
(E) two-day high-dose dexamethasone suppression test (2.0 g every 6 h for 48 h)

611. The most likely cause of Cushing's syndrome in a 65-year-old man would be

(A) basophilic pituitary adenoma
(B) adrenal adenoma
(C) adrenal carcinoma
(D) ectopic production of corticotropin-releasing hormone
(E) ectopic production of ACTH

612. In a 36-year-old woman who has had insulin-dependent diabetes mellitus since the age of 14 years, hyperkalemia is being evaluated. On physical examination her blood pressure is 146/96 mmHg. Laboratory evaluation discloses the following:

Fasting plasma glucose: 110 mg/dL
Serum creatinine: 2.2 mg/dL
Serum sodium: 135 meq/L
Serum potassium: 6.2 meq/L
Serum chloride: 116 meq/L
Serum bicarbonate: 14 meq/L

After a short ACTH infusion test, the plasma cortisol concentration increases from 14 to 26 µg/dL. After administration of 80 mg of furosemide and 3 hours of upright posture, the plasma renin activity and aldosterone concentration are unchanged from baseline values.

The most appropriate therapeutic regimen to correct the electrolyte imbalance would be

(A) administration of fludrocortisone and furosemide
(B) restriction of potassium intake
(C) administration of hydrocortisone and furosemide
(D) hemodialysis
(E) administration of potassium-binding anion-exchange resins

613. The best indicator of how well an individual's diabetes has been controlled over an extended length of time (months) is

(A) hemoglobin A_{1c} concentration
(B) glycosylated albumin concentration
(C) plasma C-peptide concentration
(D) mean of the blood sugar levels measured throughout the day
(E) 24-h urine glucose excretion

614. A 22-year-old woman who has had diabetes for 6 years now wishes to become pregnant. She takes 32 units of NPH insulin each morning, and her urine glucose values (done twice daily) are "usually trace or 1+." Her hemoglobin A$_{1c}$ level is 9.8% (normal: 5–8%). She takes oral contraceptive pills. Her physician should advise her that

(A) home glucose monitoring and a daily regimen of multiple subcutaneous injections of regular insulin are necessary now
(B) oral contraceptive agents can falsely elevate HbA$_{1c}$ levels
(C) attempts to achieve better diabetic control can wait until she has become pregnant
(D) the current insulin regimen probably will be adequate until the last trimester of pregnancy
(E) hospitalization will probably be necessary for most of her pregnancy to ensure normal delivery and perinatal survival

615. A 24-year-old man with diabetes since the age of 9 years sees his physician for a routine checkup. He has no complaints and is taking 40 units NPH and 5 units regular insulin each morning as prescribed. Funduscopic exam reveals the findings in Color Plate A. Based on these findings, his physician should recommend

(A) vitrectomy
(B) photocoagulation
(C) hypophysectomy
(D) more vigorous control of the blood sugar level
(E) followup examination in 3 months

616. A middle-aged diabetic man who has been taking chlorpropamide, 0.5 g daily, becomes confused and lethargic at home. He is brought to the emergency room, where examination is otherwise negative. Blood glucose concentration is 24 mg/dL. He is given 50 mL of a 50% intravenous glucose solution and becomes more responsive. His physician should now

(A) send the man home with instructions to decrease the dosage of chlorpropamide to 0.25 g daily
(B) send the man home with instructions to switch to tolbutamide, 0.5 g three times daily
(C) observe the man for several more hours and send him home if no further problems develop
(D) have the man eat a meal, then administer a 5% glucose solution intravenously for 12 hours, and send him home if no further problems develop
(E) have the man eat a meal, then admit him to the hospital for further observation and treatment

617. A 24-year-old pregnant woman with diabetes mellitus receiving NPH insulin has fasting blood glucose values in the 120 to 140 mg/dL range while taking 35 U in the morning. Glycosuria is present only intermittently. The most appropriate management at this time would be

(A) oral glucose tolerance test
(B) restriction of carbohydrates in the diet
(C) to increase the insulin dose if glycosuria worsens
(D) to institute intensive insulin therapy to maintain nonfasting blood glucose levels below 110 mg/dL
(E) none of the above

618. A 16-year-old girl with diabetes mellitus has morning headaches and glycosuria (3+) before breakfast. She has been receiving NPH insulin, 40 U in the morning and 28 U in the evening. She is asymptomatic during the day. The appropriate management of this patient would consist in

(A) increasing the NPH insulin dose by 5 U in the morning and evening
(B) adding 10 U of regular insulin to the NPH doses
(C) decreasing the morning NPH dose to 35 U and increasing the evening NPH dose to 33 U
(D) decreasing the evening NPH dose to 20 U
(E) restricting carbohydrate intake at dinner time

619. A patient develops hypotension following an acute myocardial infarction. All the following phenomena can contribute to the development of lactic acidosis in such a patient EXCEPT

(A) diminished hepatic uptake of lactate
(B) peripheral tissue hypoperfusion and hypoxia
(C) a fall in cellular NADH/NAD ratio
(D) accelerated tissue glycolysis and pyruvate production
(E) a decline in tissue ATP concentration

620. An 18-year-old woman fasts for 24 hours. The metabolic changes that would be expected at the end of the fasting period include all the following EXCEPT

(A) dependence by the brain on ketone metabolism
(B) breakdown of triglycerides in adipose tissue
(C) utilization of lactate, glycerol, and amino acids for hepatic gluconeogenesis
(D) a decrease in liver glycogen
(E) a fall in plasma insulin concentration and a rise in release of glucagon, cortisol, growth hormone, and epinephrine

621. A 52-year-old woman has hepatomegaly. Percutaneous liver biopsy reveals "adenocarcinoma," but the woman refuses further evaluation or treatment. A year later she presents with weight loss (13.6 kg, 30 lb) and a skin rash that has waxed and waned. Examination shows angular stomatitis and a firm, enlarged liver. An erythematous, bullous, necrotic skin rash (Color Plate B) is present on the face, perineum, and legs. Sonography reveals an enlarged pancreas. Hematologic testing shows the woman to be anemic.

The diagnostic test of choice would be

(A) serum amylase determination
(B) plasma glucagon determination
(C) plasma vasoactive intestinal polypeptide (VIP) determination
(D) plasma gastrin determination
(E) pancreatic arteriography

622. Impaired spermatogenesis associated with male infertility but unimpaired testosterone production is a common manifestation of all the following conditions affecting testicular function EXCEPT

(A) varicocele
(B) androgen resistance
(C) Klinefelter syndrome
(D) germinal cell aplasia
(E) paraplegia

623. The effectiveness of testosterone cypionate therapy in a 40-year-old man with long-standing hypogonadism resulting from total surgical castration because of bilateral seminomas at the age of 17 years can best be monitored by the assessment of

(A) plasma testosterone level
(B) plasma luteinizing hormone (LH) level
(C) plasma testosterone cypionate level
(D) change in muscle mass
(E) frequency of nocturnal erections

624. A 20-year-old swimmer is examined because of primary amenorrhea. Her height is 170 cm (67 in) and she weighs 50 kg (110 lb). Her breasts are well developed. Findings on pelvic examination are normal, and the pelvic hair appears to be normal. Cervical mucus is abundant and demonstrates ferning upon drying. Urine spot and blood tests for pregnancy are negative. She is given 10 mg of medroxyprogesterone acetate twice a day for 5 days, and 3 days later she experiences menstrual bleeding for the first time.

The most likely cause of the amenorrhea is

(A) functional hypothalamic amenorrhea
(B) 45,X gonadal dysgenesis
(C) polycystic ovarian disease
(D) chromophobe adenoma of the pituitary
(E) prolactinoma of the pituitary

625. A 21-year-old woman is examined because of secondary amenorrhea. Cyclic menses had commenced at the age of 14 years. When she was 19 years old she became pregnant and was hospitalized during the sixth month of that pregnancy because of bleeding and hypotension that proved to be the result of a spontaneous abortion with retained placental fragments; she received ten units of blood, and a dilation and curettage was performed. No menses have occurred during the two years since the hospitalization. She now wishes to become pregnant.

Findings on physical examination, including rectopelvic examination, are normal. Results on complete blood counts, SMA-12, and chest x-ray are within normal limits. Serum thyroxine (T_4) concentration is 7 μg/dL and an 8 A.M. plasma cortisol measurement is 17 μg/dL. No menstrual bleeding occurs after administration of 10 mg medroxyprogesterone acetate per day for 10 days or cyclic estrogen and progestogen (1.25 mg conjugated estrogens by mouth each day for three weeks with 10 mg medroxyprogesterone acetate per day for the last 7 days).

At this point the most appropriate diagnostic study would be

(A) CT scan of the pituitary with contrast
(B) hysterosalpingogram
(C) CT scan of the abdomen followed by wedge resection of the ovaries
(D) metyrapone test
(E) chromosomal analysis

626. A 36-year-old woman has noticed the absence of menses for the last 4 months. A pregnancy test is negative. Serum levels of luteinizing hormone and follicle-stimulating hormone are elevated, and the serum estradiol level is low. These findings suggest

(A) bilateral tubal obstruction
(B) panhypopituitarism
(C) polycystic ovarian disease
(D) premature menopause
(E) exogenous estrogen administration

627. A newborn infant with ambiguous genitalia develops vomiting and profound volume depletion. A diagnosis of congenital adrenal hyperplasia due to C-21 hydroxylase deficiency would be supported by all the following findings EXCEPT

(A) elevated urinary 17-ketosteroid concentration
(B) elevated plasma 11-deoxycortisol concentration
(C) elevated plasma 17-hydroxyprogesterone concentration
(D) elevated plasma androstenedione concentration
(E) elevated urinary pregnanediol and pregnanetriol concentrations

628. In women with gonadal dysgenesis, development of malignancy in the streak gonads is most likely when the karyotype is

(A) 46XX$_i$ (isochrome X)
(B) 46,XX
(C) 45,X
(D) 45,X/46,XY mosaicism
(E) 45X,46XX mosaicism

629. The most common presentation of primary hyperparathyroidism is

(A) peptic ulcer
(B) proximal muscle weakness
(C) osteitis fibrosa cystica
(D) calcium kidney stones
(E) asymptomatic hypercalcemia

630. The diagnosis of primary hyperparathyroidism is made in an elderly woman who has osteitis fibrosa cystica and elevated serum levels of calcium (12.0 mg/dL) and creatinine (3.5 mg/dL). The woman is not considered a surgical candidate because of pulmonary disease. The best medical treatment for hyperparathyroidism in this woman would be

(A) plicamycin
(B) estrogen
(C) phosphate
(D) diphosphonate
(E) thiazide

631. Prolonged immobilization has been associated with all the following consequences EXCEPT

(A) hypercalcemia
(B) hypercalciuria and nephrolithiasis
(C) osteoporosis
(D) soft-tissue calcifications
(E) elevation of serum parathyroid hormone levels

632. A 54-year-old man with peptic ulcer disease has been using aluminum hydroxide-containing antacids for the past several years to treat his symptoms. He complains of diffuse bone pain and progressive muscular weakness. These symptoms are most likely a result of

(A) malnutrition associated with his ulcer symptoms
(B) occult gastric malignancy
(C) aluminum-induced osteomalacia
(D) chronic phosphorus depletion
(E) aluminum intoxication

633. A 34-year-old woman has had three hospital admissions during the last year because of nephrolithiasis. Twenty-four-hour urinary calcium excretion has been above the normal range on all three occasions, and serum calcium concentrations were between 10.2 and 11.5 mg/dL. The serum phosphorus concentration was 2.4 mg/dL and the parathyroid hormone level was 229 nL eq/mL (normal less than 150 nL eq/mL).

The most appropriate management at this time would be

(A) to begin administration of prednisone, 40 mg daily, and taper the dose over a period of 4 weeks
(B) to administer thiazide diuretics to decrease calcium excretion
(C) symptomatic treatment of renal lithiasis only
(D) calcium supplementation to prevent progressive bone loss
(E) surgical exploration of the neck

634. Each of the following conditions is characteristic of the presentation of osteomalacia in adults EXCEPT which one?

(A) Bowing of the tibia
(B) Pseudofractures
(C) Long-bone pain
(D) Proximal muscle weakness
(E) Hypophosphatemia

635. During a routine checkup, a 67-year-old man is found to have a serum alkaline phosphatase activity of three times the upper limit of normal. Serum calcium and phosphorus concentrations and liver function test results are normal. He is asymptomatic. The most likely diagnosis is

(A) metastatic bone disease
(B) primary hyperparathyroidism
(C) occult plasmacytoma
(D) Paget's disease of bone
(E) osteomalacia

636. The vitamin D metabolite that regulates absorption of calcium from the gastrointestinal tract is

(A) dihydrotachysterol
(B) cholecalciferol
(C) 24,25(OH)$_2$D
(D) 1,25(OH)$_2$D
(E) 25OH vitamin D

637. A 61-year-old woman noticed severe sharp pain in her back after lifting a suitcase. A compression fracture of the T11 vertebral body is identified on x-ray examination. Routine laboratory evaluation discloses a serum calcium concentration of 8.0 mg/dL, a serum phosphorus concentration of 2.4 mg/dL, and increased serum alkaline phosphatase activity. The serum parathyroid hormone level was subsequently found to be elevated as well.

The most likely diagnosis is

(A) Paget's disease of bone
(B) ectopic parathyroid hormone secretion
(C) primary hyperparathyroidism
(D) postmenopausal osteoporosis
(E) vitamin D deficiency

638. Which of the following conditions is associated with hypocalcemia but NOT with an increased serum level of parathyroid hormone?

(A) Severe hypomagnesemia
(B) Osteomalacia secondary to vitamin D deficiency
(C) Osteomalacia secondary to vitamin D resistance
(D) Renal failure
(E) Pseudohypoparathyroidism

639. The most important regulator of serum 1,25(OH)$_2$ vitamin D concentration is

(A) serum calcium
(B) serum magnesium
(C) serum 25OH vitamin D
(D) parathyroid hormone
(E) prolactin

DIRECTIONS: Each question below contains five suggested answers. For **each** of the five alternatives of **each** item, you are to respond either YES (Y) or NO (N). In a given item all, some, or none of the alternatives may be correct.

640. Anovulatory cycles are characterized by

(A) elevated levels of plasma progesterone
(B) dysmenorrhea
(C) an absent luteal phase
(D) lack of a normal LH and FSH surge
(E) irregular uterine bleeding

641. A 25-year-old woman whose father and brother both have documented Marfan's syndrome desires counseling prior to marriage. Her clinical condition has not previously been medically evaluated. History and physical examination are uninformative. Slit-lamp examination reveals a partial subluxation of the lens in one eye. Which of the following would be appropriate to tell the patient?

(A) Advise the patient that if she becomes pregnant she should have amniocentesis to detect any chromosomal abnormalities
(B) Inform the patient that each of her sons will have a 50 percent chance of having Marfan's syndrome but that the daughters will not be affected.
(C) Inform the patient about her increased risk of development of cardiovascular disorders with pregnancy
(D) Inform the patient that if she has children with Marfan's syndrome they will be no more severely affected than she is
(E) Advise the patient that the chance of any offspring having Marfan's syndrome is miniscule provided she does not marry a first-degree relative

642. Which of the following statements regarding the pedigree analysis of an autosomally transmitted dominant disorder are true?

(A) Males and females are affected in equal proportions
(B) On average, half the siblings of an affected patient will be affected with the disorder
(C) Persons of each gender are likely to transmit the condition to male and female offspring
(D) Normal children of an affected parent will have only normal offspring
(E) Consanguinity is common among the parents of affected offspring

643. A 15-year-old boy has had hypothyroidism since early childhood. For several years, he has noticed frequent episodes of numbness and tingling of his hands, occasionally accompanied by muscle spasms. Physical examination reveals a positive Chvostek sign, short stature, and short left fourth metacarpals (absent knuckles). The boy's mother is also short and has absent knuckles. Serum calcium concentration is 7.5 mg/dL.

Further investigation of the boy's disorder would be expected to reveal

(A) antibodies to parathyroid and thyroid tissue
(B) elevated parathyroid hormone concentration
(C) diminished increase in urinary cyclic AMP in respond to parathyroid hormone administration
(D) calcification of the basal ganglia
(E) monilasis

644. The administration of medium-chain triglycerides is useful in the treatment of a variety of forms of malnutrition because the triglycerides

(A) are essential to human nutrition along with linoleic acid
(B) are absorbed directly through the portal circulation instead of via splanchnic lymphatics
(C) circulate in the blood for a longer than usual time, thus providing more calories
(D) are preferentially converted to carbohydrates and protein as compared with long-chain triglycerides
(E) can be absorbed despite a deficiency of bile acids

645. The decrease in protein requirement in patients with uremia is thought to be a result of which of the following mechanisms?

(A) Ammonia released from the breakdown of urea is used for the synthesis of nonessential amino acids by transamination
(B) The carbon skeletons of nonessential amino acids can be produced by the intermediary metabolism of glucose
(C) Essential amino acids are obtained from the recycling of unexcreted urea
(D) The metabolic rate slows, and hence the caloric requirement is decreased
(E) The turnover (catabolism) of protein is slowed

646. Protein malnutrition commonly occurs in association with energy-deficient diets because

(A) diets low in carbohydrate and fat cause acute protein malabsorption
(B) amino acids are diverted from protein synthesis into oxidative metabolism
(C) normal protein synthesis requires an adequate energy supply
(D) normal protein metabolism occurs only if fat in the diet is adequate
(E) it is common for diets to be deficient in both protein and energy

647. A 34-year-old man with alcoholic cirrhosis is admitted to the hospital for evaluation of abdominal swelling, which has become progressively worse over the last 2 weeks. On physical examination, he is noted to be cachectic; the liver is enlarged, ascites and edema are present, and stool is heme-positive. Measurement of which of the following parameters would be useful in determining the extent of the man's **protein** malnutrition?

(A) Blood ammonia concentration
(B) Serum albumin and transferrin levels
(C) Present body weight as a percentage of ideal body weight
(D) Midarm circumference and triceps skin-fold thickness
(E) Ratio of 24-hour creatinine excretion to height

648. Which of the following alterations are characteristic of combined protein-calorie starvation?

(A) Normal serum T_4, decreased serum T_3, and increased serum reverse T_3 (rT_3) levels
(B) Decreased serum insulin, glucagon, and cortisol levels
(C) Impaired cell-mediated immunity
(D) Decreased serum immunoglobulin levels and impaired humoral response to antigens
(E) Increased plasma free fatty acid and ketone levels

649. In a person suffering from severe protein starvation, which of the following conditions would increase the amount of protein needed to achieve positive nitrogen balance?

(A) Renal failure
(B) Gastrointestinal fistula
(C) Sepsis
(D) Simultaneous caloric malnutrition
(E) Thyrotoxicosis

650. In which of the following situations is total parenteral nutrition (TPN) indicated as the **first** choice to provide partial or complete nourishment?

(A) A 34-year-old man has an acute exacerbation of Crohn's disease and develops an ileocolic fistula
(B) A 70-year-old woman has chest and limb injuries and extensive burns following an airplane crash
(C) A 50-year-old woman with non-Hodgkin's lymphoma is about to receive a 4-week chemotherapy protocol known to produce severe nausea and vomiting
(D) A 53-year-old man scheduled to undergo elective surgery for gallstones will be unable to eat or drink for 5 days
(E) A 26-year-old woman is unable to swallow due to a relapse of myasthenia gravis

651. Appropriate dietary restrictions have been successful in treating individuals who have which of the following inherited metabolic disorders?

(A) Phenylketonuria
(B) Familial lipoprotein lipase deficiency
(C) Hyperprolinemia
(D) Tay-Sachs disease
(E) Galactosemia

652. In an individual with hypercholesterolemia, which of the following may be an appropriate treatment to lower serum cholesterol concentration?

(A) Cholestyramine
(B) Nicotinic acid
(C) Colestipol
(D) Probucol
(E) Low-cholesterol diet

653. Which of the following disorders are associated with premature coronary heart disease?

(A) Familial hypercholesterolemia
(B) Familial hyperalphalipoproteinemia
(C) Familial hypertriglyceridemia
(D) Familial combined hyperlipidemia
(E) Familial lipoprotein lipase deficiency

654. Hypertriglyceridemia is frequently encountered in patients with diabetes mellitus. True statements regarding this association include:

(A) Predisposition to both diseases may be independently inherited
(B) Insulin deficiency is a major factor contributing to the hypertriglyceridemia
(C) Some patients eventually need specific pharmacologic treatment for the hypertriglyceridemia
(D) Acute pancreatitis may occur with uncontrolled diabetes mellitus and elevation of the triglyceride levels
(E) Hypertriglyceridemia may resolve with adequate control of the diabetes

655. A 29-year-old obese man is referred because of hyperlipidemia. He consulted a dermatologist because of tuberous xanthomas in both elbows and yellowish discoloration of the palmar and digital creases. Serum cholesterol and triglyceride levels were 328 and 345 mg/dL, respectively. Which of the following statements regarding this patient are true?

(A) He has lipoprotein lipase deficiency
(B) Weight loss is an important feature of management to reduce his lipid levels
(C) Hypothyroidism or diabetes mellitus, or both, must be excluded by appropriate testing
(D) He is homozygous for a genetic defect of lipid metabolism
(E) Clofibrate may be useful in the management of his hyperlipidemia

656. Potential long-term complications of gastric bypass surgery in a 39-year-old, 160-kg (352-lb) man include

(A) polyarthritis
(B) progressive hepatic disease
(C) early satiety
(D) diarrhea
(E) nephrolithiasis

657. Which of the following statements accurately describe severely obese adults (more than 45 kg—100 lb—over ideal weight)?

(A) Obesity usually develops early in life
(B) Adipose cell size is increased
(C) Adipose cell number is increased
(D) Weight reduction causes adipose cells to decrease in size
(E) Weight reduction causes adipose cells to decrease in number

658. Insulin resistance in obese individuals results from which of the following phenomena?

(A) A decrease in the number of cell-surface insulin receptors
(B) Abnormal processing of proinsulin by pancreatic beta cells
(C) Circulating insulin antagonists
(D) Accelerated insulin degradation by the liver
(E) Postreceptor, intracellular defects in glucose metabolism

659. A 130-kg (286-lb) woman requests intestinal bypass surgery. Relative contraindications to such a procedure would include

(A) repeated failure of medical treatments for obesity
(B) active hepatitis or cirrhosis of the liver
(C) diabetes mellitus or hyperlipidemia
(D) renal failure
(E) pulmonary alveolar hypoventilation

660. Which of the following complications would be anticipated after an intestinal bypass operation for the treatment of morbid obesity?

(A) Chronic vomiting with volume depletion
(B) Osteomalacia
(C) Uric acid nephrolithiasis
(D) Polyarthritis
(E) Liver function abnormalities

661. Which of the following statements regarding the pathogenesis of human obesity are true?

(A) The resting metabolic rate is lower than normal in obese persons
(B) Endocrine diseases such as hypothyroidism and Cushing's syndrome are a frequent cause of obesity
(C) The energy expenditure of exercise is decreased in obese persons
(D) Genetic predisposition may be the most single important factor in obesity
(E) Decreased activity of lipoprotein lipase is the cause of obesity in some persons

662. Characteristic manifestations of Nelson's syndrome (pituitary tumor arising after bilateral adrenalectomy) include

(A) hyperpigmentation
(B) erosion of the sella turcica
(C) increased urinary 17-ketosteroid excretion
(D) failure of high doses of dexamethasone to suppress plasma cortisol levels
(E) elevated plasma ACTH levels

663. Growth hormone secretion is increased in normal persons in a number of situations, including

(A) exercise
(B) hyperglycemia
(C) infusion of levodopa
(D) infusion of arginine
(E) administration of thyrotropin-releasing hormone

664. A 45-year-old man who has noted decreased libido and sexual potency for the last 8 months is found to have a serum prolactin level of 70 ng/mL. Computed tomography of the head reveals a pituitary tumor with suprasellar extension. Appropriate management of this patient would include

(A) formal visual field testing
(B) initiation of treatment with bromocriptine, 2.5 mg daily
(C) reassurance about the return of sexual function as soon as prolactin levels return to normal
(D) initiation of prophylactic treatment with desmopressin
(E) determination of serum gonadotropin and testosterone levels

665. Low thyroidal radioactive iodine uptake (RAIU) in persons exhibiting weight loss and elevated free thyroxine index can be caused by which of the following disorders

(A) Painless thyroiditis
(B) Struma ovarii
(C) Choriocarcinoma
(D) Ingestion of exogenous levothyroxine
(E) Recent intravenous pyelography

666. Which of the following statements are true concerning the "sick euthyroid" syndrome?

(A) Thyroid hormone production is usually normal
(B) Values for free thyroxine (T_4) index may be decreased, normal, or increased
(C) Serum total T_4 concentrations are usually normal or decreased
(D) Decreased production of tri-iodothyronine (T_3) is a consistent feature of the disorder
(E) Although serum levels of thyroid-binding globulin and thyroid-binding prealbumin may be decreased, decreased protein binding of thyroid hormones is caused principally by a circulating inhibitor of binding

667. In a 33-year-old woman who recently had an upper respiratory tract infection, symptoms of thyrotoxicosis develop. Her thyroid gland is exquisitely tender and nodular. The 24-hour uptake of radioactive iodine is 2 percent. Appropriate treatment for this woman might include

(A) subtotal thyroidectomy
(B) administration of radioactive iodine
(C) administration of glucocorticoids
(D) administration of propranolol
(E) administration of aspirin

668. In a person who has Cushing's syndrome, the diagnosis of functioning adrenal carcinoma would be suggested by

(A) a palpable abdominal mass
(B) markedly increased urinary excretion of 17-ketosteroids
(C) high plasma levels of ACTH
(D) failure to suppress 17-hydroxycorticosteroid secretion with high-dose dexamethasone
(E) a doubling of urinary 17-hydroxycorticosteroid excretion after administration of metyrapone

669. A 52-year-old woman with systemic lupus erythematosus is about to be started on a long-term course of therapy with pharmacologic doses of glucocorticoids. Pretreatment evaluation should include

(A) chest x-ray and tuberculin skin test
(B) ACTH infusion test
(C) thoracic and lumbar spine films
(D) stool test for occult blood
(E) metyrapone test

670. The syndromes of congenital adrenal hyperplasia may result in which of the following disorders?

(A) Virilization
(B) Isosexual precocious puberty
(C) Male pseudohermaphroditism
(D) Hypertension
(E) Hypotension

671. Urinary 17-ketosteroid determination can be described by which of the following statements?

(A) It is a useful test to assess gonadal function
(B) It assesses the production of both adrenal and gonadal androgens
(C) It is a measurement primarily of androsterone and etiocholanolone excretion
(D) It usually is elevated in persons with untreated congenital adrenal hyperplasia due to C-21 hydroxylase deficiency
(E) Testosterone production usually contributes only about 40 percent of the value in men

672. Which of the following conditions contribute to the enhanced rate of hepatic ketogenesis common to starvation and diabetic ketoacidosis?

(A) A decline in the circulating insulin/glucagon ratio
(B) Decreased hepatic malonyl CoA concentration
(C) Increased levels of plasma free fatty acids
(D) Increased hepatic carnitine content
(E) Increased activity of hepatic carnitine acyltransferase I

673. Which of the following statements are true concerning insulin-dependent diabetes mellitus (IDDM)?

(A) Direct vertical transmission has been shown by pedigree analysis to occur with a high prevalence
(B) The concordance rate for monozygotic twins less than 40 years of age is over 80 percent
(C) The risk of IDDM is increased in individuals carrying HLA antigens B8, B15, Dw3, or Dw4
(D) Circulating islet-cell antibodies are usually present in patients with juvenile-onset IDDM studied soon after onset of symptoms
(E) Mumps virus and Coxsackie virus have been identified as possible causative agents in juvenile-onset IDDM

674. Which of the following are characteristic of hyperosmolar coma?

(A) Blood glucose concentration of 975 mg/dL
(B) Marked elevation of serum free fatty acids
(C) Association with thrombosis and bleeding from disseminated intravascular coagulation
(D) Occurrence in elderly persons with maturity-onset diabetes
(E) Best initial therapeutic response with large volumes of free water and large doses of insulin

675. The diagnosis of diabetes mellitus is certain in which of the following situations?

(A) Abnormal oral glucose tolerance in a 24-year-old woman who has been dieting
(B) Successive fasting plasma glucose concentrations of 147, 165, and 152 mg/100 mL in an asymptomatic, otherwise healthy businesswoman
(C) Hyperglycemic ketoacidosis that developed in an 18-year-old man after surgical reduction of a fractured leg
(D) Persistent asymptomatic glycosuria in a 30-year-old woman
(E) Hyperglycemic hyperosmolar coma that developed in a 73-year-old man after a stroke

676. A 45-year-old woman has had diabetes for the last 8 years and has been treated with either oral hypoglycemic agents or insulin. She has been doing well on Lente insulin for the last several months. However, in the last week she has developed symptoms of hyperglycemia. Doubling her insulin dosage does not help, and she is admitted to the hospital. Physical examination of this nonobese woman shows no sign of infection, ketoacidosis, or Cushing's syndrome. Following admission, insulin dosage is increased progressively to 240 units daily, but blood glucose concentration never falls below 350 mg/dL.

Which of the following statements regarding this woman's condition are true?

(A) IgG anti-insulin antibodies are likely to be present in high titer
(B) Cell-surface insulin receptors are likely to be decreased in number.
(C) Anti-insulin-receptor antibodies, increased erythrocyte sedimentation rate, and other signs of autoimmune disease are likely to be present
(D) Insulin desensitization procedures should be instituted
(E) Treatment should include switching to human insulin or high-dose prednisone (or both)

677. Which of the following would be associated with a poor prognosis for development of (or progression of) symptomatic renal failure in a 29-year-old woman who has had type I diabetes mellitus since the age of 14 years?

(A) Urine albumin excretion of 120 to 170 mg/24 h on three separate occasions
(B) Urine albumin excretion of 550 to 620 mg/24 h on three separate occasions
(C) Diastolic blood pressure of 110 to 123 mmHg
(D) Nocturia, 3 times per night
(E) Insulin requirement greater than 120 units per day

678. A 40-year-old physician's assistant has had episodic confusion, diaphoresis, and palpitations for the past 4 weeks. She has had several nightmares and three syncopal episodes. Fasting hypoglycemia with inappropriately elevated plasma insulin concentration is documented in the hospital. Plasma C-peptide concentration also is increased. Her physician should

(A) measure plasma insulin antibody levels
(B) measure plasma proinsulin levels
(C) measure plasma or urine sulfonylurea levels
(D) perform abdominal CT scan
(E) consult a surgeon for pancreatic surgery

679. Which of the following causes of fasting hypoglycemia are due primarily to overutilization of glucose?

(A) Carnitine deficiency
(B) Hepatoma
(C) Insulinoma
(D) Congestive heart failure from cor pulmonale
(E) Hypopituitarism

680. Testosterone replacement in a patient with Klinefelter's syndrome (47,XXY) would be indicated in order to

(A) maintain spermatogenesis
(B) prevent antisocial behavior
(C) maintain sexual potency
(D) cause disappearance of gynecomastia
(E) promote virilization

681. Treatment with physiologic doses of estrogen is indicated for all women who have

(A) premature ovarian failure
(B) inadequate luteal phase
(C) C-17 hydroxylase deficiency
(D) polycystic ovarian disease
(E) severe menopausal symptoms

682. Increased gonadal production of estrogen is characteristic of

(A) testicular feminization
(B) polycystic ovarian disease
(C) persistent follicle cyst
(D) third trimester or pregnancy
(E) arrhenoblastoma

683. Hot flashes (menopausal flushing) characteristically are associated with which of the following?

(A) Removal of testes in a 23-year-old 46,XY woman with the syndrome of complete testicular feminization
(B) Removal of the ovaries in a 26-year-old 46,XX woman with extensive pelvic inflammatory disease
(C) Removal of the streak gonads in a woman with the 46,XY form of pure gonadal dysgenesis
(D) Premature menopause
(E) Removal of the ovaries in a 23-year-old woman with bilateral dysgerminoma of the ovaries

684. A 38-year-old woman had a bilateral oophorectomy, and two months later she complains of hot flashes twice a day. The indications for estrogen replacement in this patient include

(A) suppression of hot flashes
(B) prevention of atrophic vaginitis
(C) prevention of accelerated loss of bone mass
(D) avoidance of the development of hirsutism
(E) prevention of breast atrophy

685. A 30-year-old man, father of three children, has had progressive breast enlargement during the last 6 months. He does not use any drugs. Physical examination is remarkable only for bilateral gynecomastia; testicular size is normal. Evaluation at this time should include

(A) blood sampling for SGOT and serum alkaline phosphatase and bilirubin levels
(B) blood sampling for plasma estradiol, testosterone, and LH levels
(C) a 24-hour urine collection for measurement of 17-ketosteroids
(D) chromosomal karyotype
(E) breast biopsy

686. Known causes of ambiguous genitalia include

(A) the sex-chromosome pattern XYY
(B) the mosaic sex-chromosome pattern 45,X/46,XY
(C) single gene mutations that impair androgen action
(D) hypogonadotropic hypogonadism
(E) maternal ingestion of a virilizing drug during pregnancy

687. Which of the following statements describing persons who have Klinefelter syndrome are true?

(A) They are 20 times as likely as normal men to develop breast cancer
(B) They may have a normal peripheral-blood karyotype and testes of average size
(C) They have an increased incidence of hypospadias
(D) They almost always are mentally deficient and socially maladjusted
(E) Diagnosis usually is not made until after puberty

688. A 40-year-old woman with known alcoholism is hospitalized because of dizziness and muscle aches. Serum phosphorus concentration is 0.9 mg/dL several days after admission. Clinical signs and symptoms associated with hypophosphatemia include

(A) waddling gait
(B) bone pain
(C) elevated serum creatine phosphokinase concentration
(D) hemolytic anemia
(E) congestive cardiomyopathy

689. Hypophosphatemia is associated with which of the following?

(A) Sweating
(B) Hyperventilation
(C) Use of nonabsorbable antacids
(D) Use of distally acting diuretics
(E) Junk-food diet

690. Serum concentration of 25OH vitamin D may be reduced in association with which of the following conditions?

(A) Dietary deficiency of vitamin D
(B) Chronic severe cholestatic liver disease
(C) Chronic renal failure
(D) Anticonvulsant therapy with phenobarbital or phenytoin
(E) High-dose glucocorticoid therapy

691. Which of the following statements concerning hypervitaminosis D are correct?

(A) It may result from prolonged sun exposure
(B) It usually results from a single excessive dose of vitamin D_2 or D_3
(C) Consequences include hypercalcemia, hypercalciuria, and renal impairment
(D) Anephric patients cannot develop vitamin D toxicity
(E) Serium 1,25(OH)$_2$ vitamin D levels are low to normal

692. A 60-year-old woman has low-back pain. Radiographic examination reveals diffuse demineralization and a compression fracture of the fourth lumbar vertebra. Serum calcium concentration is 11.5 mg/dL. This clinical picture is compatible with the presence of which of the following conditions?

(A) Postmenopausal osteoporosis
(B) Paget's disease
(C) Primary hyperparathyroidism
(D) Multiple myeloma
(E) Osteomalacia

DIRECTIONS: The groups of questions below consist of five lettered headings followed by several numbered items. For each numbered item choose the **one** lettered heading with which it is **most** closely associated. Each lettered heading may be used once, more than once, or not at all.

Questions 693–696

For each of the phenotypes described below, choose the disorder of sexual differentiation with which it is most likely to be associated.

(A) Complete testicular feminization
(B) C-21 hydroxylase deficiency
(C) 5α-reductase deficiency
(D) Cryptorchidism
(E) Pure gonadal dysgenesis

693. Bilateral streak gonads, female internal ducts, and female external genitalia

694. Bilateral testes, male internal ducts, and ambiguous external genitalia

695. Bilateral testes, absent internal ducts, and female external genitalia

696. Bilateral abdominal gonads, male internal ducts, and male external genitalia

Endocrine, Metabolic, and Genetic Disorders

Answers

571. The answer is B. *(Braunwald, ed 11, chap 32.)* The first step in evaluating a person found to have an enlarged sella turcica but no symptoms that can be related to a pituitary tumor is to rule out the possibility of an empty sella. A CT scan of the head is now the procedure of choice in examining for an empty sella. If an empty sella in an asymptomatic person is documented by a CT scan, no specific endocrinologic evaluation is necessary.

572. The answer is C. *(Braunwald, ed 11, chap 32. Bloom, Am J Med 47:891, 1969. Somogyi, Am J Med 26:169, 1959.)* Hypoglycemia is common in patients with Type I diabetes mellitus, particularly when aggressive efforts are made to bring the fasting glucose concentrations into the normal range and to control postprandial hyperglycemia. Hypoglycemia can worsen diabetic control, in large part by triggering the release of counterregulatory hormones, such as glucagon. This phenomenon of "hypoglycemic hyperglycemia," called the Somogyi effect, should be suspected when wide swings in blood or urine sugar levels occur over a short period of time. Other clues suggesting a Somogyi effect are worsening of diabetic control as insulin dosage is increased and increased hunger and weight gain despite worsening hyperglycemia or glycosuria. By contrast, poor control due to underdosage of insulin usually causes weight loss from caloric wastage in the urine (ketonuria and glycosuria). The correct therapy for the man described in this question is to decrease the morning dose of NPH insulin rather than to administer more or different insulin, to treat the rebound hyperglycemia, or to decrease food intake at supper.

573. The answer is D. *(Braunwald, ed 11, chaps 43, 331.)* Progestogen therapy results in secretory differentiation of an estrogen-primed proliferative endometrium, and the endometrium is sloughed following progestogen withdrawal only if it has been stimulated first by estrogen. Thus, in a woman being evaluated for secondary amenorrhea, the appearance of menses following a short course of progestogen is indicative of an estrogen-primed endometrium and is good evidence of ovarian estrogen secretion. Estrone levels do not reflect direct ovarian estrogen secretion, because estrone is derived principally from the peripheral conversion of androstenedione, which is secreted from the adrenal glands and the ovaries. A woman with amenorrhea caused by hypogonadotropic hypogonadism has deficient ovarian estrogen secretion but may demonstrate an increase in plasma estradiol following human chorionic gonadotropin (hCG) administration. Prolactin secretion is increased by estrogen stimulation, accounting for a slightly higher mean prolactin level in women compared to men. However, a normal prolactin level is not evidence of persistent estrogen secretion.

574. The answer is D. *(Braunwald, ed 11, chap 43, 331.)* In a 7-year-old girl, isosexual precocity that is associated with undetectable levels of gonadotropins and urinary 17-ketosteroid levels appropriate for her chronologic age is most likely due to an estrogen-secreting tumor. Tumor localization procedures, such as abdominal CT scanning and pelvic sonography, should be performed before laparotomy. Plasma androstenedione measurement is unlikely to be helpful, if urinary 17-ketosteroid excretion is low or normal. In idiopathic precocious puberty, a diagnosis of exclusion, urinary gonadotropins are either normal for chronologic age or elevated; in addition, if plasma gonadotropins are measured frequently during a 24-hour period, the characteristic pubertal nocturnal surge should be seen in patients with idiopathic precocious puberty.

575. The answer is B. *(Braunwald, ed 11, chaps 57, 224.)* Many autosomal dominant disorders vary in the time of onset and severity of expression. Therefore, individuals such as the two apparently unaffected siblings who are at risk for development of hereditary nephritis, even in the absence of overt evidence of renal impairment, are poor candidates as donors for a kidney. In addition, the mother is clearly a carrier and a poor candidate. The father is the best close relative to evaluate as a potential donor.

576. The answer is D. *(Braunwald, ed 11, chap 60.)* Most autosomal chromosomal trisomies cause death *in utero*. Among live-born infants with trisomies (21, 18, and 13), trisomies 18 and 13 cause death in infancy. Patients with trisomy 21 (Down's syndrome) may reach adulthood, although with a shortened life expectancy because of an increased incidence of severe infections and complications from associated malformations. On the other hand, sex chromosome trisomies are compatible with intrauterine survival and are usually associated with a normal life expectancy.

577. The answer is E. *(Braunwald, ed 11, chap 70.)* Causes of thiamine deficiency in alcoholic persons include poor dietary intake, impaired absorption and storage, and accelerated destruction of thiamine diphosphate. Both the cardiovascular and the neurologic signs of thiamine deficiency (beriberi) can become abruptly evident following the administration of glucose to thiamine-depleted, asymptomatic individuals. Nystagmus, ataxia, and confusion, often accompanied by ophthalmoplegia, are strongly suggestive of Wernicke's encephalopathy; cardiovascular involvement may be signaled by tachycardia as an early manifestation of peripheral vasodilation. Thiamine should be administered promptly—and preferably before glucose is given—to any person in whom subclinical thiamine deficiency is suspected.

578. The answer is E. *(Braunwald, ed 11, chap 75.)* The first decision regarding the administration of a dietary formula is the choice of route. In the case presented, the underlying disorder (hemorrhagic pancreatitis) and recent abdominal surgery are contraindications to enteral therapy. Both lipids and carbohydrates may be infused with amino acids to meet metabolic needs, but several considerations should be taken into account in choosing which mixture to use. First is osmolality—concentrated glucose solutions are hypertonic and cause peripheral vein thrombosis. Another factor is the metabolic state of the patient; both pancreatic insufficiency and hyperglycemia are relative contraindications to using hypertonic glucose solutions. Second, carbohydrate as the sole source of calories raises the metabolic rate and thus the production of carbon dioxide; in a patient being weaned from ventilatory assistance, giving more nonprotein calories as fat reduces CO_2 excretion. Third, lipid infusions provide essential fatty-acid requirements, and because lipids do not raise insulin levels or require insulin for metabolism they may be discontinued abruptly (e.g., if emergency surgery is needed) without risk of hypoglycemia. In summary, a regimen providing 85 percent of nonprotein calories as lipid and 15 percent as glucose is near isotonic and probably optimal in the case described.

579. The answer is D. *(Braunwald, ed 11, chap 76.)* The combination of peripheral neuritis, dermatitis, glossitis, microcytic anemia, and convulsions suggests the presence of pyridoxine deficiency. Naturally occurring pyridoxine deficiency is rare, owing to the widespread distribution of the vitamin in food. It is therefore paradoxical that clinical deficiency is frequent, because many commonly used drugs act as pyridoxine antagonists. Pyridoxal phosphate is the active cofactor for numerous enzymatic reactions in amino acid metabolism and in heme synthesis; it is also important for normal neuronal excitability. Estrogens inhibit the role of pyridoxine in tryptophan metabolism, and hydrazines such as isoniazid can inhibit various enzymes that use pyridoxine as a cofactor and thereby induce convulsions. Cycloserine and penicillamine act similarly. The appropriate management for persons receiving drugs capable of causing pyridoxine deficiency is dietary supplementation (at least 30 mg of pyridoxine daily); overt deficiency, when present, requires immediate parenteral therapy.

580. The answer is D. *(Braunwald, ed 11, chaps 229, 336.)* All conditions that increase urinary calcium excretion predispose to the formation of calcium-containing kidney stones. Some of these conditions, such as primary hyperparathyroidism and metastatic cancer, also are associated with hypercalcemia. However, in a metastatic cancer the duration of the hypercalciuria is usually insufficient to permit kidney stone formation to occur. Examples of normocalcemic hypercalciuria include idiopathic hypercalciuria, in which the defect may be either excessive intestinal calcium absorption or a renal leak of calcium, and distal renal tubular acidosis, in which hypercalciuria has been attributed to both increased bone resorption and impaired renal tubular calcium reabsorption. Hyperuricosuria may lead to formation of calcium-containing kidney stones by promoting calcium oxalate crystallization or by adsorption of inhibitors of calcium stone formation.

581. The answer is D. *(Braunwald, ed 11, chaps 270, 335, 336.)* The hypercalcemia of sarcoidosis is usually associated with disseminated disease. Therefore, almost all individuals with sarcoidosis who have hypercalcemia also have an abnormal chest x-ray (diffuse fibronodular infiltration or marked enlargement of hilar nodes, or both). This is an important point in the differential diagnosis of hypercalcemia—sarcoidosis is unlikely as a cause of hypercalcemia if the chest x-ray is normal. Hypergammaglobulinemia is another helpful clue to the presence of sarcoidosis. The hypercalcemia of sarcoidosis is thought to be the consequence of increased synthesis of $1,25(OH)_2$ vitamin D_3 and the subsequent increased intestinal absorption of calcium. Elevated serum calcium concentration in sarcoidosis causes a decreased level of serum parathyroid hormone, resulting in marked hypercalciuria.

582. The answer is C. *(Braunwald, ed 11, chap 309.)* Colchicine is useful in the treatment of acute gouty arthritis but not chronic tophaceous gout. However, it can be a useful ancillary drug in treatment of chronic gout at the start of allopurinol therapy to prevent the precipitation of acute gouty arthritis. Chronic gout can be treated either with uricosuric agents (probenecid or sulfinpyrazone) or with an inhibitor of uric acid synthesis (allopurinol). The ideal candidate for uricosuric agents is a patient under the age of 60 years who has normal renal function, a uric acid excretion of less than 700 mg per day, and no history of renal stones. Specific indications for choosing allopurinol over a uricosuric agent include the presence of uric acid nephrolithiasis, high uric acid excretion, and impairment of renal function; hence allopurinol is the appropriate initial drug in this patient. Combinations of allopurinol and uricosuric agents may be employed when uric acid levels cannot be controlled with either drug alone.

583. The answer is E. *(Braunwald, ed 11, chap 315. Miller, Annu Rev Med 31:97, 1980. Shaefer, Atherosclerosis 4:303, 1984.)* Low levels of high-density lipoprotein (HDL) have been found to be associated with diabetes mellitus, hypertriglyceridemia, and obesity. Tangier disease is a rare autosomal recessive disorder characterized by the total absence of plasma HDL. On the other hand, alcohol consumption is associated with elevations in HDL levels. Even small amounts of alcohol consumed on a regular basis (1 to 3 ounces per week) can increase plasma HDL levels.

584. The answer is E. *(Braunwald, ed 11, chap 315. Stanbury, ed 5, chap 30.)* The patient described in the question has type 5 hyperlipoproteinemia. This usually familial disorder is characterized by elevated levels of chylomicrons and VLDL. (The fact that VLDL levels are increased in the patient described is shown by the high triglyceride-to-cholesterol ratio and by the turbid intranatant layer; high levels of chylomicrons are indicated by the presence of the creamy upper layer in standing plasma.) Diabetes, pancreatitis, and hyperuricemia are common in persons with the disorder. Hypertriglyceridemia may be exacerbated by obesity, dietary factors, and alcoholism.

585. The answer is B. *(Braunwald, ed 11, chap 315.)* Whether hypertriglyceridemia in an overweight person is due to familial hypertriglyceridemia, multiple lipoprotein-type hyperlipemia, or sporadic hypertriglyceridemia, the primary mode of therapy should be weight reduction. Dietary saturated-fat content should be restricted as part of the weight reduction regimen. Hypothyroidism and diabetes mellitus, if present, should be treated, and use of alcohol and oral contraceptives should be avoided. If these measures are inadequate, drug therapy with clofibrate should be tried. Bile acid-binding resins, such as cholestyramine or colestipol, are used in the treatment of hypercholesterolemia but are not useful for treating hypertriglyceridemia.

586. The answer is C. *(Braunwald, ed 11, chap 315.)* In familial lipoprotein lipase deficiency the clearance of dietary chylomicrons is markedly impaired, causing these lipoproteins to accumulate to massive levels in plasma. The genetic defect is inherited as an autosomal recessive disorder. Typical manifestations include recurrent attacks of acute pancreatitis, eruptive xanthomas, and lipemia retinalis. Accumulation of triglycerides in the reticuloendothelial system produces hepatosplenomegaly. However, accelerated atherosclerosis does not occur in this disorder, whereas it is a prominent feature of the other types of hyperlipidemia listed.

587. The answer is D. *(Braunwald, ed 11, chap 315. Schaefer, N Engl J Med 312:1300, 1985.)* Cholestyramine and colestipol are bile acid-binding resins that decrease the reabsorption of bile acids from the intestine, thus secondarily decreasing the enterohepatic circulation of cholesterol. The liver responds to the acid depletion by increasing the synthesis of bile acids. The additional cholesterol required for bile acid synthesis is obtained by the liver by increasing the number of low density lipoprotein (LDL) receptors, which in turn lowers the plasma level of LDL. The most common side effects of these resins are constipation and bloating, although mild steatorrhea may occur when they are used in high doses.

588. The answer is A. *(Braunwald, ed 11, chap 317.)* Weight loss requires caloric deficit: the total number of calories consumed must be exceeded by the total number of calories expended as energy. The claims for various "fad" diets nothwithstanding, there is little evidence to support the efficacy of one type of hypocaloric diet over any other in achieving long-term weight loss. Basically a calorie is a calorie—whether from protein, fat, or carbohydrate. Liquid protein diets have been associated with a variety of adverse developments, including hyperuricemia, hypercholesterolemia, and sudden cardiovascular death. Total starvation diets are simpler to follow and lead to greater weight loss than hypocaloric diets, but adverse effects include increase loss of lean body mass, hypotension, and arrhythmias. Amphetamines act as weak anorexiants but are usually ineffective after several weeks; also, the risks of dependence and abuse are significant. Exercise is a useful adjunct to caloric restriction; it may increase lean body mass and improve the sense of well-being, but moderate exercise does not increase caloric expenditure sufficiently to alter the initial rate of weight loss if caloric restriction is not also undertaken.

589. The answer is A. *(Braunwald, ed 11, chap 317.)* Although only a minority of obese persons have diabetes mellitus, more than 80 percent of type II diabetics are obese. Obesity appears to be a major contributory factor to the development of diabetes, largely through its effects on insulin sensitivity. A clear relationship also exists between hypertension and obesity in adults (especially in women), though the mechanism is unclear. Hypertriglyceridemia is associated commonly with obesity and correlates with the degree of obesity; increased hepatic production of very-low density lipoproteins (VLDL) from free fatty acids is felt to be the major cause of increased triglyceride levels in obese persons, although peripheral defects in VLDL clearance may be present in some. Weight loss can reduce or reverse all these complications. The prevalence of cholelithiasis is increased with increasing adiposity, but the same cannot be said of hypothyroidism—only a small percentage of hypothyroid persons are obese, and an even smaller fraction of obese persons are hypothyroid.

590. The answer is D. *(Braunwald, ed 11, chaps 317, 327. Olefsky, Am J Physiol 243:E15, 1982.)* Obesity is the most common cause of insulin resistance. Resistance to insulin is due to a decrease in the number of cell-surface insulin receptors, decreased binding affinity for insulin, and a postreceptor intracellular defect in glucose transport. Although insulin antibodies of the immunoglobulin G type are present in almost every diabetic individual within the first 60 days of insulin therapy, they are almost never present in untreated individuals. Acanthosis nigricans is associated either with a lack of insulin receptors or with the presence of antibodies to insulin receptors but is much less common than obesity. Some nonobese persons with type 1 diabetes are insulin-resistant, but the condition disappears with aggressive insulin therapy. Up to one-third of persons with type 2 diabetes seem to have insulin resistance that is reversible with better control of the diabetes; this condition may be due to depletion of intracellular glucose-transport units.

591. The answer is B. *(Braunwald, ed 11, chap 321.)* In a woman with hyperprolactinemia and a normal-size sella, further evaluation should be directed at distinguishing among the following diagnostic possibilities: prolactin-secreting microadenoma, primary hypothyroidism, and drug-induced hyperprolactinemia. If there is no history of ingestion of drugs associated with hyperprolactinemia and if thyroid function tests are normal, then a high-resolution CT scan of the head should be obtained to look for a pituitary microadenoma. Visual-field testing in a person with a microadenoma essentially is always normal. Gonadotropin levels in persons with hyperprolactinemia and a normal sella are usually in the low to low-normal range, and their measurement adds little to the initial evaluation. Similarly, measurement of other pituitary hormones is not informative at this stage of the evaluation, and provocative tests of prolactin secretion, such as measurements of plasma prolactin following the administration of TRH or chlorpromazine, do not reliably distinguish between organic and functional (idiopathic) causes of hyperprolactinemia. Bromocriptine reduces prolactin secretion and causes cessation of galactorrhea in essentially all women with hyperprolactinemia, regardless of its etiology, and its administration is therefore of limited diagnostic use.

592. The answer is A. *(Braunwald, ed 11, chaps 321, 325.)* The adrenal glands normally produce cortisol at a rate of approximately 20 to 30 mg/day. As in the treatment of primary adrenal insufficiency, a replacement dose of hydrocortisone, 30 mg/day, should be given to all patients following transsphenoidal removal of an ACTH-secreting microadenoma; treatment should continue until the uninvolved corticotropic cells recover and secrete ACTH at a level sufficient to maintain basal glucocorticoid production. If symptoms of withdrawal from high levels of glucocorticoid develop, a transient increase in glucocorticoid dosage may be necessary. Administration of desmopressin and levothyroxine are required only if diabetes insipidus or hypothyroidism, respectively, develops postoperatively.

593. The answer is C. *(Braunwald, ed 11, chaps 321, 325.)* The absolute degree of elevation of plasma cortisol concentration is not a reliable criterion in the diagnosis of Cushing's disease. Rather, impaired suppressibility of adrenal cortisol production must be demonstrated by formal dexamethasone testing. Following administration of dexamethasone, 2 mg/day for 2 days, urinary free cortisol excretion may fall in persons with Cushing's disease but not to the degree seen in normal individuals (<20 μg/24 h). A dexamethasone regimen of 8 mg/day would cause urinary 17-hydroxycorticosteroid excretion to fall to less than 50 percent of baseline in persons with Cushing's disease. Cortisol production never increases in response to metyrapone, because this drug inhibits the final enzyme (11β-hydroxylase) in the pathway of cortisol synthesis; however, an exaggerated release of ACTH may follow metyrapone administration and result in a threefold to fivefold increase in urinary excretion of 17-hydroxycorticosteroids (predominantly 11-deoxycortisol). Patients with Cushing's disease characteristically have elevation of urinary 17-ketosteroids in addition to elevation of urinary 17-hydroxycorticosteroids.

594. The answer is E. *(Braunwald, ed 11, chaps 321, 327, 334.)* The most probable unifying explanation of the findings presented in the question would be renal failure associated with nephrotic syndrome caused by diabetic nephropathy. At this degree of renal dysfunction, secondary hyperparathyroidism is expected. Loss of binding globulins in the urine results in low total serum thyroxine and cortisol levels; in contrast, measurement of free cortisol levels following cosyntropin stimulation and of free thyroxine levels should be normal. Although calculation of the free thyroxine index (utilizing total thyroxine and resin tri-iodothyronine uptake) usually corrects for abnormalities caused by a decrease in the availability of thyroxine-binding globulin (TBG), this correction is not reliable at the extremes of TBG abnormality. Also as the result of urinary protein loss, the total measured serum calcium is depressed to a greater degree than is the ionized calcium level.

595. The answer is E. *(Braunwald, ed 11, chap 321.)* The primary empty sella syndrome is frequently diagnosed as the result of radiographic examination of the head for reasons other than suspected pituitary disease. It occurs commonly in obese multiparous women with arterial hypertension. An incomplete diaphragm sella is thought to allow an arachnoid diverticulum containing cerebrospinal fluid to protrude into the sella, which in turn displaces and compresses the pituitary gland. Pituitary function remains intact, and no further workup is indicated unless there is clinical evidence of endocrine abnormalities. Occasionally, however, hyperprolactinemia may occur as the result of stretching of the pituitary stalk or of a coincidental microprolactinoma.

ENDOCRINE, METABOLIC, AND GENETIC DISORDERS

596. The answer is B. *(Braunwald, ed 11, chap 321.)* Several features in this woman suggest the presence of hypercortisolism. Although the overnight dexamethasone suppression test (1 mg at midnight) is a useful screening test to rule out Cushing's syndrome, it may be falsely positive (failure to suppress morning cortisol rise) in obese patients. Measurement of 24-hour urinary free cortisol excretion is especially useful in these instances; if results are elevated (more than 100 μg in 24 hours), a standard two-day, low-dose dexamethasone suppression test is the next step in the evaluation. Measurement of plasma ACTH levels is usually not useful in the diagnosis of Cushing's syndrome although very high levels suggest ectopic ACTH production. Radiographic examination of the pituitary gland should not be done until a diagnosis of pituitary-dependent Cushing's syndrome has been established by laboratory testing.

597. The answer is B. *(Braunwald, ed 11, chap 321.)* A serum prolactin level above 300 ng/mL is diagnostic of a pituitary adenoma, even in a nursing woman. In fact, the serum prolactin level only rarely reaches 300 ng/mL during pregnancy and declines postpartum (with intermittent peaking with each suckling episode). Six months postpartum, basal prolactin levels are normal, and the suckling-induced rise is minimal despite continued nursing. Thus, computed tomography of the pituitary gland is indicated at this time. Suppressive treatment with bromocriptine would be indicated if the diagnosis of a pituitary adenoma is confirmed. Since bromocriptine suppresses all types of hyperprolactinemia, it cannot be used as a diagnostic test of physiologic versus pathologic hyperprolactinemia. Any delay in evaluation could allow further tumor enlargement and the risk of visual impairment resulting from optic nerve compression.

598. The answer is C. *(Braunwald, ed 11, chap 322.)* Because the secretion of growth hormone is episodic and therefore variable, random measurements of plasma growth hormone are not adequate assessments of growth hormone deficiency, and consequently provocative tests to stimulate growth hormone secretion should be utilized. In contrast, measurement of IGF-I/SM-C is a useful indicator of growth hormone status since it turns over more slowly than growth hormone itself, and hence its level reflects the mean level of growth hormone in the blood throughout the day rather than the moment-to-moment level. Measurement of the serum thyroxine concentration is useful in identification of growth retardation associated with hypothyroidism, and assessment of chromosomal karyotype is useful in identifying girls whose growth retardation is associated with gonadal dysgenesis. Assessment of bone age makes it possible to pick out discrepancies between bone age and chronologic age.

599. The answer is B. *(Braunwald, ed 11, chap 323.)* Patients with lung cancer, particularly small cell carcinoma, frequently present with the syndrome of inappropriate antidiuretic hormone (AVP, vasopressin) secretion. Indeed, more than half of patients with such tumors show evidence of inappropriate secretion of AVP, even when serum sodium concentration remains normal. AVP is produced by the tumor tissue itself and is chemically identical to arginine vasopressin secreted by the neurohypophysis. Central nervous system lesions of infectious, inflammatory, and vascular etiologies can also result in inappropriate AVP secretion, but intracerebral metastases from small cell carcinomas are not usually responsible for inappropriate AVP secretion.

600. The answer is E. *(Braunwald, ed 11, chap 323.)* Demeclocycline produces reversible renal insensitivity to endogenous vasopressin. The exact mechanism of action is unknown. The drug's effects are more consistent than those of ethanol or phenytoin, and side effects are less than with lithium. Desmopressin, a synthetic analogue of vasopressin, would worsen water intoxication in a person with chronic inappropriate vasopressin secretion.

601. The answer is D. *(Braunwald, ed 11, chap 323.)* After neurosurgical procedures or head trauma, diabetes insipidus may develop acutely. The deficiency of vasopressin may be transient and is sometimes followed by a phase of marked antidiuresis, presumably resulting from vasopressin release from damaged cells. In a significant proportion of patients complete recovery of vasopressin secretory capacity follows. Because of the changing nature of the defect, treatment with a short-acting form of vasopressin is indicated. Desmopressin has a rapid onset of action and can be administered subcutaneously. Vasopressin tannate in oil has a much prolonged action. Lypressin is available only for intranasal administration and is not suitable for use in unconscious patients. Chlorpropamide and carbamazepine are useful for long-term therapy of patients with partial defects of vasopressin secretion.

602. The answer is C. *(Braunwald, ed 11, chap 324.)* Impaired peripheral conversion of thyroxine to tri-iodothyronine (T_4 to T_3) occurs commonly in acute and chronic illnesses, in fasting and starvation, and following the administration of certain drugs. Although propylthiouracil and methimazole act similarly to cause impaired organification of iodine by thyroid glands affected by thyrotoxicosis, propylthiouracil has the additional effect of inhibiting peripheral conversion of T_4 to T_3, a property not shared by methimazole. The recognition of a similar action of dexamethasone in impairing T_4 conversion to T_3 has provided an explanation for the favorable effect of glucocorticoids in the treatment of thyroid storm. Propranolol also has a minor effect in inhibiting the conversion of T_4 to T_3. The degree of impairment of T_4 conversion to T_3 by oral cholecystography dyes is such that a compensatory increase in T_4 to greater than normal levels is frequently noted 1 to 2 weeks after ingestion of the compounds.

603. The answer is E. *(Braunwald, ed 11, chap 324.)* Surgical treatment of nontoxic goiter is most commonly undertaken for diagnostic purposes (i.e., to rule out malignancy). Enlarged thyroid glands often have a limited functional reserve capacity, and lobectomy can further compromise hormone production. The thyroid scan presented in the question demonstrates adequate concentration and diffuse distribution of the radionuclide throughout the enlarged remnant, and there is little risk of malignancy. Exogenous hormone administration can prevent or improve postsurgical "compensatory" thyroid hyperplasia, which is the likely explanation for the mass in the woman described. Ultrasonography would be useful if the scan showed irregularities of uptake.

604. The answer is D. *(Braunwald, ed 11, chap 324.)* Normal pregnancy can simulate thyrotoxicosis in regard to increased heart rate, heat intolerance, and anxiety. The test best able to exclude thyrotoxicosis in this patient would be the thyrotropin-releasing hormone (TRH) stimulation test. Testing radioactive iodine uptake (RAIU) is not always useful in diagnosing hyperthyroidism due to the wide range of normal values in the population and is not advisable in pregnancy. Similarly, the T_3 suppression test, although useful in the diagnosis of thyroid autonomy, requires RAIU tests and therefore would be contraindicated. Technetium thyroid scans and thyroid-stimulating hormone (TSH) stimulation tests are not useful in the diagnosis of hyperthyroidism.

605. The answer is B. *(Braunwald, ed 11, chap 324.)* The most appropriate treatment for Graves' disease in the third trimester of pregnancy is propylthiouracil in the minimal dosages sufficient to control the hyperthyroidism. Because levothyroxine crosses the placenta poorly, hypothyroidism may occur in the fetus if levothyroxine is combined with sufficient doses of propylthiouracil to block thyroid function in the fetus. Subtotal thyroidectomy is usually reserved for treating affected women in the second trimester. Use of radioactive iodine is contraindicated during pregnancy, because it crosses the placenta and may have deleterious effects on fetal development. Propranolol can cause fetal hypoglycemia and apnea and should not be used in treating thyrotoxicosis of pregnancy, except in emergencies.

606. The answer is C. *(Braunwald, ed 11, chaps 324, 325, 334.)* It is essential in initiating treatment for coexisting hypothyroidism and adrenal insufficiency that thyroid hormone should not be administered before glucocorticoid replacement has commenced. If this precaution is not taken, administration of thyroid hormone may result in accelerated catabolism of any residual hydrocortisone that is being secreted and thereby precipitate acute adrenal crisis. The replacement dosage of hydrocortisone should not exceed the normal adrenal secretory rate (approximately 20 to 30 mg/day). In a young individual without ischemic heart disease, full replacement of levothyroxine (between 100 and 150 µg/day) may be started at the outset of treatment. Serum thyroxine concentration should be monitored periodically to ensure adequacy of replacement. The efficacy of hydrocortisone replacement can be monitored by the patient's clinical response.

607. The answer is C. (*Braunwald, ed 11, chap 324.*) Measurement of serum TSH concentration by radioimmunoassay is useful in the diagnosis of both early and advanced primary hypothyroidism. Because of the exquisitely sensitive feedback relationship between TSH secretion and thyroid hormone levels in plasma, TSH levels in serum are increased in patients with untreated hypothyroidism of thyroidal etiology. In contrast, serum T_3 measurement and radioactive iodine uptake tests are generally poor discriminators of hypothyroidism. The TRH stimulation test is of less value in the diagnosis of hypothyroidism than in the diagnosis of hyperthyroidism. Reverse T_3 measurement, when available, is helpful in separating primary hypothyroidism from the "sick euthyroid" syndrome, since results are subnormal in patients with hypothyroidism but normal or high in association with the "sick euthyroid" syndrome.

608. The answer is E. (*Braunwald, ed 11, chap 325.*) In the case presented in the question, the development of muscle weakness, arthralgias, fatigue, and fever is likely to be the result of steroid withdrawal. Steroid withdrawal symptoms commonly appear after therapy is switched from a daily to an alternate-day regimen and ordinarily abate after a few days. If the symptoms persist, then it may be necessary to switch back to daily therapy and make the transition to alternate-day steroid treatment in stages.

609. The answer is D. (*Braunwald, ed 11, chap 325.*) In the various forms of congenital adrenal hyperplasia, including steroid C-21 hydroxylase deficiency, both pituitary and adrenal regulatory mechanisms function appropriately. The enzymatic defect in cortisol production results in an absence of the product (cortisol) necessary for feedback inhibition of ACTH secretion by the pituitary gland. ACTH in turn causes the production of increased amounts of cortisol precursors such as 17-hydroxyprogesterone which is converted to androgens by the adrenal gland. Therapy with appropriate doses of glucocorticoid causes suppression of pituitary ACTH and adrenal androgen secretion, indicating that inhibiting and stimulating control mechanisms of the hypothalamic-pituitary-adrenal axis can function normally.

610. The answer is D. (*Braunwald, ed 11, chap 325.*) In a single-dose overnight dexamethasone suppression test, which is a screening procedure in the workup of possible cortisol excess, suppression of plasma cortisol concentration to less than 5 µg/dL implies normal hypothalamic-pituitary-adrenal feedback and excludes a diagnosis of Cushing's syndrome. However, failure to suppress plasma cortisol following this procedure is not necessarily diagnostic and must be investigated further. Several factors can affect the validity of screening dexamethasone testing. For example, in 10 to 15 percent of cases obesity interferes with normal suppression of cortisol after the overnight dexamethasone test. However, obese persons uniformly show normal excretion of free cortisol in urine (<100 µg/24 h). The two-day low-dose dexamethasone test is necessary to exclude or establish the diagnosis of Cushing's syndrome in all persons with abnormal or equivocal screening tests. The high-dose test, which is reserved for patients with established Cushing's syndrome, serves to delineate the specific cause. Imaging procedures should only be performed once a diagnosis of cortisol excess is established.

611. The answer is E. (*Braunwald, ed 11, chap 325.*) The etiology of Cushing's syndrome differs in various age groups. In older men ectopic production of ACTH by nonadrenal tumors is the most frequent cause, and among the causes of ectopic ACTH production, carcinoma of the lung would be the most likely one in this patient. Pituitary-dependent Cushing's disease is more likely to occur in women and in younger men. In children under the age of 15 years, adrenal carcinoma accounts for approximately 40 percent of all cases of Cushing's syndrome. Adrenal adenomas and ectopic production of corticotropin-releasing hormone are less common causes of Cushing's syndrome at all ages.

612. The answer is A. *(Braunwald, ed 11, chap 325.)* Hyporeninemic hypoaldosteronism occurs most commonly in adults with diabetes mellitus in association with mild renal failure, metabolic acidosis, and hyperkalemia. The defect in aldosterone synthesis is almost certainly caused by hyporeninism, since in these patients aldosterone secretion increases promptly after the administration of ACTH but not after salt restriction or postural changes. Most patients respond to the administration of potent mineralocorticoid (fludrocortisone) or diuretics such as furosemide, or both, but in general mineralocorticoids should not be the sole therapeutic agents in patients with hypertension. Hemodialysis may be useful in emergency situations to correct hyperkalemia. Potassium restriction and enhancement of potassium excretion with anion-exchange resins are both likely to predispose to total-body potassium deficits.

613. The answer is A. *(Braunwald, ed 11, chap 327. Isselbacher, Update I, p 33. Brownlee, Ann Intern Med 101:527, 1984.)* Hemoglobin A_{1c} (HbA_{1c}), the most abundant minor component of human hemoglobin, is a ketoamine formed by the nonenzymatic glycosylation of the N-terminal valine on the β globin chain. Because the rate of HbA_{1c} formation is dependent on the average plasma glucose level during the lifespan of the red blood cell (nearly 120 days), HbA_{1c} levels reflect the average blood sugar for the previous weeks or months. HbA_{1c} makes up about 5 to 8 percent of the hemoglobin of persons without diabetes, whereas in persons with poorly controlled diabetes it accounts for an average of 10 to 14 percent of hemoglobin. Glycosylated albumin can serve as a monitor of diabetic control over a period up to 2 weeks. Plasma C-peptide may indicate residual beta-cell function but does not relate to diabetic control. Plasma glucose and urinary glucose levels fluctuate widely from day to day, so that measurements, no matter how valuable, reflect control only over a short period of time.

614. The answer is A. *(Braunwald, ed 11, chap 327. Gabbe, Am J Med 70:613, 1981. Jovanovic, Am J Med 71:921, 1981. Miller, N Engl J Med 304:1331, 1981.)* The prognosis for pregnancies complicated by diabetes mellitus has improved markedly, and perinatal mortality has decreased to the point that infant survival is similar to that in the population at large. This improved outcome is a result of aggressive treatment of maternal hyperglycemia and of advances in the techniques of fetal surveillance and neonatal care. When mean maternal blood glucose levels exceed 150 mg/dL in the third trimester, perinatal mortality is almost six times that associated with mean maternal glucose levels below 100 mg/dL. Congenital malformations, the leading cause of perinatal mortality in infants of diabetic pregnancies, remain an unresolved problem; such abnormalities are thought to be related to poor glucose control early in the first trimester (during early embryogenesis), a time when many women do not yet know they are pregnant. Optimal care of a diabetic woman wishing to become pregnant requires that a major attempt be made to achieve as normal a mean blood glucose concentration as possible before conception and throughout the duration of pregnancy. Hospitalization may be required for education or treatment of complications but should not be necessary for extended periods of time.

615. The answer is B. *(Braunwald, ed 11, chap 327. Diabetic Retinopathy Study Research Group, Ophthalmology 88:583, 1981.)* Dot hemorrhages and several larger lesions near the disk (caused by superficial retinal bleeding) are characteristic changes of background diabetic retinopathy. However, the presence of innumerable, fine, frondlike vessels extending around and partly covering the disk is indicative of the neovascularization of proliferative retinopathy, which requires urgent treatment. The therapy of choice is photocoagulation by xenon arc or ruby or argon laser. The Diabetic Retinopathy Study Research Group (DRSRG) has established that photocoagulation significantly improves visual prognosis in proliferative retinopathy. Tighter control of blood sugar levels has not been shown to reverse the lesions of diabetic retinopathy. Hypophysectomy is no longer used to treat proliferative retinopathy, due to the morbidity and lack of effectiveness of the procedure. Vitrectomy should be reserved for more advanced cases, such as nonresolving vitreal hemorrhage or retinal traction detachment.

616. The answer is E. *(Braunwald, ed 11, chaps 327 and 329.)* Hypoglycemia from oral hypoglycemic agents is less common than with insulin therapy, but when it occurs it can be severe and prolonged and cause confusion or coma. Immediate therapy of serious hypoglycemia requires bolus intravenous administration of a 50% glucose solution followed by constant glucose infusions until the patient can eat a meal. Oral intake of glucose is important, because intravenous glucose alone does not replenish liver glycogen. Sulfonylurea overdosage causes overutilization of glucose, so that affected persons may require considerable amounts of glucose to remain conscious. Mild glycosuria is one indication of adequate infusion rates; frequent capillary glucose measurements also may be helpful. Hypoglycemia from the use of sulfonylurea agents may last for several days, especially with chlorpropamide, and patients may lapse back into coma if glucose infusions are stopped prematurely. Hospitalization is mandatory in cases of serious hypoglycemia.

617. The answer is D. *(Braunwald, ed 11, chap 327. Freinkel, N Engl J Med 313:96, 1985.)* A fasting blood glucose level of 120 to 140 mg/dL represents reasonable blood sugar control of a nonpregnant diabetic patient, but during pregnancy stringent control of diabetes is a mandatory goal. Maintenance of plasma glucose values below 100 mg/dL, especially during the last weeks of pregnancy, is associated with a reduction in perinatal mortality. An oral glucose tolerance test in this patient serves no purpose since the diagnosis of diabetes mellitus is already established. Glycosuria at these relatively low blood levels of glucose reflects the lowered renal threshold for glucose reabsorption typical of pregnancy, and measurement of glycosuria does not provide insight into the adequacy of treatment. Carbohydrate restriction is contraindicated during pregnancy because it necessitates caloric restriction and thus predisposes to the development of ketosis, which has been associated with fetal wastage.

618. The answer is D. *(Braunwald, ed 11, chap 327. Wilson, Ann Intern Med 98:219, 1983. Cryer, N Engl J Med 313:232, 1985.)* Nocturnal hypoglycemia occurs not infrequently in insulin-dependent diabetic patients under aggressive treatment with insulin. During sleep, the typical symptoms of hypoglycemia go unnoticed unless witnessed by other persons. More frequently, manifestations of early morning hypoglycemia are nightmares, morning headaches, tiredness and, on occasion, intellectual deterioration. In this patient any increase in the insulin dose or restriction of caloric intake would lead to worsening of the symptoms of nocturnal hypoglycemia. Conversely, a reduction in the evening insulin dose (initially by 10 percent of the total daily dose) will probably lead to the resolution of early morning hypoglycemia and result in improved control of the diabetes.

619. The answer is C. *(Braunwald, ed 11, chap 328.)* Myocardial infarction with hypotension is a common cause of lactic acidosis with hypoxia. When blood flow to peripheral tissue is diminished and oxygen delivery is inadequate, several metabolic changes occur. NADH, which is produced by the oxidation of glucose, free fatty acids, and acetyl CoA, cannot be reoxidized by the electron transport pathway to NAD. As a result, the NADH/NAD ratio in both cytosolic and mitochondrial compartments increases. ATP cannot be generated, and tissue ATP levels decline; ADP and AMP levels rise. Phosphofructokinase is activated, and glycogen breakdown and glycolysis rapidly increase. These latter changes markedly enhance production of pyruvate, which in turn is reduced to lactic acid due to the high NADH/NAD ratio. The net effect is peripheral overproduction of lactic acid. In addition, hypoperfusion of the liver results in impaired hepatic lactate uptake and metabolism.

620. The answer is A. *(Braunwald, ed 11, chap 329.)* The catabolic changes that occur during fasting vary with the length of the fast. Early on, a slight drop in plasma glucose concentration causes insulin levels to fall and increases the release of counterregulatory hormones, such as glucagon, cortisol, epinephrine, and growth hormone; in this way, plasma glucose levels are sustained within a safe range. Glucagon increases hepatic cyclic AMP, which activates glycogen phosphorylase (and hence stimulates glycogenolysis) and inhibits glycogen synthetase. It also suppresses glycolysis and enhances gluconeogenesis by blocking phosphofructokinase and stimulating fructose diphosphatase, respectively. The effect is to make the liver an organ of net glucose production; however, because hepatic glycogen stores are limited, glycogen breakdown can sustain plasma glucose levels for only 12 to 24 hours. After this period, new glucose must be produced from peripheral precursors, such as glycerol, lactate, and especially amino acids (notably alanine). In adipose tissue, lipolysis of stored triglycerides liberates free fatty acids, which are either used in liver for ketone body production or oxidized in peripheral tissues. Fatty acid oxidation also provides the energy for hepatic gluconeogenesis. The brain continues to metabolize glucose for several days of fasting, after which time ketone bodies become a major substrate.

621. The answer is B. *(Braunwald, ed 11, chap 329. Wilson, ed 7, chap 34. Freedberg, N Engl J Med 292:1117, 1975.)* The combination of weight loss, anemia, and a bullous skin eruption in a patient with hepatic metastases and evidence of a pancreatic lesion is highly suggestive of a glucagonoma. This tumor of pancreatic alpha cells is usually malignant; metastasizes early; often occurs in middle-aged women; and is accompanied by hyperglycemia, painful stomatitis and cheilosis, hypoaminoacidemia, and a characteristic skin rash—necrolytic migratory erythema. With appropriate histologic techniques, the diagnosis of a pancreatic alpha-cell tumor can be established by liver biopsy, but marked plasma hyperglucagonemia is pathognomonic. Arteriography may demonstrate a pancreatic tumor but is not diagnostic. Treatment is early surgical removal; chemotherapy of metastatic disease is usually ineffective.

622. The answer is C. *(Braunwald, ed 11, chap 330.)* Impaired testicular function in adults can be due to pituitary disease or disorders that affect the testes directly. Although some abnormalities affect Leydig cell or seminiferous tubule function selectively, most testicular diseases impair both functions. For example, disorders that affect Leydig cell function usually also impair sperm production as a result of diminished testosterone production. Conditions that may be manifested by infertility alone include germinal cell aplasia, cryptorchidism, varicocele, radiation exposure, cyclophosphamide therapy, autoimmunity, febrile illness, and paraplegia. Although Leydig cell function initially is sufficient to maintain testosterone levels in the normal range in young men with Klinefelter syndrome, it is only at the expense of elevated LH levels, and deficiency in androgen production usually supervenes during the course of the disorder.

623. The answer is A. *(Braunwald, ed 11, chap 330.)* Testosterone esters are hydrolyzed by esterases in the blood as they are absorbed from the oily depots in which they are administered, and, as a consequence, the esters themselves can rarely be detected in blood. Therefore, effectiveness of therapy with agents such as testosterone cypionate can be monitored by measuring the plasma levels of testosterone itself. In men with recent onset of hypogonadism, plasma LH levels should be suppressed into the normal range by testosterone, but when LH levels have been high for many years, LH secretion becomes semiautonomous and may not return to the normal range for many months or years after the restoration of blood testosterone levels to normal. The frequency of nocturnal erections may or may not reflect plasma testosterone levels on a day-to-day or week-to-week basis, and muscle mass depends on factors in addition to plasma testosterone levels, including exercise level.

624. The answer is C. *(Braunwald, ed 11, chap 331. Wilson, ed 7, chap 9.)* The fact that withdrawal bleeding occurred after the administration of progestogen indicates that estrogen was being produced. Women with chronic anovulation who react in this way are said to be in the state of "estrus" because of acyclic production of estrogen. This diagnostic response clearly excludes those causes of amenorrhea associated with suppression of ovarian function, including pituitary disease, either functional or organic, and conditions associated with streak gonads. The most likely cause of amenorrhea in such a situation is polycystic ovarian disease (PCOD) in which the ovaries produce androgens that can be converted to estrogens (largely estrone) in extraglandular tissues. In most women with PCOD, menarche occurs at the expected time, and amenorrhea supervenes after a variable time. However, in some women this disorder has an early onset and may cause primary amenorrhea. Other causes of anovulation in the presence of estrogen include estrogen-secreting tumors of the ovary and adrenal tumors.

625. The answer is B. *(Braunwald, ed 11, chap 331.)* Asherman's syndrome, destruction of the endometrium, occurs after vigorous curettage, usually in association with postpartum hemorrhage or therapeutic abortion. The diagnosis is confirmed by hysterosalpingography or by direct visualization of the scarred endometrium using a hysteroscope. Treatment consists of dilation and curettage, followed by the insertion of an intrauterine device for 8 weeks.

626. The answer is D. *(Braunwald, ed 11, chap 331.)* Low circulating levels of estrogens coupled with elevated gonadotropin levels exclude the presence of pituitary disease and indicate primary ovarian failure, which is premature at this patient's age. Bilateral tubal obstruction would cause infertility but not amenorrhea. Polycystic ovarian disease is associated with typical physical findings of weight gain

ENDOCRINE, METABOLIC, AND GENETIC DISORDERS

and hirsutism, an earlier age of onset, and elevated circulating levels of estrogens. Exogenous administration of estrogens would lead to suppression of gonadotropin secretion.

627. The answer is B. *(Braunwald, ed 11, chap 333.)* The clinical situation described in the question is characteristic of congenital adrenal hyperplasia due to deficiency of either C-21 hydroxylase or 3β-ol-dehydrogenase. Urinary 17-ketosteroids are elevated in both disorders, whereas urinary pregnanediol and pregnanetriol and plasma 17-hydroxyprogesterone and androstenedione levels are elevated in association with C-21 hydroxylase deficiency. Plasma 11-deoxycortisol is elevated in C-11 hydroxylase deficiency, a disorder producing hypertension due to overproduction of mineralocorticoids and consequently not associated with vomiting and volume depletion.

628. The answer is D. *(Braunwald, ed 11, chap 333.)* Tumors of the streak gonads are unusual in the common forms of gonadal dysgenesis, including those associated with normal karyotypes (46,XX), X-chromosome deletion (45,X), structurally abnormal X chromosomes (46, XX$_i$), and X chromosome mosaicism (45,X/46,XX). However, malignant tumors of the streaks (so-called gonadoblastomas) are common when gonadal dysgenesis is associated with cell lines containing Y chromosomes or fragments of Y chromosomes. Consequently, the gonadal streaks should be resected whenever a Y chromosome is present in a woman with gonadal dysgenesis.

629. The answer is E. *(Braunwald, ed 11, chap 336.)* Individuals who have hyperparathyroidism can present with manifestations of hypercalcemia—e.g., peptic ulcer, muscle weakness, kidney stones—or symptoms of osteitis fibrosa cystica, a form of bone involvement characteristic of the disease. However, with the widespread application of biochemical screening as a routine tool in patient evaluation, more and more patients are diagnosed early in the course of the disease, when it is manifested only by asymptomatic hypercalcemia. At present, this is the most common source of diagnosing hyperparathyroidism.

630. The answer is B. *(Braunwald, ed 11, chap 336.)* Unless contraindicated by a history of thromboembolic phenomena, severe hypertension, or breast cancer, estrogen therapy provides a useful means for controlling hypercalcemia and protecting the skeleton in postmenopausal women who have hyperparathyroidism but are not good operative candidates. Plicamycin, though also of benefit, is administered as weekly intravenous injections and has cumulative toxic effects on the kidneys, liver, and bone marrow; however, it would be a good choice for treatment of hypercalcemic emergencies if saline and furosemide were ineffective or contraindicated. Phosphate promotes the deposition of calcium into the skeleton, but long-term use in persons with renal insufficiency would cause a buildup in serum phosphorus levels and thereby promote soft-tissue calcification. Oral diphosphonate has not been demonstrated to have a sustained effect in controlling the hypercalcemia of primary hyperparathyroidism, perhaps because it retards bone formation as well as bone resorption. Thiazides would exacerbate hypercalcemia by increasing renal calcium reabsorption.

631. The answer is E. *(Braunwald, ed 11, chap 336.)* Remodeling of bone is physiologically responsive to mechanical forces. The early response to immobilization is an increase in bone resorption; bone formation remains normal or decreases. Prolonged immobilization may lead to hypercalcemia, especially in persons with high rates of bone turnover (e.g., persons who have Paget's disease or young persons undergoing rapid growth). Excess calcium entering the circulation results in both hypercalciuria, which can cause nephrolithiasis, and soft-tissue calcification. Although the reason for enhanced bone resorption following immobilization is not completely understood, secretion of parathyroid hormone is suppressed. Hypercalcemia and hypercalciuria resolve when immobilized subjects become ambulatory; parathyroidectomy is unnecessary.

632. The answer is D. *(Braunwald, ed 11, chap 336. Carmichael, Am J Med 76:1137, 1984. Ryan, Am J Med 77:501, 1984.)* A direct effect of ingestion of aluminum in patients with renal failure is severe, unresponsive osteomalacia caused by its deposition at the site of osteoid mineralization. However, aluminum accumulation does not occur in patients with normal renal function, and the effects of long-term ingestion of aluminum hydroxide-containing antacids in such patients are a result of phosphorus depletion—that is, the binding of phosphorus by aluminum within the intestine prevents its absorption. In the absence of more specific symptoms, malnutrition is unlikely. Osteomalacia has been reported in association with benign tumors of mesenchymal origin (oncogenous osteomalacia) but not with gastric carcinomas.

633. The answer is E. *(Braunwald, ed 11, chap 336.)* Patients with primary hyperparathyroidism are usually asymptomatic, and mild degrees of hypercalcemia in such patients can usually be managed with adequate hydration. Whether observation alone is appropriate in these patients is controversial, especially when the diagnosis is made at a young age, since surveillance of renal function and bone status is lifelong and cumbersome. On the other hand, definitive treatment is clearly indicated when complications arise. In this patient, hypercalcemia and nephrolithiasis constitute a clear-cut indication for surgical treatment of the hyperparathyroidism. An additional reason would be to prevent bone loss in this young woman which would place her at an increased risk for development of skeletal complications at a later time. Glucocorticoids are usually ineffective in the management of primary hyperparathyroidism and would affect bone metabolism negatively, besides producing other serious side effects when administered on a long-term basis. Thiazide diuretics or calcium supplementation are contraindicated in this patient because of the risk of inducing hypercalcemia.

634. The answer is A. *(Braunwald, ed 11, chap 337.)* Osteomalacia and rickets both are characterized by defective mineralization of bone; osteomalacia affects the adult skeleton, and rickets impairs the developing skeleton. Muscle weakness, hypocalcemia, hypophosphatemia, skeletal pain, and pseudofractures are cardinal features of both forms of osteomalacia. Bowing of the tibia, although common in children who have rickets, is not prominent in affected adults.

635. The answer is D. *(Braunwald, ed 11, chaps 337, 338.)* Paget's disease of bone is relatively common, and the incidence increases with age. An estimated prevalence of 3 percent in persons over the age of 40 years is a generally accepted figure. Most frequently, the disease is asymptomatic and diagnosed only when the typical sclerotic bones are incidentally detected on x-ray examinations done for other reasons or when an increased alkaline phosphatase activity is recognized on routine laboratory measurements. The etiology is unknown, but increased bone resorption followed by intensive bone repair is thought to be the mechanism causing increased bone density and increased serum alkaline phosphatase activity as a marker of osteoblast activity. Since increased mineralization of bone takes place (although in an abnormal pattern), hypercalcemia is not present unless a severely affected patient becomes immobilized. Hypercalcemia, in fact, would be an expected finding in a patient with primary hyperparathyroidism, bone metastases, or plasmacytoma, the latter typically producing no increase in the alkaline phosphatase activity. Osteomalacia resulting from vitamin D deficiency is associated with bone pain and hypophosphatemia; normal or decreased serum calcium concentrations produces secondary hyperparathyroidism, further aggravating the defective bone mineralization.

636. The answer is D. *(Braunwald, ed 11, chap 338.)* The most potent vitamin D metabolite in regulating absorption of calcium by the gastrointestinal tract is $1,25(OH)_2D$. Indeed, it is likely that vitamin D (cholecalciferol) and its 25OH derivative become active only after conversion in the kidney to $1,25(OH)_2D$. The 3-hydroxyl group on dihydrotachysterol enhances its capacity to stimulate calcium absorption, but not as much as 1-hydroxylation. When high serum calcium concentration causes decreased parathyroid hormone secretion or when serum phosphorus concentration is high, $24,25(OH)_2D$ is preferentially synthesized by the kidney. Although present in the serum in concentrations considerably higher than that of $1,25(OH)_2D$, $24,25(OH)_2D$ only weakly stimulates intestinal calcium absorption. However, it may have preferential effects on bone mineralization.

ENDOCRINE, METABOLIC, AND GENETIC DISORDERS

637. The answer is E. *(Braunwald, ed 11, chap 337.)* The combination of hypocalcemia, hypophosphatemia, and elevated serum parathyroid hormone levels, and bone fractures is consistent with a diagnosis of osteomalacia in this patient. In the absence of other gastrointestinal or renal abnormalities leading to malabsorption or increased renal loss of calcium or phosphorus, vitamin D deficiency is likely to be present. Inadequate intake of vitamin D and calcium together with limited exposure to the sun are frequent in this age group. Postmenopausal osteoporosis is associated with vertebral and hip fractures as well, but laboratory abnormalities are not present. Primary hyperparathyroidism is associated with increased serum calcium concentration, as is ectopic parathyroid hormone secretion (although existence of the latter has been questioned). Paget's disease of bone does not produce hypocalcemia, and it causes typical sclerotic changes on x-ray examination.

638. The answer is A. *(Braunwald, ed 11, chap 338.)* In most conditions in which hypocalcemia is present—e.g., osteomalacia, renal failure, and parathyroid hormone-resistance states (pseudohypoparathyroidism)—the concentration of circulating parathyroid hormone (PTH) is increased as assessed by radioimmunoassay. However, the syndrome of hypocalcemia with severe hypomagnesemia (<0.8 meq/L) is associated with a state of functional hypoparathyroidism. This severe degree of hypomagnesemia, most commonly associated with alcoholism and steatorrhea, may blunt or totally block PTH secretion. Magnesium deficiency also may be associated with reduced peripheral responsiveness to PTH. Correction of hypomagnesemia over several days restores normal parathyroid secretion and responsiveness.

639. The answer is D. *(Braunwald, ed 11, chap 338.)* A major function of parathyroid hormone is to act as a trophic hormone to regulate the rate of formation of $1,25(OH)_2$ vitamin D. The mechanism by which parathyroid hormone exerts this effect may be secondary to its effects on phosphorus metabolism. Other hormones, including prolactin and estrogen, also may play a role in stimulating the production of $1,25(OH)_2$ vitamin D.

640. The answer is A-N, B-N, C-Y, D-Y, E-Y. *(Braunwald, ed 11, chaps 43, 331.)* The luteal phase of the menstrual cycle follows ovulation and is characterized by an increase in progesterone secretion by the corpus luteum. With anovulatory cycles the corpus luteum does not form, and progesterone levels remain low. Furthermore, with anovulatory cycles the characteristic surge of LH and FSH at midcycle is absent, and menses are usually painless. Irregular estrogen breakthrough bleeding that occurs with anovulatory cycles is the consequence of persistent ovarian estradiol secretion and an absence of luteal-phase progesterone secretion.

641. The answer is A-N, B-N, C-Y, D-N, E-N. *(Braunwald, ed 11, chaps 57, 319.)* Marfan's syndrome is inherited as an autosomal dominant trait, and since both sexes are affected equally, half of the offspring of an affected individual are at risk. Between 15 and 30 percent of cases may result from new mutations. The ocular findings in this patient indicate that she is affected. Thus, she will transmit the disease to half of her offspring on average, although "skipped generations" are not infrequent, probably because of variability in the expression of the disease. For the same reason, it is incorrect to assume that her children would be less severely affected. Because of the autosomal dominant pattern of inheritance, consanguinity is not required to produce clinically affected offspring. Chromosomal complement is normal in patients with Marfan's syndrome, and no abnormality would be detected by karyotype analysis of amniotic cells. The risk of development of cardiovascular disorders during pregnancy is increased in women with Marfan's syndrome because of the predisposition to aortic dilatation and mitral valve prolapse. An echocardiogram is useful in detecting these abnormalities.

642. The answer is A-Y, B-Y, C-Y, D-Y, E-N. *(Braunwald, ed 11, chap 57.)* Since the gene responsible for an autosomally transmitted dominant disorder is located on one of the 22 autosomes, no predilection for either sex exists; on average, both sexes are affected equally, and half the offspring of an affected patient (and hence half the siblings) are affected. For the same reason, male-to-male transmission can occur. Since dominantly inherited disorders are manifested in the heterozygous state, unaffected persons are not carriers of the defective gene and cannot transmit it. Consanguinity among parents of affected offspring is not common, and new mutation seems to be the usual mechanism in affected patients without a family history of the disorder.

643. The answer is A-N, B-Y, C-Y, D-Y, E-N. *(Braunwald, ed 11, chaps 67, 336.)* Familial hypocalcemia, short stature, and abnormalities of the metacarpal and metatarsal bones are characteristic features of pseudohypoparathyroidism. The underlying defect is renal resistance to the action of parathyroid hormone; although plasma levels of parathyroid hormone are elevated, urinary cyclic AMP is low, and there is a diminished response of urinary cyclic AMP to the exogenous administration of the hormone. The basal ganglia are frequently calcified. No antibodies to parathyroid tissue can be demonstrated, and, unlike the situation in idiopathic hypoparathyroidism, the frequency of monilial infection is not increased. Hypothyroidism is common in persons with pseudohypoparathyroidism, usually the result of resistance to thyroid-stimulating hormone due to the same defect in membrane adenylate cyclase that causes resistance to parathyroid hormone.

644. The answer is A-N, B-Y, C-N, D-N, E-Y. *(Braunwald, ed 11, chap 70.)* Medium-chain triglycerides (12 to 14 carbons in length) are absorbed directly into the portal circulation and do not require emulsification with bile acids as do the rest of dietary fats before they can be absorbed into the intestinal lymph as chylomicrons. The metabolism of medium-chain triglycerides is faster, in part, because they are rapidly cleared from the portal blood by the liver. Although useful in providing adequate fat intake and hence adequate caloric intake in patients with biliary insufficiency or other forms of fat malabsorption, they are not essential for human nutrition.

645. The answer is A-Y, B-Y, C-N, D-N, E-N. *(Braunwald, ed 11, chap 70.)* Between 25 and 40 percent of urea formed by the liver is hydrolyzed by bacteria within the colon, and the nitrogen is recycled as ammonia for the synthesis of nonessential amino acids. Since the urinary excretion of urea is severely compromised in patients with uremia, the amount of recycled ammonia increases proportionately. The intermediary metabolism of glucose provides carbon skeletons for nonessential amino acids. Thus, patients with uremia can meet their protein requirements by receiving a limited amount of protein rich in essential amino acids ("Giovanetti" diet). Otherwise, energy requirements in these patients are unchanged or even increased by accompanying features such as anemia.

646. The answer is A-N, B-Y, C-Y, D-N, E-Y. *(Braunwald, ed 11, chap 70.)* Whenever caloric intake is deficient, amino acids are utilized as energy substrates and for gluconeogenesis to maintain an adequate blood level of glucose, especially important for metabolism of the brain. Thus, protein synthesis is compromised when energy requirements are not met by nonprotein calories. Stated in another way, energy undernutrition predisposes to protein starvation even when the protein supply is otherwise adequate. Nevertheless, it should be kept in mind that diets deficient in energy are frequently deficient in protein as well. Carbohydrates have a protein-sparing effect if given in sufficient quantities, but this effect does not hold true for fat. Low carbohydrate and fat diets do not produce a selective protein malabsorption, although generalized malabsorption occurs in patients with severe chronic malnutrition.

647. The answer is A-N, B-Y, C-N, D-Y, E-Y. *(Braunwald, ed 11, chap 71. Baker, N Engl J Med 306:969, 1982.)* Several methods are useful in assessing protein undernutrition. Clinically, the ratio of 24-hour urinary creatinine excretion to height is the most sensitive and practical measure of muscle mass; it is decreased in the presence of protein malnutrition. Reduced blood levels of proteins synthesized by the liver, such as albumin and transferrin, are also characteristic findings with protein starvation. Anthropometric assessment of midarm circumference and triceps skin-fold thickness are measures of the mass of muscle and adipose tissue, respectively. While in many instances calculation of body weight as a percentage of ideal body weight is a good measure of lean body mass plus adipose tissue, the presence of ascites and edema makes this assessment unreliable. Blood ammonia levels may indicate protein overload from intestinal causes (e.g., gastrointestinal bleeding) but are not helpful in assessing protein nutrition. The combination of a careful clinical history and a thorough examination is also a reproducible and valid technique to evaluate nutritional status; however, many cachectic individuals are unable to provide a detailed history.

648. The answer is A-Y, B-N, C-Y, D-N, E-Y. *(Braunwald, ed 11, chap 72. Saudek, Am J Med 60:117, 1976.)* Protein-calorie undernutrition affects the function of nearly every organ. Physiologic adaptations to caloric deficiency include a fall in plasma insulin concentration coupled with a rise in glucagon and cortisol levels. This mechanism, which protects against hypoglycemia, permits liberation of amino acids from muscle and of free fatty acids from adipose tissue, thereby providing carbon chains for hepatic gluconeogenesis and ketogenesis, respectively. In addition, ketones and free fatty acids are oxidized directly in many tissues and provide the energy for hepatic gluconeogenesis. Thyroid hormone metabolism is also changed: 5'-deiodination of T_4 is decreased, so that serum T_4 concentration remains the same or rises slightly and serum T_3 concentration declines. The 5'-deiodination of reverse T_3 (rT_3) is also reduced, causing serum levels of rT_3, which is metabolically inert, to rise significantly. Cell-mediated immunity is impaired (as evidenced by cutaneous anergy), although serum immunoglobulin levels and humoral response to antigens are preserved.

649. The answer is A-N, B-Y, C-Y, D-Y, E-Y. *(Braunwald, ed 11, chaps 74, 75.)* In most malnourished persons, positive nitrogen balance can be achieved by providing 1 g of amino acids per kilogram of ideal body weight. However, in the presence of abnormal protein losses (e.g., from burn exudates, pancreatic secretions, or gastrointestinal fistula) or hypermetabolic states (sepsis, trauma, hyperthyroidism), additional protein intake must be provided. Likewise, daily protein requirements are increased in the presence of caloric deficiency, because amino acids are used for oxidative metabolism and gluconeogenesis. Renal insufficiency and hepatic insufficiency are examples of "nitrogen accumulation diseases." When the kidneys are unable to excrete urea, ammonia may be used for the net synthesis of nonessential amino acids; thus, the need for nonessential nitrogen is reduced. In hepatic failure, amino acid catabolism is decreased, so that even normal protein intake may be deleterious.

650. The answer is A-Y, B-Y, C-Y, D-N, E-N. *(Braunwald, ed 11, chaps 74, 75.)* As a general rule, when patients cannot eat a normal diet, cannot absorb an oral diet efficiently, or deteriorate in health with oral feeding, total parenteral nutrition (TPN) is needed to provide partial or complete nourishment. Bowel rest, a frequent indication for TPN, is important in treating exacerbations of inflammatory bowel disease, intestinal fistulas, and pancreatitis. All persons with profound anorexia, vomiting, and mucosal inflammation from cancer chemotherapy can benefit from TPN. Persons who are markedly hypermetabolic due to severe trauma, burns, or sepsis, for example, also may be helped by supplemental parenteral nutrition, even when some oral intake is possible. Well-nourished patients who are not expected to be able to eat for 10 to 14 days should receive TPN to avoid excess wasting and malnutrition. It is unclear whether the decrease in negative nitrogen balance that results from administration for a week or less of TPN to otherwise healthy people is of clinical significance. Patients who are unable to swallow for long periods of time (e.g., due to stroke, neuromuscular disorders, or coma) are best treated with enteral feedings.

651. The answer is A-Y, B-Y, C-N, D-N, E-Y. *(Braunwald, ed 11, chap 305.)* Several inborn errors of metabolism can be treated successfully by the appropriate dietary restriction of a substrate or its precursors. Mental retardation and other problems associated with galactosemia and phenylketonuria can be prevented by reduced intake of galactose or phenylalanine, respectively, during childhood. Restriction of neutral fats can prevent pancreatitis in persons with lipoprotein lipase deficiency. Neither hyperprolinemia nor Tay-Sachs disease is treatable by dietary management.

652. The correct answer is A-Y, B-Y, C-Y, D-Y, E-Y. *(Braunwald, ed 11, chap 315.)* Appropriate therapy for individuals who have familial hypercholesterolemia should begin with a diet that is low in cholesterol and saturated fats and high in polyunsaturated fats. The administration of nicotinic acid and bile acid-binding resins, such as cholestyramine or colestipol, may be required if diet alone is insufficient therapy. Probucol also can be effective in lowering serum cholesterol levels when other measures are inadequate.

653. The answer is A-Y, B-N, C-Y, D-Y, E-N. *(Braunwald, ed 11, chap 315. Motulsky, N Engl J Med 294:823, 1976.)* Genetic analysis of survivors of myocardial infarction indicates that 20 percent of those persons less than 60 years of age have some form of inherited hyperlipidemia. Familial hypercholesterolemia, familial hypertriglyceridemia, and familial combined hyperlipidemia are the three most common primary hyperlipidemias. Inherited in an autosomal dominant manner, these disorders are associated with a fivefold to tenfold increase in the risk of developing premature coronary atherosclerosis. Familial hyperalphalipoproteinemia is characterized by elevated levels of high-density lipoprotein (HDL); it is associated with a slightly increased longevity and confers an apparent protection against myocardial infarction. Familial lipoprotein lipase deficiency is a rare autosomal recessive disorder.

654. The answer is A-Y, B-Y, C-Y, D-Y, E-Y. *(Braunwald, ed 11, chap 315.)* Diabetic patients with insulin deficiency may show massive elevation of the serum level of triglycerides, with the concomitant risk of development of acute pancreatitis. Adequate insulin replacement restores lipoprotein lipase activity and decreases hepatic production of very low density lipoproteins by impairing fatty acid mobilization from the adipose tissue. However, hypertriglyceridemia also occurs in well-controlled diabetic patients (generally obese) in whom it may be present as an independently inherited trait as shown by family studies. Specific drug therapy may be required in this group of patients when diet and adequate control of the diabetic state fail to return triglyceride levels to normal.

655. The answer is A-N, B-Y, C-Y, D-Y, E-Y. *(Braunwald, ed 11, chap 315. Brewer, Ann Intern Med 98:623, 1983.)* This patient has familial type III hyperlipoproteinemia with typical tuberoeruptive and palmar xanthomas. The basic defect in type III hyperlipoproteinemia is an abnormal form of apoprotein E (E_2) which has a lower affinity for its liver receptor, thus impairing the rate of clearance of chylomicron remnants and intermediate density lipoprotein (IDL) from the circulation. Heterozygotes for the E_2 allele (e.g., E_1/E_2, E_3/E_2) do not have hyperlipidemia. Since the incidence of the E_2/E_2 genotype in the general population is 1 in 100, but the incidence of type III hyperlipoproteinemia is only 1 in 10,000, other factors contribute to the expression of the genetic defect. Thus, obesity, hypothyroidism, and diabetes mellitus must be sought and treated accordingly. Clofibrate is usually effective when drug therapy is required in these patients.

656. The answer is A-N, B-N, C-Y, D-N, E-N. *(Braunwald, ed 11, chap 317. Bray, Diabetes 26:1072, 1977.)* The failure of traditional medical therapies for morbid obesity has provided the impetus for the development of bypass surgery. The initial common bypass operation was jejunoileal bypass. Although weight loss is usually rapid and long-lasting, there are serious postoperative complications, including wound infection (2 to 5 percent), thromboembolism (1 to 5 percent), and death (4 percent). Medical sequelae include diarrhea in all patients, polyarthritis due to circulating immune complexes (6 percent), progressive liver disease (2 to 4 percent), and nephrolithiasis due to calcium malabsorption with secondary hyperoxaluria (3 to 10 percent). Gastric surgery—either bypass or plication—leads to limitation of food intake by delaying gastric emptying and providing a smaller reservoir, which result in early satiety. Both types of gastric procedures, by maintaining intestinal continuity, can promote significant weight loss without causing malabsorption, diarrhea, or hepatic dysfunction.

657. The answer is A-Y, B-Y, C-Y, D-Y, E-N. *(Braunwald, ed 11, chap 317. Felig, chap 21. Wilson, ed 7, chap 27.)* Human obesity is due to overexpansion of adipose tissue, either from an increase in adipocyte size (hypertrophic obesity) or from an increase in both cell number and size (hypercellular-hypertrophic obesity). Most persons with mild to moderate obesity have hypertrophic obesity; the characteristic onset is during adult life ("middle-age spread"). By contrast, persons with severe obesity usually have both hypertrophy and hyperplasia of adipose cells. Fat-cell hypercellularity is most likely to develop during one of two periods: in utero or early infancy or at or shortly before the time of puberty. Hence, individuals with this type of obesity frequently give a history of onset early in life. Adipose hypercellularity seems to be a permanent, irreversible phenomenon; weight reduction, even to a significant degree, decreases adipocyte size but not number.

ENDOCRINE, METABOLIC, AND GENETIC DISORDERS

658. The answer is A-Y, B-N, C-N, D-N, E-Y. *(Braunwald, ed 11, chap 317. Olefsky, Am J Med 70:151, 1981.)* Increased insulin secretion is a characteristic feature of obesity, and the combination of normal or elevated blood sugar concentration with hyperinsulinemia indicates that an insulin-resistant state is present. Tissue insensitivity to insulin is common in obesity and appears to have two components: a decreased number of tissue insulin receptors and, with more severe insulin resistance, a postreceptor intracellular defect in glucose metabolism. Circulating insulin antagonists have not been implicated in the insulin resistance of obesity. Both the formation of insulin and the rate of insulin degradation are normal in obese persons.

659. The answer is A-N, B-Y, C-N, C-Y, E-N. *(Braunwald, ed 11, chap 317. Bray, Diabetes 26:1072, 1977.)* Intestinal bypass surgery is a last-resort treatment for morbidly obese persons who have not lost weight with traditional medical therapies. The presence of certain complications of obesity—e.g., diabetes, hypertriglyceridemia, hypertension, osteoarthritis, and alveolar hypoventilation—may provide further impetus to consider surgery. Most centers restrict the operation to persons between the ages of 18 and 40 years; older persons usually are excluded because of increased postoperative morbidity. Complications of jejunoileal bypass surgery include renal failure, nephrolithiasis, and progressive liver disease; therefore, significant renal or hepatic disease usually is considered a contraindication to this procedure.

660. The answer is A-N, B-Y, C-N, D-Y, E-Y. *(Braunwald, ed 11, chap 317.)* Jejunum-ileal bypass has been used in the past as an effective means of reducing weight in patients with severe obesity resistant to medical and diet therapies. Besides decreasing the total absorptive area of the small bowel, steatorrhea frequently occurs, causing malabsorption of fat-soluble vitamins, including vitamin D. Increased amounts of fatty acids in the gut lumen complex intestinal calcium, thus decreasing calcium absorption and secondarily causing hyperabsorption of oxalate, which leads to hyperoxaluria and oxalate nephrolithiasis. Hepatic dysfunction is thought to result from essential amino acid deficiency or absorption of hepatotoxic substances from the excluded bowel, or both. The associated polyarthritis is thought to be mediated by immune complexes.

661. The answer is A-N, B-N, C-N, D-Y, E-N. *(Braunwald, ed 11, chap 317. Stunkard, N Engl J Med 314:193, 1986.)* Basal metabolic rates in obese persons are normal when the results are expressed as a function of fat-free body weight. Similarly, depending on the type of exercise performed, energy expenditure is normal or even increased in obese persons because of extra body mass. Although weight gain does occur in patients with hypothyroidism, the gain is usually modest and is a result of fluid retention in connective tissues rich in mucopolysaccharides. The obesity associated with Cushing's syndrome is centripetal in type and is usually accompanied by other manifestations of the disease such as cutaneous striae, muscle weakness, and hypertension. The genetic background is probably more important than environmental factors in the development of human obesity. Overactivity of lipoprotein lipase rather than its deficiency has been suggested as a pathogenetic mechanism in rodent and human obesity, but the importance of this is still unclear.

662. The answer is A-Y, B-Y, C-N, D-N, E-Y. *(Braunwald, ed 11, chap 321.)* The development of a pituitary adenoma in a patient who has undergone bilateral adrenalectomy for the treatment of Cushing's disease is termed Nelson's syndrome. This disorder is characterized by hyperpigmentation, erosion of the sella turcica, and high plasma ACTH levels. Because of adrenalectomy, urinary 17-ketosteroid excretion usually is low; plasma cortisol levels are determined by the regimen of replacement therapy.

663. The answer is A-Y, B-N, C-Y, D-Y, E-N. *(Braunwald, ed 11, chap 321.)* Hypoglycemia, exercise, administration of levodopa, and intravenous arginine infusion all stimulate growth hormone secretion in normal subjects. These factors commonly serve as the basis for stimulation tests to measure reserve capacities for growth hormone secretion and consequently to assess the functional capacity of the pituitary gland. Hyperglycemia suppresses growth hormone secretion, and thyrotropin-releasing hormone does not release growth hormone in normal subjects; these stimuli, however, may cause a paradoxical increase in plasma growth hormone concentration in persons with acromegaly.

664. The answer is A-Y, B-N, C-N, D-N, E-Y. *(Braunwald, ed 11, chap 321. Snyder, Endocr Rev 6:552, 1985.)* Serum prolactin levels correlate with tumor size in patients with macroprolactinomas. Thus, the prolactin level in this patient is lower than that expected in association with a large pituitary prolactinoma, and the modest hyperprolactinemia probably reflects impaired delivery of dopamine from the hypothalamus resulting from mechanical effects of the tumor. Since the patient has no clinical evidence of acromegaly, hyperthyroidism, or Cushing's syndrome, measurement of serum gonadotropin and testosterone levels would be useful to assess the mechanism of the sexual dysfunction or to rule out the presence of a gonadotropin-producing pituitary adenoma, or both. Paradoxically, gonadotropin-secreting tumors usually cause hypogonadotropic hypogonadism because they produce isolated α or β subunits of luteinizing hormone (LH) instead of intact, bioactive LH. Evaluation for other pituitary hormone deficiencies is also indicated. Treatment with desmopressin is not indicated unless diabetes insipidus ensues. The use of bromocriptine would be confusing in this patient because it would suppress the elevated prolactin levels without affecting tumor behavior. Formal visual testing is mandatory in every patient with a pituitary macroadenoma.

665. The answer is A-Y, B-Y, C-N, D-Y, E-Y. *(Braunwald, ed 11, chap 324.)* Radioactive iodine uptake (RAIU) is often a useful test in distinguishing among the various causes of hyperthyroidism. Elevation of RAIU above the normal range usually indicates thyroid hyperfunction (some persons with hyperthyroidism have a normal or low RAIU). Painless thyroiditis is a variant of chronic lymphocytic thyroiditis associated with transient thyrotoxicosis from release of preformed hormone. Radiographic contrast studies, such as intravenous pyelography and oral cholecystography, use organic media that release iodide and thus serve as sources for dilution of administered radioactive iodine; as a result, RAIU may be falsely low for as long as 6 months. Thyrotoxicosis factitia is the term used to designate thyrotoxicosis resulting from ingestion of thyroid hormones. Ingestion of liothyronine (T_3) results in a low serum thyroxine (T_4) concentration, while ingestion of levothyroxine leads to elevations of both T_4 and T_3. In either case, feedback of exogenous thyroid hormone decreases TSH secretion and lowers RAIU. Struma ovarii, which is an ovarian tumor with thyroid-like tissue that releases thyroid hormone, is a rare cause of thyrotoxicosis. Measurement of RAIU over the thyroid gland would not, of course, detect the abdominal source of increased RAIU in women affected with struma ovarii. Choriocarcinoma releases factors with TSH-like activity that enhance uptake of radioactive iodine.

666. The answer is A-Y, B-Y, C-Y, D-Y, E-Y. *(Braunwald, ed 11, chap 324.)* The changes in thyroid hormone economy termed the "sick euthyroid" syndrome may be induced by a variety of illnesses, traumas, and stresses. Depending upon the severity and duration of the stress, these changes lead to alterations in the free and, eventually, in the concentration of total circulating thyroid hormones. Decreased production of T_3 resulting from inhibition of the peripheral 5'-monodeiodination of T_4 is a consistent feature. A decrease in the protein binding of T_4 and T_3 also occurs, and as a consequence the percentage of free T_4 usually increases. In more seriously ill patients, abnormalities of hormone binding to protein increase still further so that serum T_4 concentrations decrease into the hypothyroid range, most commonly the consequence of an inhibition of thyroid hormone binding to protein. Such inhibition is likely on the basis of an increase in quantity of a circulating fatty acid.

667. The answer is A-N, B-N, C-Y, D-Y, E-Y. *(Braunwald, ed 11, chap 324.)* The woman described has subacute thyroiditis, which seems to have a viral etiology. The tenderness may respond to aspirin therapy, and, in more severe cases, the use of glucocorticoids is generally efficacious in treatment, although its use is associated with a high recurrence rate. Hyperthyroidism, when it occurs in association with subacute thyroiditis, is usually transient and is best controlled symptomatically with propranolol or phenobarbital, or both. Subtotal thyroidecotomy and radioactive iodine therapy are never appropriate therapy for such acute thyroiditis.

668. The answer is A-Y, B-Y, C-N, D-Y, E-N. *(Braunwald, ed 11, chap 325.)* Adrenal carcinomas are likely to present as abdominal masses and secrete large amounts of adrenal androgens, which results in markedly elevated urinary 17-ketosteroid excretion. Neoplastic secretion of adrenal steroids characteristically is not suppressed with high doses (2 mg every 6 hours) of dexamethasone, because it is not regulated by ACTH. Indeed, ACTH levels are usually immeasurably low in persons with adrenal carcinoma. Testing with metyrapone (750 mg every 4 hours for a day) usually does not result in an increase in urinary 17-hydroxycorticosteroids or plasma 11-deoxycortisol because of the prolonged suppression of ACTH secretion by the autonomous adrenal tumor. In contrast, patients with pituitary-dependent Cushing's syndrome show normal response to metyrapone.

669. The answer is A-Y, B-N, C-Y, D-Y, E-N. *(Braunwald, ed 11, chap 325.)* Complications of long-term treatment with high doses of corticosteroids include the development or acceleration of osteoporosis and depression of immune function. Whether high-dose steroids can induce frank peptic ulceration is not established, but persons with preexisting ulcer disease may have exacerbations while on steroid therapy. Detection of preexisting abnormalities before the start of steroid therapy allows clinicians to institute appropriate treatment concurrently with the institution of steroid therapy. Testing the integrity of the hypothalamic-pituitary-adrenal axis is unwarranted prior to the initiation of chronic high-dose steroid therapy.

670. The answer is A-Y, B-Y, C-Y, D-Y, E-Y. *(Braunwald, ed 11, chaps 325, 333.)* The syndromes of congenital adrenal hyperplasia may result in all of the following: virilization in females (due to C-21 hydroxylase or C-11 hydroxylase deficiency); isosexual precocious puberty in male individuals (C-21 hydroxylase or C-11 hydroxylase deficiency); male pseudohermaphroditism (3β-ol-dehydrogenase, C-17 hydroxylase, or 20, 22-desmolase deficiency); hypertension due to salt retention (C-11 hydroxylase or C-17 hydroxylase deficiency); and hypotension secondary to renal salt wasting (C-21 hydroxylase, 3β-ol-dehydrogenase, or 20, 22-desmolase deficiency.)

671. The answer is A-N, B-Y, C-Y, D-Y, E-Y. *(Braunwald, ed 11, chaps 325, 333.)* Urinary 17-ketosteroid determination, a venerable procedure in endocrinology, measures the metabolites of weak adrenal and gonadal androgens. It is not a specific test for assessment of gonadal function and is a poor means of assessing the potent testicular androgen testosterone (only about 40 percent of urinary levels of 17-ketosteroids in men comes from production of testosterone). Although it is not the most sensitive indicator of congenital adrenal hyperplasia, urinary excretion of 17-ketosteroids usually is elevated in affected untreated individuals.

672. The answer is A-Y, B-Y, C-Y, D-Y, E-Y. *(Braunwald, ed 11, chap 327. McGarry, Annu Rev Biochem 49:395, 1980.)* The insulin-to-glucagon ratio determines the rate of ketogenesis by the liver. A fall in insulin increases adipose-cell lipolysis, with the resultant liberation of free fatty acids, the substrate for ketone body synthesis. In the liver, carnitine acyltransferase I is the critical mitochondrial enzyme necessary to transport free fatty acids from the cytosol into the mitochondrial matrix, where they are oxidized to ketone bodies. Glucagon stimulates ketogenesis by increasing hepatic carnitine levels and decreasing liver malonyl CoA concentrations. Carnitine is required for this movement of free fatty acids into the mitochondria, and malonyl CoA, the first committed intermediate in the synthesis of fatty acids from glucose, is a powerful competitive inhibitor of carnitine acyltransferase I.

673. The answer is A-N, B-N, C-Y, D-Y, E-Y. *(Braunwald, ed 11, chap 327. Yoon, N Engl J Med 300:1173, 1979.)* There is considerable disagreement regarding the genetics of diabetes mellitus, but certain aspects appear to be clearcut. Genetic factors are probably permissive for the development of IDDM and related more directly to the development of noninsulin-dependent diabetes mellitus (NIDDM). The genetic locus for diabetes appears to be located near the HLA genes on the sixth chromosome. The presence of HLA antigens B8 or B15 increases the risk for developing IDDM nearly threefold, antigens Dw3 and Dw4 fourfold to fivefold, and antigen combinations (e.g., B8/B15) up to tenfold. However, homozygosity for a high-risk allele (e.g., Dw3/Dw3) does not increase the risk further. The concordance rate for monozygotic twins under 40 years of age is less than 50 percent, while for those twins older than 40 years it approaches the expected 100 percent. Pedigree analysis has shown a very low prevalence of vertical transmission for NIDDM. The onset of juvenile diabetes has a seasonal variation and may follow mumps, hepatitis, or Coxsackie virus infections, among others. These infections in genetically predisposed persons are theorized to produce an immune response with the development of cytotoxic islet-cell antibodies, which complete the destruction of the beta cells. This theory would explain why circulating islet cell antibodies are usually detectable soon after the onset of IDDM.

674. The answer is A-Y, B-N, C-Y, D-Y, E-N. *(Braunwald, ed 11, chap 327. Arieff, Medicine 51:73, 1972. Feig, N Engl J Med 297:1444, 1977. Carroll, Diabetes Care 6:579, 1983.)* Diabetic hyperosmolar nonketotic coma is a medical emergency usually occurring as a complication of maturity-onset diabetes. Typically, affected persons are elderly (often living alone or in a nursing home), have a history of recent stroke or infection, and are unable to drink sufficient water to balance urinary fluid losses. These factors combine to cause sustained hyperglycemic diuresis with profound volume depletion and decreased urine output. Presenting features often include signs of circulatory compromise as well as central nervous system manifestations ranging from confusion or seizures to coma. Ketoacidosis is absent, perhaps because portal-vein insulin concentration is high enough to prevent full activation of hepatic ketogenesis. Serum levels of free fatty acids are generally lower than in diabetic ketoacidosis, and although hypertonicity is marked, measured serum sodium concentration is kept from being significantly elevated by the profound hyperglycemia. Infections are common, and disseminated intravascular coagulation can occur as a result of elevated plamsa viscosity (both bleeding and in situ thrombosis have been reported). Although administration of free water eventually becomes necessary, the treatment of salt deficits has highest initial therapeutic priority. Several liters of isotonic saline should be given over the first 2 hours, followed by half-normal saline, and then a 5% glucose solution when blood glucose levels approach normal. Hypotonic fluids should not be used initially, because most of the water enters the intracellular compartment—possibly leading to cerebral edema—rather than remaining in the plasma and interstitial spaces, where it is needed to support the circulation. Insulin also is required but usually in lower doses than in diabetic ketoacidosis.

675. The answer is A-N, B-Y, C-Y, D-N, E-Y. *(Braunwald, ed 11, chap 327.)* The occurrence of hyperglycemic ketoacidosis or hyperglycemic hyperosmolar coma is diagnostic of diabetes mellitus. Similarly, persistent fasting hyperglycemia (glucose concentration greater than 140 mg/100 mL), even if asymptomatic, has been recommended by the National Diabetes Data Group as a criterion for the diagnosis of diabetes. On the other hand, abnormal glucose tolerance—whether after eating or occurring after a standard "glucose tolerance test"— can be caused by many factors (e.g., anxiety, infection or other illness, lack of exercise, or inadequate diet). Likewise, glycosuria may have renal as well as endocrinologic causes. Therefore, these two conditions cannot be considered diagnostic of diabetes.

676. The answer is A-Y, B-N, C-N, D-N, E-Y. *(Braunwald, ed 11, chap 327. Wilson, ed 7, chap 26. Flier, N Engl J Med 306:1537, 1982.)* Chronic insulin resistance is defined as a need for more than 200 units of insulin per day for several days in the absence of infection or ketoacidosis. This definition was based on the assumption that the normal human pancreas produces this much insulin daily; in fact, normal daily insulin production is probably 30 to 40 units, so that relative resistance is present when more than this amount is required to control blood sugar levels. The most common causes of insulin resistance are obesity and anti-insulin antibodies of the IgG type. Antibodies develop within 60 days of initiation of insulin therapy in nearly all diabetic persons. It is assumed that the binding of insulin by these antibodies is the major cause of severe insulin resistance, but the correlation between antibody titer and resistance is not always close. Uncontrolled hyperglycemia is the major consequence of insulin resistance, though ketoacidosis also may result. A history of discontinuous insulin use is frequent, and concomitant insulin allergy occurs in a minority of affected persons. Treatment should start by increasing the dosage of insulin and then prescribing pure human insulin (although antibodies can also develop to human insulin, presumably because of denaturation of some molecules during manufacture). Most patients require high doses of steroids, which frequently begin to take effect in a few days.

Acanthosis nigricans is a cutaneous disorder associated with two types of insulin resistance: type A, in which young women show accelerated growth, evidence of virilization, and decreased numbers of insulin receptors; and type B, in which older women have anti-insulin-receptor antibodies and other symptoms and signs of autoimmune disease (arthralgias, positive assay for antinuclear antibody, and others). The absence of acanthosis nigricans in the woman described in the question makes it unlikely that decreased numbers of insulin receptors or the presence of anti-insulin-receptor antibodies is playing a role in her insulin resistance.

677. The answer is A-Y, B-Y, C-Y, D-N, E-N. *(Braunwald, ed 11, chap 327.)* Approximately 40 percent of patients with type I diabetes mellitus sustain diabetic nephropathy. Progression of renal disease is markedly accelerated by hypertension, and even mild degrees of hypertension in diabetic patients should be treated aggressively. A hallmark of diabetic nephropathy is the presence of so-called macroproteinuria (excretion of more than 550 mg/24 h), and once this phase is reached there is a steady decline in renal function. So-called microalbuminuria, the excretion of 30 to 300 mg of albumin per day, is also statistically predictive of progression of renal disease. In contrast, nocturia is usually a manifestation of undertreatment of diabetes and is an indication not of renal failure but of an osmotic diuresis. There is no clear-cut relation between insulin requirement and the development of any of the long-term complications of diabetes, including nephropathy; the development of these complications correlates better with the duration rather than the severity of diabetes mellitus.

678. The answer is A-N, B-Y, C-Y, D-N, E-N. *(Braunwald, ed 11 chap 329. Jordan, Arch Intern Med 137:390, 1977. Scarlett, N Engl J Med 297:1029, 1977. Bauman, JAMA 252:2730, 1984.)* Because factitious hypoglycemia due to insulin injection or sulfonylurea ingestion is common, the finding of hyperinsulinemia associated with a low blood sugar concentration can no longer be considered diagnostic of an islet cell tumor (insulinoma). Suspicion of factitious disease should be especially high in medical personnel and in families of diabetics. The alpha and beta subunits of insulin are cleaved from proinsulin in the beta cell and released in equimolar amounts with the connecting (C) peptide; elevation of plasma C-peptide levels signifies endogenous hyperinsulinemia, because exogenous insulin administration suppresses beta-cell function. Therefore, the triad of fasting hypoglycemia, hyperinsulinemia, and elevated plasma C-peptide levels is consistent with either endogenous hyperinsulinemia or ingestion of a sulfonylurea; documentation of the latter in urine or plasma would be diagnostic. Proinsulin usually is released into the circulation in small quantities. However, in patients with insulinoma, proinsulin concentration frequently exceeds 20 percent of total insulin; ingestion of a sulfonylurea, on the other hand, does not cause a disproportionate elevation of plasma proinsulin levels. Insulin antibody measurements in this case would not be expected to be helpful—antibodies may not develop for several months after the start of insulin injections, and the high C-peptide levels essentially rule out an exogenous source of insulin. However, under some circumstances antibodies to specific species of insulin can be identified and hence establish that exogenous insulin has been taken. Attempts to localize an islet cell tumor by radiologic means should only be done once factitious types of hypoglycemia are excluded.

679. The answer is A-Y, B-Y, C-Y, D-N, E-N. *(Braunwald, ed 11, chap 329.)* Hypoglycemia due to overutilization of glucose can be associated either with high or low insulin levels. Hypoglycemia associated with hyperinsulinism can occur in persons who have pancreatic insulinoma or who take exogenous insulin or ingest sulfonylurea drugs. Low plasma insulin levels can be associated with overutilization of glucose; examples include large, solid extrapancreatic tumors (e.g., hepatoma and sarcoma), in which high levels of insulin-like growth factors may play a role, and systemic carnitine deficiency, in which peripheral tissues are unable to use free fatty acids for energy production and the liver cannot synthesize ketone bodies. Underproduction of glucose may occur with acquired liver disease, such as hepatic congestion due to right-sided heart failure or viral hepatitis, or with hormone deficiencies, such as adrenal insufficiency and hypopituitarism.

680. The answer is A-N, B-N, C-Y, D-N, E-Y. *(Braunwald, ed 11, chap 330. Wilson, ed 7, chap 10.)* Klinefelter's syndrome is frequently not diagnosed in patients until the time of expected puberty or during adult life when incomplete virilization or some other manifestation of androgen deficiency first becomes apparent. Testosterone replacement is likely to promote virilization and to restore potency in these patients. However, if gynecomastia is already present, testosterone replacement therapy does not produce regression of the breast tissue, and it may even aggravate the gynecomastia. Surgical resection of the breast is usually necessary in this situation. Since the basic testicular lesion consists of progressive hyalinization of the seminiferous tubules, spermatogenic function is irreversibly impaired, and no form of hormonal therapy is effective in maintaining spermatogenesis. Even in normal persons, testosterone treatment produces hypospermia because of the inhibition of gonadotropin production. Although antisocial behavior may be a part of the Klinefelter syndrome, it is unlikely to be a manifestation of androgen deficiency and is not correctable by testosterone replacement.

681. The answer is A-Y, B-N, C-Y, D-N, E-Y. *(Braunwald, ed 11, chap 331.)* All women with premature ovarian failure should receive estrogen replacement. Treatment should be continued through the time of expected menopause to prevent acceleration of osteoporosis. Persons with C-17 hydroxylase deficiency remain sexually infantile because of an enzymatic block in biosynthesis of androgen and estrogen. Both genotypic males and females with C-17 hydroxylase deficiency have unambiguously female phenotypes and therefore require estrogen to effect sexual maturation. Women with an inadequate luteal phase have normal estrogen production, as evidenced by the presence of ovulatory cycles; progesterone production by the corpus luteum is deficient. Women with polycystic ovarian disease are hyperestrogenic, the result of extraglandular estrogen formation from androgen produced in increased amount by the ovaries; oral contraceptives are administered to some affected women to inhibit ovarian steroid synthesis and thus to diminish the degree of hirsutism. Most menopausal women have only mild to moderate symptoms of vasomotor instability and therefore do not require administration of estrogen to control these symptoms. More severe menopausal symptoms warrant a course of estrogen therapy.

682. The answer is A-Y, B-N, C-Y, D-N, E-N. *(Braunwald, ed 11, chaps 331, 333.)* In individuals with testicular feminization, estradiol secretion by the testes is markedly increased (but not to the level produced by normal ovaries); the mechanism is lack of suppression of luteinizing hormone by testosterone and consequent increased stimulation of gonadal testosterone and estradiol secretion. Ovaries containing follicle cysts may be a source of increased estrogen production, particularly during the postmenopausal years, when gonadotropin levels are very high. The increase in estrogen production characteristic of polycystic ovarian disease is the consequence of peripheral conversion of androstenedione to estrogen and not of direct gonadal production. During the third trimester of pregnancy estrogen production is increased because of formation of estrogen by the placenta rather than by the ovary. Arrhenoblastoma is a virilizing ovarian tumor and does not secrete estrogen.

683. The answer is A-Y, B-Y, C-N, D-Y, E-Y. *(Braunwald, ed 11, chaps 331, 333.)* The pathogenesis of hot flashes is uncertain, but in some manner it is related to estrogen deprivation. There is a close temporal relationship between the timing of the hot flash and the onset of pulses of luteinizing hormone (LH) secretion, and suggestions have been made that the flash itself is caused by alterations in metabolism of catecholamines, catecholestrogens, endorphins, or neurotensin. However, the most striking feature is that the symptoms are preceded by a decrease in estrogen secretion, so that the hot flashes commonly result after the removal of estrogen-secreting tissues, including estrogen-secreting testes in patients with testicular feminization, normal ovaries from premenopausal women, and estrogen-secreting tumors of the ovaries (dysgerminomas). Likewise, menopause at all ages commonly causes symptoms that include hot flashes, whereas removal of gonads or gonadal streaks in women who have never had estrogen secretion from the ovaries, as in women with gonadal dysgenesis, does not cause hot flashes.

684. The answer is A-Y, B-Y, C-Y, D-N, E-Y. *(Braunwald, ed 11, chap 331. Judd, Ann Intern Med 98:195, 1983.)* In this young woman with surgical castration, estrogen replacement therapy is indicated to relieve the vasomotor instability and to prevent the atrophy of estrogen target tissues such as the breast and urogenital epithelium. The beneficial effects of estrogens on bone metabolism and calcium balance constitute another indication for replacement therapy, especially in patients at high risk for postmenopausal development of osteoporosis (menopause at a young age in thin, white women). Hirsutism is a manifestation of androgen excess rather than of estrogen deficiency. Treatment with estrogen at physiologic or pharmacologic doses should be cyclic and include administration of progestogen during the last 10 days of the cycle to diminish the risk of development of endometrial hyperplasia and carcinoma of the uterus.

685. The answer is A-Y, B-Y, C-Y, D-N, E-N. *(Braunwald, ed 11, chap 332.)* Pathologic gynecomastia develops when the effective testosterone-to-estrogen ratio is decreased, due either to diminished testosterone production (as in primary testicular failure) or to increased estrogen production. The latter may arise from direct estradiol secretion by a testis stimulated by luteinizing hormone or human chorionic gonadotropin or from an increase in peripheral aromatization of precursor steroids, most notably androstenedione. Elevated androstenedione levels may result from increased secretion by an adrenal tumor (leading to an elevated level of urinary 17-ketosteroids) or decreased hepatic clearance in individuals with chronic liver disease. A variety of drugs, including diethylstilbestrol, heroin, digitalis, spironolactone, cimetidine, isoniazid, and tricyclic antidepressants, also can cause gynecomastia. In the case presented in the question, the history of paternity and the otherwise-normal physical examination speak against the necessity of obtaining a karyotype, and the bilateral breast enlargement essentially excludes the presence of carcinoma and, thus, the need for biopsy.

686. The answer is A-N, B-Y, C-Y, D-N, E-Y. *(Braunwald, ed 11, chap 333.)* Ambiguous genitalia results when androgen production (or action) is defective in a male fetus or when androgen production is enhanced in a female fetus. Such aberrations can arise from a variety of causes. The most common cause is congenital adrenal hyperplasia, followed by mixed gonadal dysgenesis, which is a nonfamilial aberration of the sex chromosomes that interferes with normal sexual development, including 45,X/46,XY mosaicism. Examples of single gene mutations leading to abnormal sexual differentiation are the Reifenstein syndrome, in which genetic male individuals have incompletely developed male genitalia because of androgen resistance, and 5α-reductase deficiency, in which testosterone cannot be converted to dihydrotestosterone. The use in the past of progestational agents to treat pregnant women presenting with threatened abortion was associated with variable degrees of hypospadias in male offspring. Hypogonadotropic hypogonadism is associated with microphallus in male infants but not with hypospadias or abnormal sexual differentiation. Men whose chromosome pattern is 47,XYY are anatomically normal.

687. The answer is A-Y, B-Y, C-N, D-N, E-Y. *(Braunwald, ed 11, chap 333.)* Phenotypic men who have two or more X chromosomes have Klinefelter syndrome. Although the diagnosis of Klinefelter syndrome may be suspected prepubertally due to the increased length of the lower body segment, most affected individuals first present postpubertally with signs of decreased testosterone production and small testes. The risk of breast cancer is 20 times that of normal men (and one-fifth that of women), presumably the consequence of long-term estrogen stimulation of the breast. Mosaic chromosome patterns (46,XY/47,XXY) are found in 10 percent of affected individuals, 70 percent of whom display the mosaicism only in the testes, which may be normal in size. Hypospadias is not increased in incidence in affected persons. Although mental deficiency and social maladjustment occur with increased frequency in persons with Klinefelter syndrome, most patients with the disorder have normal mental and social competence.

688. The answer is A-Y, B-Y, C-Y, D-Y, E-Y. *(Braunwald, ed 11, chap 335.)* Persistent hypophosphatemia is characterized by varying degrees of anorexia, dizziness, bone pain, proximal muscle weakness, and waddling gait. Severe hypophosphatemia may result in rhabdomyolysis, which is heralded by a sharp elevation in serum creatine phosphokinase concentration; hemolytic anemia, which is probably the consequence of reduced levels of 2,3-diphosphoglycerate and ATP in erythrocytes; and severe congestive cardiomyopathy. Persons with alcoholism may develop severe hypophosphatemia shortly after hospitalization, probably related to the combined effects of glucose administration and phosphorus deficiency due to diminished intake. Correction of phosphorus deficits leads to prompt reversal of the abnormalities.

689. The answer is A-N, B-Y, C-Y, D-N, E-N. *(Braunwald, ed 11, chap 335).* Because dietary phosphorus is so ubiquitous and its absorption is so efficient, phosphorus deficiency from poor intake alone is unusual. However, hypophosphatemia can arise if absorption is prevented by some means, such as the administration of nonabsorbable antacids, which bind phosphorus and block its absorption from the gastrointestinal tract. Significant but rapidly reversible hypophosphatemia may accompany the respiratory alkalosis of hyperventilation. Little phosphorus is lost in sweat. In the kidney, phosphorus is reabsorbed efficiently in the proximal tubule; therefore, diuretics that act proximally are phosphaturic (their use may result in hypophosphatemia), whereas distally acting diuretics are not.

690. The answer is A-Y, B-Y, C-N, D-Y, E-Y. *(Braunwald, ed 11, chap 335.)* Measuring the serum concentration of 25OH vitamin D, the major circulating form of vitamin D, can be used to assess the adequacy of dietary intake and absorption of the vitamin. (Vitamin D also is made in the skin in the presence of sunlight.) Once ingested or synthesized, vitamin D is metabolized to 25OH vitamin D in the liver. This reaction is not tightly regulated, and an increase in dietary intake or endogenous production of vitamin D is reflected by linear elevations of serum 25OH vitamin D levels. Levels are reduced in severe chronic parenchymal and cholestatic liver disease but usually are normal in renal failure. Anticonvulsant drugs and glucocorticoids induce hepatic microsomal enzymes, which metabolize vitamin D and 25OH vitamin D into inactive products; this phenomenon, along with other complex effects on calcium metabolism, helps to explain why these drugs cause osteopenia.

691. The answer is A-N, B-N, C-Y, D-N, E-Y. *(Braunwald, ed 11, chaps 335, 337.)* Vitamin D toxicity generally occurs after chronic ingestion of large doses of vitamin D_2 or D_3 (usually in excess of 50,000 to 100,000 IU daily for months). Ingestion of a single large dose of vitamin D_2 or D_3 does not cause acute toxicity, because excessive quantities are stored in body fat and released slowly into the bloodstream. Some vitamin D metabolites, such as $1,25(OH)_2$ vitamin D, could conceivably cause toxicity after a single overdose. Hypervitaminosis D has not been reported following prolonged sun exposure, partly because the vitamin is released slowly from the skin after conversion from previtamin D. Hypervitaminosis D causes hypercalcemia, hypercalciuria, and soft-tissue calcification, particularly in the kidneys. It is believed that high circulating levels of 25OH vitamin D directly stimulate intestinal calcium absorption and bone resorption, since toxicity can occur in anephric individuals. In fact, even in normal individuals with hypervitaminosis D serum $1,25(OH)_2$ vitamin D levels are low to normal (presumably because of suppression of parathyroid hormone production and renal damage).

692. The answer is A-N, B-N, C-Y, D-Y, E-N. *(Braunwald, ed 11, chap 337.)* The presenting findings in both primary hyperparathyroidism and multiple myeloma can include hypercalcemia and vertebral compression fractures. The absence of several key features—anemia, elevated erythrocyte sedimentation rate, abnormal serum protein electrophoresis, and Bence Jones proteinuria—is helpful in eliminating the possibility of multiple myeloma. If doubt remains as to the diagnosis of myeloma, a marrow aspiration should be performed. The presence of hypercalcemia makes unlikely the diagnoses of osteomalacia, which is associated with hypocalcemia, and of osteoporosis and Paget's disease, which are associated with normal blood calcium values.

693–696. The answers are: 693-E, 694-C, 695-A, 696-D. *(Braunwald, ed 11, chap 333.)* Sexual differentiation in the male fetus is dependent on testicular differentiation, testicular function, and response of target tissues to the hormones elaborated by the fetal testis, testosterone and müllerian regression factor. Target-tissue response (i.e., differentiation into male genital structures) depends not only on testosterone but also on its 5α-reduced metabolite, dihydrotestosterone. Infants born with complete testicular feminization have testes that function normally, but because of abnormal intracellular androgen receptors the wolffian ducts do not differentiate and the external genitalia are female in appearance. Regression of the müllerian ducts, however, occurs normally due to the action of müllerian regression factor secreted by the fetal testis. Males with 5α-reductase deficiency have absent or ambiguously developed prostate gland and external genitalia, the structures dependent on dihydrotestosterone for normal differentiation. Most males with cryptorchidism are normally virilized, suggesting intact fetal testicular function; however, an as yet unidentified testicular factor that is responsible for normal testicular descent may be deficient in these individuals. Pure gonadal dysgenesis occurs in individuals with a uniform 46,XY or 46,XX chromosomal complement and is often familial; the bilateral streak gonads and female internal ducts and external genitalia are similar to those associated with gonadal dysgenesis, but the somatic features of the Turner phenotype are absent.

DERMATOLOGIC DISORDERS

DIRECTIONS: Each question below contains five suggested answers. Choose the **one best** response to each question.

Questions 697–698

After several weeks of tetracycline treatment for acne, an obese 20-year-old man develops a scaling groin rash with satellite pustules. He has been applying nonprescription ointments for "jock itch" without relief. A potassium hydroxide preparation of the pustules and scales reveals budding yeasts and nonseptate and nonbranching pseudohyphae.

697. The most likely diagnosis in the case described above is

(A) tinea cruris
(B) moniliasis
(C) nonspecific intertrigo
(D) intertriginous psoriasis
(E) tinea versicolor

698. Which of the following therapeutic measures would NOT be appropriate for the man presented?

(A) Hydrocortisone cream (1%)
(B) Nystatin cream
(C) Miconazole cream
(D) Clotrimazole cream
(E) Discontinuation of tetracycline therapy

699. A 7-year-old girl is brought to the local emergency room after having a generalized seizure during which she lost consciousness. No history of head trauma can be elicited from her family and friends. A paternal uncle is mentally retarded and has had seizures. On examination, numerous brown spots—each greater than 3 cm and similar to those in Color Plate C—are present on the torso and extremities; one spot is 5 cm in size. Many smaller lesions, 1 mm or less are noted, especially in the axillary areas. The most likely diagnosis is

(A) Peutz-Jeghers syndrome
(B) Gardner's syndrome
(C) neurofibromatosis
(D) xeroderma pigmentosum
(E) hemochromatosis

700. A 45-year-old man has recently noted an increase in his shoe size. His wedding ring, which had always been loose, is now difficult to remove. He says that small pieces of meat frequently lodge between his teeth while he is eating dinner. He also remarks that he is sweating and urinating more, that he is more thirsty than usual, and that his skin is oily. Physical examination is remarkable for an enlarged tongue (as shown in Color Plate D), prominent jaw, and dark, velvety areas beneath his axillae. The most likely diagnosis is

(A) primary amyloidosis
(B) hypothyroidism
(C) acromegaly
(D) iron-deficiency anemia
(E) adult-onset diabetes mellitus

701. A 55-year-old Japanese businessman visiting the United States had been in excellent health until 6 months ago, when he first noted mild upper abdominal fullness after meals. On examination the man is noted to have hyperpigmented, heaped-up velvety lesions (as shown in Color Plate E) confined to the neck, axillae, and groin. Which of the following conditions have NOT been associated with the skin findings presented?

(A) Cushing's syndrome
(B) Massive obesity
(C) Acromegaly
(D) Adenocarcinoma of the stomach
(E) Addison's disease

702. A skin lesion (as shown in Color Plate F) is found on an 80-year-old woman hospitalized for stroke. She states the lesion has been present for 2 years but has gradually increased in size. Topical steroids were ineffective in treating the lesion 18 months ago. The most likely diagnosis is

(A) atopic dermatitis
(B) contact dermatitis
(C) seborrheic dermatitis
(D) Paget's disease of the nipple
(E) psoriasis

703. A 70-year-old man of Irish extraction returns to his physician for a routine check of his blood pressure. He is a vigorous retired executive who except for mild hypertension is healthy. After his examination, as he is getting dressed, he states that his wife has been nagging him to mention a spot on his nose (as shown in Color Plate G). He is certain that this lesion, which has been present for several years, is of no significance. The most likely diagnosis for this lesion is

(A) dermal nevus
(B) sebaceous hyperplasia
(C) clear cell acanthoma
(D) xanthoma
(E) basal cell carcinoma

704. A 52-year-old woman sees her physician for an "insurance physical." Physical examination reveals only a pigmented lesion (as shown in Color Plate H) present on one foot. The woman states that the lesion apparently was present at birth and does not itch or bleed; it is, however, not as homogeneous in color as it used to be. Which of the following statements about the condition described is true?

(A) Bleeding and tenderness would be the first signs of malignant degeneration
(B) It is unlikely that the lesion, present since birth, is malignant
(C) It would be dangerous to perform an incisional biopsy of this lesion
(D) Change in color of the lesion is a suspicious sign for potential malignancy
(E) Early diagnosis of this lesion would not affect prognosis

705. A 17-year-old girl complains of pain during chewing and tender lesions on the sides of her fingers. Shallow yellow to gray ulcerations with erythematous halos are present on her tongue, hard palate, and buccal mucosa. On the dorsal and lateral surfaces of her fingers are oval vesicles with a surrounding ring of erythema (as shown in Color Plate I). Her 5-year-old sister had a similar eruption last week and is now well. The most likely diagnosis is

(A) bullous erythema multiforme
(B) herpes simplex
(C) hand-foot-and mouth disease
(D) Behçet's syndrome
(E) gonococcemia

706. For the last 2 days, a 24-year-old woman has had fever and pain in the left wrist, right ankle, and left knee. Nine painful skin lesions are present on the distal extremities, predominantly about the joints (as shown in color Plate J). The most likely diagnosis is

(A) herpes simplex
(B) meningococcemia
(C) gonococcemia
(D) erythema multiforme
(E) anthrax

DERMATOLOGIC DISORDERS

Questions 707–708

A 42 year old obese male is admitted to the hospital for severe right upper quadrant pain suggestive of cholecystitis. During the first two days of hospitalization he is afebrile, has normal white blood cell counts, liver function tests, and oral cholecystogram. On the third day clusters of small vesicles are noted on the right upper abdomen extending laterally around to the right side of his back (as shown in Color Plate K). His right upper quadrant pain becomes more intense.

707. A helpful diagnostic test to determine the cause of his pain would be

(A) percutaneous liver biopsy
(B) right upper quadrant ultrasound
(C) Giemsa stain of cellular material from base of a vesicle
(D) endoscopic retrograde cholangiopancreatography (ERCP)
(E) exploratory laparotomy

708. Appropriate therapy for this condition would include

(A) cholecystectomy
(B) intravenous antibiotic therapy
(C) topical acyclovir
(D) topical fluorinated steroids
(E) none of the above

709. A 21-year-old woman is hospitalized for the treatment of a painful ulcer that has been present on her right lower leg for the last 4 weeks. The lesion began as a painful reddish-purple nodule, then rapidly broke down and enlarged (see Color Plate L). Bacterial cultures did not yield a significant pathogen, and a 2-week course of oral dicloxacillin, 250 mg four times daily, was not helpful. The lesion border now is undermined with a violaceous rim; biopsy is consistent with pyoderma gangrenosum. The lesion described is associated with all the following disorders EXCEPT

(A) ulcerative colitis
(B) regional enteritis
(C) multiple myeloma
(D) rheumatoid arthritis
(E) pernicious anema

Questions 710–711

A 26-year-old man from Cape Cod sees his physician because of a 3-week history of an expanding, slightly burning ring of redness (as shown in Color Plate M) that first surrounded a red papule on the posterior neck. He complains of headaches, generalized muscle aches, anorexia, and malaise. On examination, he is noted to be febrile (38.3°C—101°F); his rash is slightly raised and slightly tender and displays central clearing but no scaling, even after vigorous scraping.

710. Which of the following vectors has been strongly associated with the type of rash described above?

(A) Kissing bug
(B) Spider
(C) Flea
(D) Tick
(E) Housefly

711. After 6 weeks of observation without treatment, the rash and systemic signs and symptoms disappear. Two months later, however, the man develops acute arthritis of his shoulders and knees. Joint and bone x-rays are normal, and serologic studies for systemic lupus erythematosus and rheumatoid arthritis are negative. The man's joint complaints resolve wtihout therapy in a week, but during the next 3 months he has three similar episodes of asymmetrical arthritis of the knees, elbows, and shoulders, each episode lasting 5 to 7 days and responding to therapy with aspirin. Between episodes, he has been entirely asymptomatic, and neither joint deformities nor persistent synovitis has occurred. The most likely diagnosos for the man described is

(A) sarcoidosis with arthritis
(B) Lyme arthritis
(C) Reiter's syndrome
(D) systemic lupus erythematosus
(E) Still's disease

712. A 38-year-old male notes the development of three asymptomatic reddish brown indurated plaques and nodules (as shown in Color Plate N). One is located anterior to his right ear, one on the upper back, and one on the lower leg. These lesions have been slowly enlarging. He has a "butterfly" rash on his face. He also complains of persistent lymphadenopathy, weight loss, and chronic diarrhea. A nonhealing perirectal ulcer has been a problem. In addition, he had recently been hospitalized for pneumocystis pneumonia. Which of the following statements are *not* true about the above condition.

(A) Severe seborrheic dermatitis of the face is common in this condition
(B) Bactrim rashes occur in 5 to 10 percent of patients
(C) The patient should be advised not to donate blood
(D) Candida infections are a frequent problem
(E) This patient is at increased risk to develop lymphoma.

DIRECTIONS: Each question below contains five suggested answers. For **each** of the five alternatives of **each** item, you are to respond either YES (Y) or NO (N). In a given item all, some, or none of the alternatives may be correct.

713. A 50-year-old man has had 3 months of stiffness and pain in both wrists, his right knee, left elbow, back, and the distal interphalangeal joints of several fingers of both hands. On examination, he has the skin findings shown in Color Plate O. Which of the following statements about this case are true?

(A) An oral psoralen compound plus long-wave ultraviolet light would likely be effective therapy for the skin lesions
(B) Weekly oral methotrexate administration would likely be effective therapy for both the skin lesions and arthritis
(C) Treatment with prednisone, 40 mg daily for 4 weeks, would likely be effective
(D) The incidence of hyperuricemia in persons with this disease is greater than that in the unaffected population
(E) The prevalence of arthritis in persons with this disease is higher than that in the unaffected population

714. A 35-year-old woman visits her doctor for her yearly checkup. Physical examination is unremarkable except for white patches (as shown in Color Plate P) involving her face, hands, torso, anus, and genitalia. The white spots have been present for 2 years. This dermatologic condition has been associated with which of the following diseases?

(A) Diabetes mellitus
(B) Pernicious anemia
(C) Addison's disease
(D) Hyperthyroidism
(E) Hypoparathyroidism

715. A 9-month-old baby has a generalized seizure at home. Emergency examination and laboratory studies are unremarkable, with the exception of three hypopigmented macules on the back. Family history of genetic or neurologic disorders is negative. Follow-up examination of the parents and two older siblings is unremarkable. The baby's physician should inform the parents that

(A) the child most likely will have normal mental development
(B) the child may develop an acne-like condition
(C) the child will develop neurofibromas
(D) subsequent children, if they have them, probably would be normal
(E) they should seek genetic counseling

716. A 35-year-old man has had recurrent diarrhea for at least 5 years. About 7 years ago many reddish-brown macules appeared on his torso and extremities (see Color Plate Q.) Rubbing these lesions gently results in the formation of a wheal. He also has been bothered by severe generalized itching, which is made worse when he takes aspirin for his frequent headaches. He has lost 11.4 kg (25 lb) in the last few months. Reasonable measures in his management would include

(A) reassurance that his disease is likely to disappear spontaneously
(B) bone survey and liver scan for evaluation of systemic involvement
(C) prescription of oral disodium cromoglycate for diarrhea
(D) prescription of codeine for his headaches
(E) genetic counseling

717. A 22-year-old man presents to the local emergency room with a 3-day history of tarry stools. He has had similar episodes lasting 3 to 5 days for the last 3 years, and in the last 5 years he has been hospitalized three times for episodes of abdominal pain. Examination is entirely normal except for perioral skin lesions (as shown in Color Plate R), which have been present since infancy; similar lesions appear on the bucal mucosa, fingertips, and nose. Commonly associated with the disorder described are

(A) a positive family history of similar pigmentation
(B) multiple sebaceous and desmoid cysts of the skin
(C) colon carcinoma
(D) intussusception
(E) hamartomatous polyps in the small intestine

DIRECTIONS: Each question below contains five suggested answers. Choose **one or more** of the responses to each question.

Questions 718–719

A 55-year-old female noted the onset of skin fragility on the back of her hands six months ago. Occasional tense blisters are noted at these sites (see color plate S). The blisters heal with the formation of tiny inclusion cysts (milia). Increased facial hair on the upper cheeks and a violaceous color periocularly is noted. The skin appears entirely normal in non-sun exposed areas. She has smoked two packs of cigarettes per day for 20 years and has consumed a six pack of beer daily for years.

718. Laboratory findings might include the following

(A) elevated SGOT
(B) elevated serum iron
(C) elevated urinary uroporphyrin and coproporphyrin
(D) elevated immunoglobulin E
(E) anemia

719. Effective treatments might include

(A) oral ferrous sulfate
(B) serial phlebotomy
(C) oral estrogens
(D) oral hexachlorobenzene
(E) oral chloroquine

Dermatologic Disorders

Answers

697. The answer is B. *(Braunwald, ed 11, chap 48.)* Moniliasis commonly occurs in warm, moist areas, such as the axillae, groin, and beneath the breasts. Predisposing factors include obesity, diabetes mellitus, pregnancy, and use of broad-spectrum antibiotics, oral contraceptives, or local and systemic steroids. The presence of satellite pustules distinguishes moniliasis from tinea cruris. Potassium hydroxide preparations assist in the differential diagnosis—budding yeast and pseudohyphae are diagnostic for moniliasis.

698. The answer is A. *(Braunwald, ed 11, chap 48.)* Nystatin, a polyene antibiotic, is quite effective in eradicating monilial infection. Clotrimazole, one of the new imidazoles, has broad-spectrum activity against both yeast and fungi and is useful if mixed infection is present or if the diagnosis is in doubt. A related drug, miconazole, also is an effective treatment of moniliasis. Use of hydrocortisone would allow yeast to flourish. In the case described, stopping the tetracycline would eliminate one of the predisposing factors.

699. The answer is C. *(Braunwald, ed 11, chap 52. Miller, Lancet 2:1071–1072, 1978.)* Flat, brown spots, called café au lait spots, are areas of increased pigmentation produced by clones of genetically programmed melanocytes. Café au lait spots, which can vary in size from several millimeters up to 15 cm in diameter, occur in both neurofibromatosis (von Recklinghausen's disease) and Albright's disease (polyostotic fibrous dysplasia), as well as in some normal individuals. One or two spots at least 0.5 cm in diameter appear in 25 percent of normal children, but three or more spots of the same size occur in only 0.6 percent. About 9 percent of college-age persons have at least one spot 1.5 cm in size or greater. Of those persons with neurofibromatosis, 95 percent have at least one spot 1.5 cm or larger, and 78 percent have six or more spots. Because individuals who have Albright's disease rarely have more than four macules, the presence of six or more spots 1.5 cm or greater in size, especially in the presence of axillary freckling, is strongly suggestive of neurofibromatosis.

700. The answer is C. *(Braunwald, ed 11, chap 321.)* Acromegaly is an insidious disorder that usually has been present for many years before the diagnosis is established. Cutaneous signs are diverse and include acanthosis nigricans, acne vulgaris, oiliness, increased sweating, diffuse thickening of skin, and enlargement of the tongue. Glucose intolerance is also a typical finding. Primary amyloidosis and some forms of hypothyroidism can cause enlargement of the tongue but not the other findings. Increases in the size of the feet, fingers, and jaw (as reflected by more space between teeth) are signs in an adult of increased growth hormone activity.

701. The answer is E. *(Braunwald, ed 11, chap 300.)* Acanthosis nigricans is a skin disease associated with a number of disorders. The skin, which is thrown up into folds, appears velvety and hyperpigmented (brown to black) grossly and papillomatous microscopically. The lesions appear on the flexural areas of the neck, axillae, groin, antecubital fossae, and occasionally around the areolae, periumbilical and perianal areas, lips, buccal mucosa, and over the surfaces of the palms, elbows, knees, and interphalangeal joints. The disorder may be hereditary or appear in association with obesity or an endocrinopathy (acromegaly, Stein-Leventhal syndrome, diabetes mellitus, Cushing's syndrome, but **not** adrenal insufficiency). Drugs such as nicotinic acid also can produce the condition. When acanthosis nigricans develops in a nonobese adult, neoplasia, particularly gastric adenocarcinoma, must be suspected.

702. The answer is D. *(Braunwald, ed 11, chap 300. Ashikari, Cancer 26:680, 1970.)* Paget's disease of the nipple is associated with a scaling, weeping, well-circumscribed crusted plaque clinically similar to eczematous dermatitis but unresponsive to treatment with corticosteroids. It represents an intraepidermal carcinoma, and the histologic picture of "clear cells" filled with mucopolysaccharide is specific for the disease. A skin lesion is invariably associated with a primary intraductal or parenchymal carcinoma of the breast. The lesion often obliterates normal nipple architecture.

703. The answer is E. *(Braunwald, ed 11, chap 301.)* Basal cell carcinoma is the most common malignancy occurring in the United States. The typical appearance is that of a slowly enlarging, pearly translucent papule with rolled borders and overlying telangiectasias. As the lesion enlarges, central ulceration may occur (rodent ulcer). Sun-exposed areas are most commonly involved—about 90 percent of tumors occur on the head and neck—and fair-skinned individuals are at greatest risk. Dermal nevi, which occur commonly on the faces of adults, lack the translucency seen in basal cell carcinoma. Sebaceous hyperplasia usually is smaller and has a distinct yellowish color. Diagnosis of basal cell carcinoma is easily established by punch or incisional biopsy.

704. The answer is D. *(Braunwald, ed 11, chap 302.)* The characteristics distinguishing superficial spreading malignant melanoma from a normal mole include irregularity of its border and variegation of color. Instead of the homogeneous color and regular borders of a "normal" mole, the lesion shows disorderliness and irregularity. The first changes noted by persons who develop melanoma in a preexisting mole are a "darkening" in color or a change in the borders of the lesion. Irregularity of the borders in an expanding, darkening mole is melanoma until proven otherwise; biopsy should be done promptly, because early diagnosis and excision reduce the mortality rate.

705. The answer is C. *(Braunwald, ed 11, chap 194. Fitzpatrick, Dermatology in General Medicine, ed 3, chap 188.)* Although hand-foot-and mouth disease usually affects children under the age of 10 years, especially preschoolers, the disease has been noted in adults with or without contact with affected children. The responsible agent is a coxsackievirus. The differential diagnosis includes aphthous ulcers, herpangina, herpes simplex, and erythema multiforme. Characteristically, the prodromal phase of hand-foot-and-mouth disease features malaise and upper respiratory-tract symptoms; then, acute ulcerative stomatitis, mild pyrexia, and vesiculation of hands, feet, and buttocks occur. Vesicles in the oral cavity rapidly become ulcerated; tongue, gums, buccal mucous membrane, palate, and pharynx can all be involved. The cutaneous vesicles frequently are oval in shape and have an erythematous halo. Recovery occurs without specific treatment in 7 to 10 days.

706. The answer is C. *(Braunwald, ed 11, chap 104.)* The skin lesions of disseminated gonococcal infection occur on the distal extremities, usually around joints, and appear within a week of the onset of joint symptoms. The lesions, which may number as many as 20 (average: 4 or 5), often are painful, and each crop of new lesions is associated with a temperature rise. Lesions begin as a red macule or purpuric spot and then develop into a papule, a vesicle, and, finally, a pustule. Organisms rarely are cultured from the skin lesions; they can be demonstrated occasionally on Gram stain and more regularly with immunofluorescent techniques. Herpes simplex typically occurs as grouped vesicles. Skin lesions of meningococcemia consist of red macules that quickly become petechial or purpuric; migratory polyarthralgias and tenosynovitis are atypical. Erythema multiforme requires "iris" lesions for diagnosis. Anthrax consists of a single pimple or papule on exposed parts of the body; the lesion

DERMATOLOGIC DISORDERS

rapidly enlarges, developing into a vesicle that is surrounded by edema and later undergoes hemorrhagic necrosis, ulceration, and eschar formation.

707. The answer is C. *(Braunwald, ed 11, chap 135.)* The differential diagnosis of grouped vesicular eruptions includes contact dermatitis and herpetic infections. Microscopic examination of the cellular material from the base of a fresh vesicle (less than 2 days old is best) stained with Giemsa reveals pathopneumonic multinucleated giant cells diagnostic of a herpes virus infection (varicella, zoster, or simplex). Unilateral dermatomal involvement establishes the diagnosis of shingles (herpes zoster). Neuralgia associated with zoster may precede the appearance of the cutaneous eruption and mimic myocardial infarction or acute cholecystitis.

708. The answer is E. *(Braunwald, ed 11, chap 135.)* Herpes zoster will not respond to topical acyclovir. Oral or intravenous acyclovir may be helpful if dissemination occurs. Antibiotic therapy is indicated only for significant secondary bacterial infection. There is no evidence that fluorinated topical steroids are of help although systemic steroids are sometimes employed in the hope that the frequency of post herpetic neuralgia might be reduced. Most patients will respond to conservative therapy which should include adequate oral pain medication, and topical wet to dry saline or aluminum acetate (Domeboro) soaks to help dry up the vesicles and reduce the likelihood of secondary bacterial infection.

709. The answer is E. *(Braunwald, ed 11, chap 239.)* Pyoderma gangrenosum is most closely associated with ulcerative colitis and regional enteritis. Its association with rheumatoid arthritis also is well recognized, and it can accompany a variety of myeloproliferative disorders, such as myelogenous and myeloblastic leukemia, myeloma, myeloid metaplasia, monoclonal gammopathy, and polycythemia vera. Bacterial cultures and skin biopsies should be done in an evaluation for sepsis, vasculitis, or leukemia cutis. However, diagnosis of pyoderma gangrenosum is not made by biopsy.

710. The answer is D. *(Braunwald, ed 11, chap 278.)* An expanding erythematous rash not associated with scaling is characteristic of erythema chronicum migrans. The disease first appears weeks to months after a tick bite. The lesion begins as a red macule at the site of the bite; the borders of the lesion then expand to form a red ring, with central clearing, as wide as 20 to 30 cm or more in diameter. Occasionally, secondary rings may occur within the original one. The lesion may itch or burn and may be accompanied by fever, headache, vomiting, fatigue, and regional adenopathy.

711. The answer is B. *(Braunwald, ed 11, chap 278. Burgdorfer, Science 216:1317–1319, 1982.)* Acute recurrent arthritis not associated with joint damage should suggest the possibility of Lyme arthritis. Present evidence implicates the spirochete as the etiologic factor. Prompt treatment with oral antibiotics as soon as the diagnosis is made is indicated. The arthritis is sometimes monoarticular, often asymmetrical and migratory; the knee joints most commonly are involved. Attacks are separated by gradually lengthening intervals: 1 to 3 weeks at first, later as much as 1 to 3 years. Acute attacks, which may be associated with fever, sometimes are preceded by a few days to several weeks by erythema chronicum migrans. The other syndromes listed in the question are not typically recurrent, nor are they as short-lived as Lyme arthritis or as asymptomatic between flare-ups.

712. The answer is B. *(Braunwald, ed 11, chap 257. Mathes, J Am Acad Dermatol 13:947, 1985. Penneys, J Am Acad Dermatol 13:845, 1985.)* Patients with acquired immunodeficiency syndrome (AIDS) have many cutaneous manifestations including, as in this case, Kaposi's sarcoma, prominent seborrheic dermatitis, and perirectal herpes simplex. Other common skin manifestations include monilia, dermatophytosis, warts, and molluscus contagiosum. Bactrim-induced drug rashes are extremely common in AIDS patients. Not only is the risk for Kaposi's sarcoma increased, but the risk for lymphoma as well. In AIDS patients, early lesions of Kaposi's sarcoma may not be impressive. In the appropriate setting a high index of suspicion and careful skin biopsy will make the diagnosis.

713. The answer is A-Y, B-Y, C-N, D-Y, E-Y. *(Braunwald, ed 11, chap 48.)* Psoriasis is manifested by silvery and scaly thick red plaques. Serum uric acid levels are elevated in 10 to 20 percent of affected persons, probably as a result of the high epidermal turnover rate, which causes accelerated synthesis and degradation of nucleoproteins. There are several forms of psoriatic arthritis, including asymmetrical interphalangeal joint involvement similar to that seen in rheumatoid arthritis and a severe destructive polyarthritis often associated with spondylitis. Oral methoxsalen, a psoralen compound, in conjunction with long-wave ultraviolet light (PUVA) offers the possibility of excellent control of the skin lesions. Methotrexate, which also is effective in treating psoriasis, is reserved for adults with severe disease. Treatment with systemic corticosteroids is contraindicated.

714. The answer is A-Y, B-Y, C-Y, D-Y, E-Y. *(Braunwald, ed 11, chap 51.)* The photographed skin lesions are depigmented macules of vitiligo. Vitiliginous macules are completely lacking in pigment and are histologically devoid of melanocytes. This disorder is believed to be transmitted as an autosomal dominant trait with incomplete penetrance. Although the majority of cases of vitiligo are not associated with other disease processes, an association has been described between vitiligo and several disorders, including diabetes mellitus, pernicious anemia, hyperthyroidism, hypothyroidism, Addison's disease, alopecia areata, and hypoparathyroidism.

715. The answer is A-N, B-Y, C-N, D-Y, E-Y. *(Braunwald, ed 11, chap 51.)* Tuberous sclerosis is a relatively uncommon disorder (5 to 7/100,000) in which a diverse combination of features is noted (seizures, mental retardation, adenoma sebaceum, periungual fibromas, connective tissue nevi, and hypopigmented macules). The hypopigmented macules, present in 98 percent of cases, may be the earliest and only physical finding at initial presentation. Wood's lamp examination (with long-wave ultraviolet light) of affected children and their families may make previously unrecognized hypopigmented areas discernible. Although inherited as an autosomal dominant gene, tuberous sclerosis usually is the result of spontaneous mutations.

716. The answer is A-N, B-Y, C-Y, D-N, E-Y. *(Braunwald, ed 11, chap 51.)* Urticaria pigmentosa is a disorder of mast cells. The development of a wheal on gentle stroking of a pigmented macule (Darier's sign) is a useful diagnostic maneuver. Prognosis is said to worsen with age of onset: half the patients who develop multiple lesions by 4 years of age are disease-free by adolescence. Onset in adulthood is more ominous, with active skin lesions persisting indefinitely; systemic mastocytosis, which may have a fatal outcome, occurs frequently in affected adults. Symptomatic improvement has been reported with oral disodium cromoglycate. Affected persons should be warned to avoid substances and environmental factors known to cause mast-cell degranulation (e.g., cold, heat, trauma, or the ingestion of alcohol, aspirin, or morphine-opium alkaloid drugs). Although the disorder is usually an isolated event, familial disease occurs, indicating autosomal dominant inheritance in some cases.

717. The answer is A-Y, B-N, C-N, D-Y, E-Y. *(Braunwald, ed 11, chap 300.)* Peutz–Jeghers syndrome, an autosomal dominant disorder that first appears during infancy or early childhood, is characterized by distinctive freckle-like pigmentation of the buccal mucosa and skin. The buccal mucosal pigmentation, not unlike that associated with Addison's disease, persists throughout life; pigmentation about the face, lips, and distal extremities may fade with age. The distinctive pigmentation is an important indicator of the presence of hamartomatous polyps, which arise predominantly in the ileum and jejunum. The polyps, which typically become clinically symptomatic during the second decade of life, may also occur throughout the colon, appendix, rectum, stomach, and duodenum. Fewer than 2 percent of persons with Peutz–Jeghers syndrome develop malignancy related to the polyps; in contrast, Gardner's syndrome, an autosomal dominant disorder consisting of adenomatous polyps of the colon and associated with epidermal inclusion cysts, osteomas, and fibrous tissue proliferation, leads to colonic malignancy in 45 percent of cases.

718. The answers are A, B, C.   719. The answers are B, D. *(Braunwald, ed 11, chap 312.)* Porphyria cutanea tarda results from a derangement of hepatic porphyrin metabolism usually induced by a toxin (alcohol, hexachlorobenzene, etc.) The condition is associated with iron overload and has been effectively treated with serial phlebotomy or with oral chlorquine (mechanism unknown). Laboratory findings usually include elevation of hematocrit, serum iron, hepatic transaminases, and urinary uro- and coproporphyrins. The elevation of porphyrins in the circulation leads to the development of phototoxic tense blisters in sun-exposed areas which heal with milia formation. Increased facial hair, increased skin fragility in sun-exposed areas and periocular violaceous skin coloration are also frequently found. Estrogen use has also been reported as a precipitant in the disorder.

DISORDERS OF THE NERVOUS SYSTEM AND MUSCLES

DIRECTIONS: Each question below contains five suggested answers. Choose the **one best** response to each question

720. A 70-year-old man complains of loss of energy, trouble concentrating, decreased appetite, and insomnia. He has lost considerable weight since his last visit and appears disheveled. It would be most appropriate initially to

(A) suspect that he has depression, and inquire whether he has frequent crying spells and has thought about suicide
(B) examine his stool for occult blood and schedule tests to search for a malignancy
(C) order tests to determine reversible causes of dementia
(D) refer the patient to a psychiatric clinic
(E) engage a social worker to help with basic home skills

721. Biologic factors associated with depression include

(A) derangement in pituitary-adrenal function
(B) a higher-than-normal incidence of epileptiform activity on electroencephalography
(C) abnormalities of dopamine metabolism reflected in elevated dopamine β-hydroxylase levels
(D) increased levels of γ-aminobutyric acid (GABA) in the cerebrospinal fluid after probenecid loading
(E) suppression of serum cortisol levels with small doses of dexamethasone

722. The function of the muscle spindle is to furnish the central nervous system with information concerning

(A) muscle tension
(B) muscle length
(C) muscle tone
(D) joint flexion
(E) joint extension

723. For the last 5 weeks, a 35-year-old woman has had episodes of intense vertigo lasting several hours. Each episode is associated with tinnitus and a sense of fullness in her right ear; during the attacks, she prefers to lie on her left side. Examination during an attack shows that she has fine rotatory nystagmus, which is maximal on gaze to the left. There are no ocular palsies, cranial-nerve signs, or long-tract signs. An audiogram shows a high-tone hearing loss in the right ear, with recruitment but no tone decay.

The most likely diagnosis in the case described is

(A) labyrinthitis
(B) Ménière's disease
(C) vertebral-basilar insufficiency
(D) acoustic neurinoma
(E) multiple sclerosis

724. A 29-year-old woman who uses oral contraceptives comes to the emergency room because when she looked in the mirror this morning, her face was twisted. It felt numb and swollen. Eating breakfast, she found that her food tasted different because it drooled out of the right side of her mouth when she swallowed. Neurologic examination discloses only a dense right facial paresis equally involving the frontalis, orbicularis oculi, and orbicularis oris. Finger rubbing is appreciated as louder in the right ear than in the left. The physician should

(A) instruct the patient in using a patch over the right eye during sleep
(B) recommend that she discontinue use of oral contraceptives
(C) order brainstem auditory evoked potentials to assess her hearing asymmetry
(D) inform her that her chances of substantial improvement within several weeks are only about 40 percent
(E) order an echocardiogram to rule out mitral valve prolapse as a source of emboli

725. The distinctive tetrad of symptoms of the narcolepsy-cataplexy syndrome includes all the following EXCEPT

(A) uncontrollable daytime sleepiness
(B) sudden brief episodes of loss of muscle tone
(C) paralysis upon falling asleep
(D) confusional episodes
(E) hallucinations at the onset of sleep or wakening

726. A man brought into an emergency room is unresponsive and is displaying posturing. Pupils are 4 mm in size and react to light. No eye movements occur with head turning (oculocephalic maneuver) or with ice-water irrigation of the ear canals. The most likely diagnosis is

(A) brain death
(B) hysteria-conversion coma
(C) brainstem hemorrhage
(D) drug ingestion
(E) bilateral internal carotid artery occlusion

727. A patient with previous spells of diplopia, ataxia, dysarthria, and dizziness becomes acutely comatose. The most likely cause is

(A) basilar artery thrombosis
(B) subarachnoid hemorrhage
(C) carotid occlusion
(D) cerebellar hemorrhage
(E) pontine hemorrhage

728. Evoked-potential testing is most useful in diagnosing

(A) brainstem involvement in stroke
(B) a clinically occult lesion in multiple sclerosis
(C) large hemispheral strokes
(D) spinal cord compression
(E) shearing of white matter tracts after head injury

729. A normal pattern-shift visual evoked response is most useful and specific in diagnosing

(A) malingering
(B) Jakob-Creutzfeldt disease
(C) pituitary tumor
(D) brainstem glioma
(E) temporal arteritis

730. All the following statements are true of typical absence seizures in children EXCEPT

(A) they frequently present as learning disability
(B) they are associated with a characteristic electroencephalographic pattern
(C) they generally are not associated with other neurologic abnormalities
(D) phenytoin is the treatment of choice
(E) one-third of affected children outgrow the condition

731. A 25-year-old weight lifter comes to the emergency room frightened by recent headaches. He recently read a newspaper article about cerebral aneurysms. He reports 5 to 10 sudden, severe headaches, all occurring during coitus, each lasting about one hour. The physician should

(A) recommend that the patient seek psychiatric help for his sexual dysfunction
(B) perform a CT scan with contrast and schedule four-vessel cerebral angiography to search for an aneurysm or arteriovenous malformation
(C) inform the patient that coital headache is a benign clinical syndrome that may be helped by administration of propranol, 20 mg three times a day
(D) tell the patient to report back to the emergency room for a cerebrospinal fluid examination and CT scan without contrast to search for subarachnoid blood
(E) determine whether other members of his family have a history of migraine

732. While wrestling with his young son, a 32-year-old man suddenly develops a severe headache then lapses into unconsciousness. Examination in the emergency room reveals retinal hemorrhages, nuchal rigidity, and normal eye movements on passive head rotation. The best initial diagnostic measure would be

(A) lumbar puncture
(B) skull x-rays
(C) CT scan of the head
(D) radionuclide brain scan
(E) bilateral carotid and vertebral angiography

733. The most common site for hypertensive brain hemorrhage is the

(A) pons
(B) central white matter
(C) cerebellar hemispheres
(D) putamen
(E) thalamus

734. Depression may be mistaken for dementia because of the hypokinetic state, poor attention span, and loss of impulse control common to both conditions. However, a major distinguishing feature of dementia would be

(A) anorexia
(B) headache
(C) multiple somatic complaints
(D) impaired performance on memory tests
(E) prominent release reflexes

735. A man has dyslexia without dysgraphia—i.e., he can write but not read. Auditory comprehension is only slightly impaired. This man's symptoms most likely are due to a lesion or lesions in

(A) the left frontal lobe, posterior to Broca's area
(B) the left temporal lobe, near Wernicke's area
(C) both temporal lobes
(D) the left parietooccipital region
(E) both parietooccipital regions

736. Which of the following would help to confirm the diagnosis of syncope in a patient with sudden loss of consciousness?

(A) A brief period of tonic-clonic movements at the time of falling
(B) An aura of a strange odor prior to falling
(C) Sudden return to normal mental function upon awakening, though feeling physically weak
(D) Urinary incontinence
(E) Laceration of the tongue

737. A physician confronted with a comatose patient with a severe head injury would be best advised to

(A) perform a skull and neurologic examination, obtain a CT scan of the head, and recommend burr holes if the pupils are enlarged
(B) stabilize the neck, administer mannitol and steroids, and obtain a CT scan
(C) treat hypotension, ensure airway patency, perform a skull and neurologic examination, and obtain a CT scan
(D) treat hypoxia and hypotension, raise the head, and obtain a CT scan
(E) stabilize the neck, obtain neck and skull x-rays, and recommend burr holes if the pupils are enlarged

738. In addition to blindness, temporal arteritis may cause

(A) alopecia
(B) migraine-like visual displays
(C) diplopia
(D) loss of consciousness
(E) Raynaud's phenomenon

739. Which of the following brain tumors tends to occur in immunosuppressed individuals, arise in periventricular regions, and respond both clinically and radiographically to corticosteroid therapy?

(A) Glioblastoma
(B) Ependymoma
(C) Meningioma
(D) Medulloblastoma
(E) Histiocytic lymphoma

740. Distant systemic cancer most likely would produce which of the following neurologic syndromes?

(A) Myasthenia gravis
(B) Noninflammatory myopathy
(C) Cranial nerve palsies
(D) Generalized neuropathy
(E) Grand mal seizures

741. Septic cerebral emboli can be described by which of the following statements?

(A) Anaerobes commonly predominate
(B) Staphylococci commonly predominate
(C) Meningitis commonly is present
(D) Microbiologic diagnosis can be made by Gram stain of cerebrospinal fluid
(E) None of the above

742. A person who has right hemiparesis from stroke would be LEAST likely to display

(A) left facial weakness
(B) left-gaze paresis
(C) inability to calculate
(D) left-right confusion
(E) ignoring of the deficit

743. Lumbar back pain may be caused by all of the following EXCEPT

(A) metastatic carcinoma of the prostate
(B) retroperitoneal hemorrhage in a patient on a regimen of warfarin
(C) expanding abdominal aneurysm
(D) pancreatitis
(E) diphtheritic polyneuropathy

744. For the last several days a college student has had back pain in the midlumbar area, difficulty in starting urination, and paresthesias in the feet. On examination, temperature is 38.3°C (101°F); straight leg raising produces pain, slight hip weakness is present, and Babinski signs are absent. The physician should

(A) perform a lumbar puncture
(B) obtain spine films and a bone scan
(C) obtain blood cultures and start antibiotic therapy
(D) obtain urinalysis and retroperitoneal ultrasound
(E) arrange for emergency myelography or CT scan of the spine

745. Elevated levels of gamma globulin in cerebrospinal fluid are associated with

(A) subacute sclerosing panencephalitis
(B) Jakob-Creutzfeldt disease
(C) progressive multifocal leukoencephalopathy
(D) paracarcinomatous encephalopathy
(E) western equine encephalitis

746. For the last 6 weeks, a 64-year-old woman has had a headache and difficulty reading. Her husband has noted a mild but progressive intellectual decline in his wife during this period. On examination, she has grasping reactions and myoclonic jerks when loud noises occur. CT scan and cerebrospinal fluid examination are normal.
 The most likely diagnosis is

(A) multiple sclerosis
(B) Alzheimer's disease
(C) bilateral subdural hematoma
(D) Jakob-Creutzfeldt disease
(E) subacute sclerosing panencephalitis

747. The most common presenting finding or symptom of multiple sclerosis is

(A) internuclear ophthalmoplegia
(B) transverse myelitis
(C) cerebellar ataxia
(D) optic neuritis
(E) urinary retention

748. A 28-year-old woman complains of horizontal diplopia. Examination shows only a lag in adduction of the left eye with nystagmus in the abducting right eye. The most appropriate workup would include

(A) electroencephalography and CT scan with contrast infusion
(B) cerebral angiography and formal visual-field testing
(C) lumbar puncture and evoked potentials
(D) electronystagmography and electroencephalography
(E) none of the above

749. A 19-year-old man with a history of childhood jaundice presents with nervousness, drooling, rigidity of the limbs, and a fixed vacuous smile. Physical examination reveals hepatosplenomegaly and a coarse "wing-beating" tremor of his outstretched arms. On the basis of this information, his physician should first

(A) perform a liver biopsy
(B) ask for an ophthalmologic consultation
(C) obtain CT scans of the abdomen and cranium
(D) order serum calcium and phosphate concentrations
(E) order measurement of serum and urinary porphyrins

750. Initial therapy for persons with increased intracranial pressure would include

(A) beta-adrenergic blockers
(B) phenytoin
(C) mechanical ventilation to achieve high airway pressures
(D) hyperosmolar dehydration
(E) intravenous fluids

751. A 59-year-old man who has alcoholic cirrhosis but has been abstinent for 10 years has progressive dysarthria, tongue dystonia, shuffling gait, and fast tremor that worsens as his hand moves toward a target. The disease process causing these symptoms most likely is

(A) Wilson's disease
(B) acquired hepatocerebral degeneration
(C) Wernicke's disease
(D) Marchiafava-Bignami disease
(E) paracarcinomatous syndrome

752. The most likely diagnosis for a patient with impotence and urinary incontinence who, over years, sustains a tremor at rest, bradykinesia, rigidity, severe orthostatic hypotension, and anhidrosis is

(A) an autonomic form of the Landry-Guillain-Barré syndrome
(B) the Shy-Drager syndrome
(C) guanethidine intoxication
(D) micturition syncope
(E) Parkinson's disease

753. Lower brachial plexus injuries commonly occur during certain surgical procedures or in association with apical lung tumors. These injuries most typically cause

(A) weakness of thumb abduction and opposition
(B) ulnar hand numbness and a "claw hand" deformity
(C) ulnar hand numbness and inability to flex the elbow
(D) weakness of shoulder abduction and a patch of numbness over the triceps
(E) wrist drop and numbness over the dorsal hand between the thumb and index finger

754. A 42-year-old man, who has had difficulty concentrating on his job lately, comes to medical attention because of irregular, jerky movements of his extremities and fingers. A sister and an uncle died in mental institutions, and his mother became demented in middle age. The most likely diagnosis is

(A) alcoholic cerebral degeneration
(B) Huntington's chorea
(C) Wilson's disease
(D) Hallevorden-Spatz disease
(E) Gilles de la Tourette's disease

755. A 67-year-old woman appears to have parkinsonian rigidity but no tremor. In addition, she is completely unable to look down and has difficulty looking up. No improvement is seen after treatment with carbidopa-levodopa (Sinemet). The most likely diagnosis is

(A) atypical parkinsonism
(B) postencephalitic parkinsonism
(C) striatonigral degeneration
(D) progressive supranuclear palsy
(E) drug-induced parkinsonism and oculogyric crisis

756. Syringomyelia is characterized by all the following EXCEPT

(A) thoracic scoliosis
(B) ataxia
(C) muscle atrophy in the hands
(D) loss of pain sensation in the shoulders
(E) preservation of sense of touch

757. A 30-year-old man comes to the emergency room because for the last 3 days he has had progressive weakness of his legs, sensory loss ascending from his toes to the level of his umbilicus, and urinary retention. Examination reveals a central scotoma, absent knee and ankle jerks, and diminished pinprick sensation in the legs and abdomen up to the umbilicus. Cerebrospinal fluid contains 40 lymphocytes/mm^3 and a protein concentration of 72 mg/dL.

This clinical picture is LEAST consistent with which of the following diagnoses?

(A) Acute idiopathic polyneuritis
(B) Acute necrotizing myelitis
(C) Postvaccinal myelitis
(D) Postinfectious myelitis
(E) Multiple sclerosis

758. Bitemporal hemianopsia is most commonly due to

(A) saccular aneurysm of the distal internal carotid artery
(B) craniopharyngioma
(C) meningioma
(D) metastatic carcinoma
(E) suprasellar extension of a pituitary tumor

759. Which of the following findings may be associated with acute idiopathic polyneuritis?

(A) Cerebrospinal fluid pleocytosis
(B) Meningeal irritation
(C) Fever
(D) Unilateral foot drop
(E) Anesthesia of the legs

760. A 60-year-old mildly obese woman complains of a very bothersome burning pain on the anterolateral aspect of her right thigh from the groin almost as far distally as the knee. Examination shows reduction of sensation to touch and pinprick in the affected area. There is no loss of muscle strength and reflexes are normal.

The most likely diagnosis is

(A) ruptured intervertebral disk
(B) femoral hernia
(C) nutritional neuropathy
(D) compression of the lateral femoral cutaneous nerve
(E) disruption of the lumbosacral plexus

761. The major pathologic feature of idiopathic inflammatory polyneuropathy (Guillain-Barré syndrome) is

(A) loss of anterior horn cells
(B) destruction of axons
(C) inflammation of sensory ganglia
(D) wallerian degeneration
(E) segmental demyelination

762. Cataracts, frontal baldness, testicular atrophy, and muscle weakness and wasting occur in association with

(A) myotonic dystrophy
(B) limb-girdle dystrophy
(C) pseudohypertrophic dystrophy
(D) facioscapulohumeral dystrophy
(E) myotonia congenita

763. The form of muscular dystrophy most likely to be encountered in persons older than 50 years of age is

(A) facioscapulohumeral dystrophy
(B) oculopharyngeal dystrophy
(C) myotonic dystrophy
(D) Duchenne's dystrophy
(E) limb-girdle dystrophy

764. Delayed relaxation of a muscle after voluntary contraction is characteristic of certain dystrophic diseases and periodic paralysis. This phenomenon is called

(A) myokymia
(B) myoedema
(C) myotonia
(D) contracture
(E) fibrillation

765. A 65-year-old woman with diabetes mellitus has a three-month history of sacral pain. In the last month a burning pain progressively developed over the lateral aspect of her left foot followed by loss of sensation and weakness of plantar flexion and dorsiflexion. Electromyography showed fibrillations in left gastrocnemius, extensor hallucis, and quadriceps muscles. Nerve conduction was normal in the legs. A myelogram showed normal results. Now she complains that her knee "gives out" while walking; she has an absence of left knee and ankle jerks.

Her physician should

(A) inform the patient that normal results on her myelogram makes a diabetic neuropathy the most likely diagnosis
(B) arrange for a pelvic examination and schedule a CT scan of the pelvis to search for a malignancy compressing or infiltrating the lumbarsacral plexus
(C) arrange for a repeat myelogram because of new quadriceps weakness
(D) arrange for a CT scan of the head to search for an expanding mass over the right sensorimotor strip that would affect the foot and leg
(E) reexamine her at 2-month intervals to determine progression of her condition

766. The weakness associated with myasthenia gravis is due to which of the following disorders in the neuromuscular junction?

(A) Reduced acetylcholine in presynaptic vesicles
(B) Presynaptic block in release of acetylcholine
(C) Presence of antibodies against presynaptic membranes
(D) Degradation and blockage of postsynaptic receptors
(E) Damage of postsynaptic membranes by T lymphocytes

767. Familial periodic paralysis is described by which of the following statements?

(A) Weakness develops instantaneously during attacks
(B) Weakness can be overcome by electrical stimulation
(C) Serum potassium levels typically are less than 2.5 meq/L
(D) Cardiac muscle may be involved
(E) Affected persons may have myotonia between attacks

768. A 35-year-old man comes to the emergency room at midnight because he has awakened from sleep three nights in a row with severe pain in and above his left eye. In addition he noted unusual tearing, nasal stuffiness, and a sense of swelling over his left cheek. Neurologic evaluation reveals left ptosis and miosis that disappear after the headache resolves. The most appropriate action is to

(A) obtain an emergency CT scan and if results are normal, perform a lumbar puncture to search for evidence of subarachnoid hemorrhage
(B) reassure the patient that he has a characteristic clinical syndrome called cluster headache. It is benign and frequently responds to administration of ergotamine or lithium
(C) refer the patient to an ophthalmologist for evaluation of eye pain and pupillary change
(D) inform the patient that he has "classic migraine" and administer ergotamine, 1 mg four times a day
(E) evaluate diabetes mellitus in the patient

769. A 27-year-old man seeks advice because he has noticed fasciculations in his calf muscles. He has no other complaints. Examination shows that muscle bulk and strength, tendon and plantar reflexes, and sensory function are all normal. He should undergo

(A) muscle biopsy
(B) sural nerve biopsy
(C) myelography
(D) electromyography
(E) none of the above

770. Which of the following statements concerning porphyric neuropathy is true?

(A) It is always associated with confusion or seizures
(B) It predominantly involves the sensory system
(C) It is symmetrical, and weakness is often more proximal than distal
(D) It causes elevated protein concentration in cerebrospinal fluid
(E) It is associated with inflammation of nerves

771. A patient has a total right hemianesthesia at the time of cerebral infarction. One year later he complains of constant severe burning pain with occasional sharp jabs of pain in the left side of his face and left arm. The chronic pain syndrome is most likely

(A) part of a biologic depressive syndrome secondary to a right parietal lobe stroke
(B) caused by a lesion in the spinal cord affecting the right spinal spinothalamic tract
(C) a debilitating sequela of right thalamic infarction known as the Déjerine-Roussy syndrome
(D) secondary to a shoulder-hand syndrome involving the side affected by the stroke
(E) tic douloureux

DIRECTIONS: Each question below contains five suggested answers. For **each** of the five alternatives of **each** item you are to respond YES (Y) or NO (N). In a given item all, some, or none of the alternatives may be correct.

772. Weakness is a prominent symptom in which of the following disorders?

(A) Polymyositis
(B) Polymyalgia rheumatica
(C) Polyneuritis
(D) Botulism
(E) Subacute combined degeneration

773. Progressive gait disability in elderly individuals may be due to

(A) normal-pressure hydrocephalus
(B) cervical spondylosis
(C) subdural hematoma
(D) carotid stenosis
(E) subacute combined degeneration

774. Which of the following disorders are associated with the rapid-eye-movement (REM) phase of sleep?

(A) Night terrors
(B) Narcolepsy
(C) Cluster headache
(D) Somnambulism
(E) Nocturnal epilepsy

775. In the acute workup of newly comatose persons, CT scanning would be helpful in establishing a diagnosis of

(A) subarachnoid hemorrhage
(B) brain death
(C) brainstem infarction
(D) middle cerebral artery infarction
(E) subdural hematoma

776. Seizure discharges in the temporal lobe may manifest as

(A) facial paresthesias
(B) foot twitching
(C) vertigo
(D) intense fear
(E) déjà vu

777. Useful tests for myasthenia gravis would include which of the following?

(A) Repetitive motor-nerve stimulation
(B) Single-fiber electromyography
(C) Muscle biopsy
(D) Nerve conduction studies
(E) Curare challenge testing

778. Which of the following would be consistent with a diagnosis of muscle spasm in a patient with low back pain?

(A) Limitation of flexion of the spine
(B) Scoliosis or straightening of the normal lordosis as noted on x-ray films
(C) Urinary retention and obstipation
(D) Sudden onset while bending over shoveling snow
(E) Absence of ankle reflex with radiating pain

779. The destruction of all motor nerves supplying a muscle would result in

(A) fasciculations
(B) fibrillations
(C) hypotonia
(D) atrophy
(E) loss of response to electrical stimulations of short duration (faradic stimuli)

780. Medical illnesses associated with focal occlusive stroke include

(A) polycythemia
(B) hyperproteinemia
(C) sickle cell disease
(D) cirrhosis
(E) idiopathic thrombocytosis

781. Which of the following statements about optic neuritis are true?

(A) Papillitis associated with optic neuritis is difficult to distinguish from papilledema
(B) As in papilledema, visual acuity is spared in patients with disc swelling caused by papillitis
(C) The pupil of an eye with optic neuritis usually has a better constriction to light shown in the normal eye than to direct light in the affected eye
(D) A young adult with optic neuritis has a 30 percent to 40 percent chance for development of multiple sclerosis
(E) Optic disc pallor is a frequent sequela of optic neuritis

782. Dialysis encephalopathy can be described by which of the following statements?

(A) It is a progressive disorder
(B) Dysarthria is a characteristic sign
(C) Dementia is a key feature
(D) Myoclonus can be treated with clonazepam
(E) Cerebrospinal fluid analysis reveals characteristic abnormalities

783. Peripheral nerve damage caused by diabetes may result in

(A) relapsing weakness
(B) distal sensory neuropathy
(C) incontinence
(D) foot drop
(E) ophthalmoplegia

784. Chronically progressive spinal cord disease with sensory and motor signs evolving over years may be due to

(A) spinocerebellar degeneration
(B) multiple sclerosis
(C) cervical spondylosis
(D) lumbar disk disease
(E) amyotrophic lateral sclerosis

785. A person with long-standing alcoholism develops bilateral lateral-rectus (sixth-nerve) palsies. Diagnostic considerations would include

(A) brainstem hemorrhage
(B) subdural hematoma
(C) orbital fractures
(D) neurosyphilis
(E) Wernicke's encephalopathy

786. Which of the following disorders usually produce a sensory level on neurologic examination?

(A) Myelopathy due to vitamin-B_{12} deficiency
(B) Neoplastic cord compression
(C) Vertebral dislocation and cord compression
(D) Acute myelitis
(E) Spinal epidural abscess

787. A 60-year-old man comes to the emergency room with sudden onset of a neurologic deficit. After examining the patient the physician orders cerebral angiography. Results show occlusion of the left vertebral artery from its origin to where it joins the basilar. The right vertebral artery, basilar artery, and both carotid arteries are patent. Examination in the emergency room probably disclosed

(A) left hemiparesis sparing the face
(B) deviation of the uvula to the right on phonation
(C) left appendicular ataxia
(D) left internuclear ophthalmoplegia
(E) diminished pain and temperature sensation in the right arm and leg

788. Which of the following may occur ipsilateral to a disease process within the cavernous sinus?

(A) Ptosis
(B) Numbness of the brow
(C) Numbness of the chin
(D) Marked decrease in visual acuity
(E) Inability to elevate the eye

DIRECTIONS: The groups of questions below consist of four or five lettered headings followed by several numbered items. For each numbered item choose the **one** lettered heading with which it is **most** closely associated. Each lettered heading may be used once, more than once, or not at all.

Questions 789–792

For each clinical syndrome described below, select the most likely site of disk protrusion.

(A) L2-L3 interspace
(B) L3-L4 interspace
(C) L4-L5 interspace
(D) L5-S1 interspace
(E) S1-S2 interspace

789. Sciatica, inability to walk on toes, and depressed ankle tendon reflex

790. Sciatica, weakness of foot inversion, and hallux extensor weakness

791. Sciatica, foot drop, and normal reflexes

792. Hip flexion weakness, knee extension weakness, and diminished knee tendon reflex

Questions 793–797

For each of the following conditions, select the region of the brain most likely affected by a pathologic process

(A) Frontal lobe
(B) Temporal lobe
(C) Dominant parietal lobe
(D) Nondominant parietal lobe
(E) Occipital lobe

793. Wernicke's aphasia

794. Apathy and lack of initiative and spontaneity

795. Acalculia

796. Inability to recognize faces

797. Dense homonymous hemianopsia

Questions 798–801

For each cause of acute ascending motor paralysis listed below, select the finding or condition with which it is most likely to be associated.

(A) Prodrome of mild respiratory or gastrointestinal infection
(B) Presence of polymorphonuclear leukocytes in the cerebrospinal fluid
(C) Paralysis of the larynx
(D) Meningoencephalitis
(E) Psychosis

798. Infectious mononucleosis

799. Diphtheria

800. Porphyria

801. Acute idiopathic polyneuritis

Questions 802–806

Match each anatomic landmark to the appropriate sensory dermatomal level

(A) C2
(B) T2
(C) T4
(D) T10
(E) L5

802. Posterior scalp

803. Nipple

804. Axilla

805. Umbilicus

806. Great toe

Questions 807–812

For each systemic side effect listed below, choose the anticonvulsant drug with which it is most likely to be associated.

(A) Phenobarbital
(B) Phenytoin
(C) Carbamazepine
(D) Valproic acid
(E) Clonazepam

807. Hirsutism

808. Gum hyperplasia

809. Leukopenia

810. Osteomalacia

811. Lymphadenopathy

812. Acute hepatic failure

Questions 813–816

For each presumed function in the appreciation of pain listed below, select the associated nervous system structure.

(A) Nucleus of the ventralis posterolateralis (VPL)
(B) Type C primary sensory afferents
(C) Nucleus raphe magnus
(D) Medial thalamus, periaqueductal gray, nucleus raphe
(E) Parietal sensory cortex

813. Projects to the spinal cord and inhibits nociceptive responses in dorsal horn neurons

814. Contains high density of opiate receptors

815. Terminal field of the direct spinothalamic pathway

816. Releases substance P

Questions 817–821

For each abnormality of eye movement listed below, select the associated lesion.

(A) Lesion in the low pons surrounding the left abducens (sixth nerve) nucleus including the left pontine gaze center
(B) Lesion in the right frontal lobe
(C) Lesion in the left upper pons affecting the medial longitudinal fasciculus
(D) Unilateral left labyrinthine dysfunction
(E) Midbrain lesion affecting the rostral interstitial nucleus of the medial longitudinal fasciculus

817. Absence of vertical gaze

818. Inability to move the eyes to the left of midline

819. Tendency to keep the eyes to the right of midline

820. Saw-toothed jerk nystagmus with slow phase to the left and quick corrective movements to the right

821. Inability to adduct the left eye past the midline and nystagmus in the right eye when abducted

Question 822–826

All the following drugs are used in the treatment of parkinsonism and are associated with characteristic side effects. For each side effect listed below, choose the drug with which it is most likely to be associated.

(A) Carbidopa-levodopa (Sinemet)
(B) Benztropine mesylate (Cogentin)
(C) Amantadine (Symmetrel)
(D) Propranolol (Inderal)
(E) Methylphenidate (Ritalin)

822. Dry mouth

823. Skin changes

824. Asthma

825. Pedal edema

826. Dyskinesias

Questions 827–831

Progressive supranuclear palsy (Steele-Richardson-Olszewski syndrome) in its early stages is often difficult to distinguish from Parkinson's disease. For each characteristic listed below that occurs early in the course of the illness, determine whether it is likely to be found in

(A) Progressive supranuclear palsy
(B) Parkinson's disease
(C) Both
(D) Neither

827. Masked facies and hypophonic speech

828. Loss of saccadic eye movements, downward before horizontal

829. Tremor, 3 Hz

830. Frequent falls unexplained by rigidity or other neurologic signs

831. Dementia

Questions 832–835

In several neurodegenerative diseases, loss of a particular group of neurons is associated with decreased levels of a particular neurotransmitter or enzyme, or both, involved in neurotransmitter biochemistry. Match the neuronal group listed below that is selectively lost in a given disease with the substance whose level is decreased.

(A) Medium-sized spiny neurons in the striatum
(B) Neurons of the nucleus basalis of Meynert
(C) Cerebellar Purkinje cells
(D) Neurons of the substantia nigra

832. Choline-acetyl transferase

833. Glutamic acid decarboxylase

834. Dopamine

835. Glutamic acid dehydrogenase

Disorders of the Nervous System and Muscles

Answers

720. The answer is A. *(Braunwald, ed 11, chaps 10, 364.)* None of the actions listed is inappropriate. Malignancy, endocrine disorders, and Alzheimer's disease are frequent causes of depressive symptoms. The majority of depressed patients present to their physicians with the somatic complaints listed. In a major depression the most immediate threat to the patient's health is suicide. The risk needs to be assessed by direct questioning, and appropriate safety precautions then taken.

721. The answer is A. *(Braunwald, ed 11, chap 11.)* Endogenous depression can be distinguished from reactive depression in some cases by the dexamethasone suppression test. In this procedure, the integrity of the hypothalamic-pituitary-adrenal axis is tested by response to low doses (1 or 2 mg) of dexamethasone. Normally, suppression of endogenous cortisol production would be expected to last at least 24 hours; in endogenous depression, however, suppression is overcome rapidly. Retesting after treatment had produced clinical improvement typically is associated with reversion to a suppression response. Biochemical theories of depression mainly involve deficiencies of norepinephrine and its metabolites. Dopamine metabolism appears to be normal. No EEG abnormalities have been associated with depression.

722. The answer is B. *(Braunwald, ed 11, chaps 15, 354.)* Muscle spindles are bundles of small striated muscle fibers encased in a connective-tissue capsule around which are coiled specialized sensory nerve endings. Dispersed throughout each muscle, spindles send subliminal afferent impulses that aid the central nervous system in monitoring changes in muscle length. Joint capsule receptors are responsible for conscious proprioception; muscle tension is monitored by Golgi tendon organs.

723. The answer is B. *(Braunwald, ed 11, chap 14.)* The symptoms and signs described in the question are most consistent with Ménière's disease. In this disorder, paroxysmal vertigo due to labyrinthine lesions is associated with nausea, vomiting, rotatory nystagmus, tinnitus, high-tone hearing loss with recruitment, and, most characteristically, fullness in the ear. Labyrinthitis would be an unlikely diagnosis in the case presented because of the hearing loss and multiple episodes. Vertebral-basilar insufficiency and multiple sclerosis typically are associated with brainstem signs. Acoustic neurinoma only rarely causes vertigo as its initial symptom, and the vertigo it causes is mild and intermittent.

724. The answer is A. *(Braunwald, ed 11, chap 352.)* The abrupt appearance of an isolated peripheral facial palsy, which may include ipsilateral hyperacusis resulting from involvement of fibers to the stapedius and loss of taste on the anterior two thirds of the tongue resulting from involvement of the fibers of the chorda tympani, is most often idiopathic, i.e., Bell's palsy. If the patient is unable to close the eye, artificial tears may be helpful during the day to prevent drying, and the eye should be patched at night to prevent corneal abrasion. Excellent recovery occurs in 80 percent of such cases. Oral contraceptives and mitral valve prolapse are not associated with causes of such a clinical picture. Evoked potentials are not helpful diagnostically.

725. The answer is D. (*Braunwald, ed 11, chap 20.*) Narcolepsy is uncontrollable daytime sleepiness, and cataplexy is sudden, brief loss of muscle tone. Sleep paralysis and hypnagogic hallucinations are common in persons with narcolepsy. A properly performed sleep electroencephalogram is useful in supporting a diagnosis of narcolepsy—REM sleep occurs much earlier in sleep than normal in affected individuals. (False-positive tests can occur if the subject has recently been sleeping, awakens briefly, and then falls asleep again for the test.) Confusion and epileptic disorders are not part of the narcolepsy-cataplexy syndrome.

726. The answer is D. (*Braunwald, ed 11, chap 21.*) In a comatose person, reactive pupils and the absence of eye movements in response to head turning or ice-water irrigation of the ear canals signify metabolic suppression of brainstem neurons. The major distinction that must be made is between true unresponsiveness and a "locked-in" stroke state, in which eye movements also may be obliterated. In brain death, pupils are unreactive. A person unresponsive due to a conversion reaction cannot voluntarily suppress the nystagmus induced by caloric irrigation, although tonic eye movements can be suppressed by gaze fixation. Pontine hemorrhage is associated with small pupils. Bilateral infarcts in a carotid distribution may cause coma, but oculocephalic movements are normal.

727. The answer is A. (*Braunwald, ed 11, chap 21.*) Patients with basilar artery stenosis frequently have spells of ischemic brainstem dysfunction prior to a catastrophic stroke caused by arterial thrombosis. Timely anticoagulation and allowing a higher blood pressure can arrest the progression of this potentially fatal stroke. Acute coma can occur in association with each of the cerebrovascular accidents mentioned except carotid occlusion. Subarachnoid hemorrhage causes an acute increase in intracranial pressure that reduces blood flow to the brain. Unilateral cortical infarction does not cause coma, but damage to brainstem structures via infarction or compression will cause coma.

728. The answer is B. (*Braunwald, ed 11, chap 341.*) The testing of evoked potentials is of greatest utility in detecting subclinical spinal cord and optic nerve lesions. Up to two-thirds of persons who have multiple sclerosis have neurologic deficits evident on visual or peroneal somatic evoked potentials but **not** on physical examination. Such a "second lesion" frequently establishes the diagnosis of multiple sclerosis. Evoked potentials may be abnormal in the other conditions listed in the question.

729. The answer is A. (*Braunwald, ed 11, chap 341.*) Because visual acuity even as poor as 20/200 would not produce an abnormal pattern-shift visual evoked potential, the test may be used to support a diagnosis of hysterical blindness or malingering. By alteration of the check sizes on the displayed pattern and variation in the pattern's distance from the eyes, the technique can be refined to provide an accurate measure of acuity. Papilledema does not affect the test, unless it causes severe optic atrophy. Temporal arteritis and pituitary tumor may be associated with an abnormal evoked response if the optic nerve is affected.

730. The answer is D. (*Braunwald, ed 11, chap 342.*) Absence, or petit mal, seizures are distinguished from complex partial seizures in a number of ways, including lack of an aura, a characteristic 3-Hz rhythmic EEG pattern during a spell, and immediate recovery. Because of their brevity and subtlety, absence seizures frequently go unrecognized until an affected child begins school and performs poorly. The prognosis is good: one-third outgrow the disorder, one-third have a milder form in adulthood, and one-third have easily controlled generalized seizures. Ethosuximide (Zarotin), not phenytoin, is the drug of choice.

731. The answer is C. (*Braunwald, ed 11, chap 6.*) Errors made in the investigation of patients with sudden onset of severe headache can result in catastrophic subarachnoid hemorrhage from a ruptured aneurysm. Patients frequently have "warning" bleeding that causes severe headache and brings them for medical attention. Sudden headache during physical exertion is a presentation of ruptured intracranial aneurysm. A careful cerebrospinal fluid examination is the most sensitive test, but a noncontrast CT scan may show the subarachnoid blood and make the lumbar puncture unnecessary. A patient with a reasonable suspicion for aneurysmal bleeding should not be sent home to wait for other symptoms because the next symptom is often a catastrophic subarachnoid hemorrhage. In the patient described, however, the repeated onset of headache with coitus is characteristic of a benign coital headache

DISORDERS OF THE NERVOUS SYSTEM AND MUSCLES

syndrome. If faced with only a single sudden coital headache, then an investigation for a cerebral aneurysm would be appropriate. The family history of migraine is usually not helpful for the diagnosis of coital headache.

732. The answer is C. *(Braunwald, ed 11, chap 343.)* The clinical picture presented in the question suggests acute subarachnoid hemorrhage, either from a ruptured saccular aneurysm or from an arteriovenous malformation. A CT scan of the head, done initially without infusion of contrast material, would be more likely than the other procedures listed to demonstrate the presence of blood in the subarachnoid space and possibly in the ventricles as well. In addition, a CT scan also can detect the presence of hydrocephalus and intracerebral hematoma, two conditions that, in the presence of coma, may require surgical intervention. Skull films are not likely to be informative in this case, although in the presence of a large arteriovenous malformation they may show intracranial calcification. Lumbar puncture as a means of establishing the presence of intracranial bleeding is rendered less useful and is possibly dangerous in this instance by the finding of retinal hemorrhages, a sign of acute intracranial hemorrhage. A radionuclide scan would have little to offer in this set of circumstances, and angiography would be premature.

733. The answer is D. *(Braunwald, ed 11, chap 343.)* Half of all episodes of hypertensive intracerebral hemorrhage occur in the putamen and the adjacent internal capsule. Other sites, in decreasing order of frequency, are the thalamus, cerebellar hemispheres, and pons. Hemorrhages in the subcortical white matter are not generally associated with hypertension and should prompt a search for a bleeding diathesis or an underlying brain lesion. The diagnosis of brain hemorrhage is suggested by clinical signs and confirmed by CT scan; lumbar puncture no longer is recommended.

734. The answer is E. *(Braunwald, ed 11, chaps 11, 12.)* The presence of grasp or suck responses, though not diagnostic of dementia, do indicate a loss of neurons and thus support the diagnosis of dementia. Somatic complaints, including headache, are common in both dementia and depression, although they tend to be more persistent in depression. Memory may be impaired in persons with depression, because of lack of attention to tasks, as well as in persons with dementia; immediate recall is usually poor in severe depression, whereas it is often good in dementia.

735. The answer is D. *(Braunwald, ed 11, chaps 22, 343.)* The man described in the question develops dyslexia (without dysgraphia) and slight impairment in auditory comprehension. This syndrome is not uncommon and generally results from an embolus to the left parietooccipital region. It also frequently develops as part of a larger stroke involving the middle cerebral artery and occasionally after cardic arrest with border-zone infarction.

736. The answer is C. *(Braunwald, ed 11, chap 12.)* Patients with loss of consciousness resulting from a seizure usually have mental confusion, headache, and drowsiness postictally, whereas the patient with a brief syncopal spell recovers fully as soon as the blood pressure returns to normal. Auras, urinary incontinence, and a laceration of the tongue are clues that the cause of the loss of consciousness was a seizure.

737. The answer is C. *(Braunwald, ed 11, chap 344.)* Treatment of hypotension, control of the airway, and a search for lesions that raise intracranial pressure are the first priorities in managing persons with severe head trauma. Skull x-rays have been largely replaced by CT scans, because contusions and hemorrhages are better seen by CT scanning. Although stabilization of the neck is very important, the other treatment choices mentioned in the question are not.

738. The answer is C. *(Braunwald, ed 11, chaps 269, 343.)* Diplopia is not unusual in persons with temporal arteritis and may occur even in those persons experiencing visual loss. The site of pathology—muscle or nerve—is still unsettled. Less common symptoms are jaw claudication and pharyngeal ulcer from infarction.

739. The answer is E. *(Braunwald, ed 11, chap 345.)* Histiocytic lymphoma of the brain (reticulum cell sarcoma) is increasingly common as a sporadic tumor and occurs frequently in immunosuppressed patients, such as renal transplant recipients. Its clinical sensitivity to corticosteroids can mistakenly suggest a diagnosis of multiple sclerosis, and its complete disappearance or dramatic improvement on CT scan after steroid therapy is baffling. Most histiocytic lymphomas of the brain are very radiosensitive.

740. The answer is D. *(Braunwald, ed 11, chaps 345, 358.)* The neuromuscular disease produced by distant cancer, Eaton-Lambert syndrome, differs from myasthenia gravis in that the ocular muscles are spared. In addition, there is an incremental response in power when an affected muscle is stimulated rapidly; the opposite effect occurs in myasthenia gravis. The relationship between cancer and polymyositis and dermatomyositis still is controversial, but a noninflammatory myopathy has not been related to tumors. Cranial nerve palsies are invariably related to carcinomatous meningitis rather than to distant effects.

741. The answer is A. *(Braunwald, ed 11, chap 346.)* Septic cerebral emboli originate in infected left-sided heart valves, liver abscesses, and other similar lesions. More than one type of organism generally are involved, and anaerobes, such as *Streptococcus, Bacteroides, Fusobacterium, Veillonella, Proprionibacterium,* and *Actinomyces,* are common. Although culture from a resulting abscess may be negative, Gram stain of pus (not cerebrospinal fluid) can be useful.

742. The answer is E. *(Braunwald, ed 11, chap 343.)* Before assuming that a stroke is due to hemispheral disease, clinicians should search for contralateral brainstem signs. Right hemiparesis with either left facial weakness or left-gaze paresis indicates a pontine stroke, which generally is due to basilar artery branch disease. Inability to calculate (acalculia) and left-right confusion with dysgraphia are part of the Gerstmann syndrome of left parietal stroke and may occur with right hemiparesis. Minimizing or ignoring the deficit is most typical of a right-brain lesion and is associated with a left hemiparesis.

743. The answer is E. *(Braunwald, ed 11, chap 7.)* Lumbar back pain is frequently associated with each of the first four medical conditions described. The patient with lumbar back pain should therefore be given careful abdominal and pelvic examinations; spine films are necessary to detect destructive bone lesions that may cause referred pain to the buttock or leg. Laboratory evaluation should include blood count and determinations of serum calcium, alkaline phosphatase, and acid phosphatase (in elderly males) concentrations. Diphtheria toxin causes a painless, demyelinative neuropathy which can simulate the Landry-Guillain-Barré syndrome. Aching muscular pain occurs commonly in Landry-Guillain-Barré patients.

744. The answer is E. *(Braunwald, ed 11, chaps 346, 353.)* Spinal epidural abscess, a neurologic emergency, is currently best diagnosed by myelography, which would demonstrate a blocked flow of dye in the spinal subarachnoid space. Lumbar puncture would show a high protein content and cell count but would not establish the diagnosis and may in fact be harmful. Babinski signs are absent in the case described because lumbar pain indicates an abscess overlying the cauda equina, which is made up of peripheral nerves, rather than the spinal cord.

745. The answer is A. *(Braunwald, ed 11, chap 347.)* An increase in the gamma globulin fraction of cerebrospinal fluid (CSF) protein is commonly, but not invariably, associated with multiple sclerosis and occurs in nearly all cases of subacute sclerosing panencephalitis. Slow-virus infections, such as Jakob-Creutzfeldt disease, do not alter CSF chemistries. Viral encephalitis may cause elevated levels of total protein, but CSF gamma globulin levels generally are normal.

746. The answer is D. *(Braunwald, ed 11, chaps 347, 350.)* Very few diseases cause rapid dementia, noticeable in a period of weeks. Among them are depression, metabolic encephalopathy, encephalitis, poisoning, Binswanger's disease (white-matter infarction), and Jakob-Creutzfeldt disease. (Alzheimer's disease has a more insidious onset.) Jakob-Creutzfeldt disease is a slow-virus infection that causes a spongiform change in the cerebral cortex; it is characterized by rapid dementia, startle myoclonus, and, frequently, signs of occipital and cerebellar disease. CT scan and cerebrospinal fluid examination are nearly always normal in affected persons; after a period of time electroencephalography shows rapid synchronous sharp waves, a diagnostic finding.

747. The answer is D. *(Braunwald, ed 11, chap 348.)* Optic neuritis is the initial symptom in approximately 40 percent of individuals who eventually are diagnosed as having multiple sclerosis. This rapidly developing ophthalmologic disorder is associated with partial or total loss of vision, pain on motion of the involved eye, scotoma affecting macular vision, and a variety of other visual-field defects. Ophthalmoscopically visible optic papillitis occurs in about half of cases.

748. The answer is C. *(Braunwald, ed 11, chap 348.)* By far the most common cause of unilateral internuclear ophthalmoplegia is multiple sclerosis. Preferred diagnostic tests for multiple sclerosis are lumbar puncture to check particularly for an elevated immunoglobulin G fraction and evoked potentials to search for an occult second lesion in the nervous system (the demonstration of a second lesion makes the diagnosis of multiple sclerosis definite). The workup can be performed on an outpatient basis. Magnetic resonance imaging may also reveal occult white matter lesions.

749. The answer is B. *(Braunwald, ed 11, chap 349.)* The syndrome described in the question is most strongly suggestive of Wilson's disease. Diagnosis can be confirmed by the demonstration of a Kayser-Fleischer ring on slit-lamp ophthalmologic examination. A careful family history often uncovers other cases. Laboratory findings associated with Wilson's disease include low serum copper and ceruloplasmin levels and, more consistently, elevated urinary copper excretion. Early in the course of the illness the most reliable diagnostic finding is high copper content in a biopsy sample of liver tissue.

750. The answer is D. *(Braunwald, ed 11, chap 344.)* Hyperosmolar dehydration with mannitol or an equivalent agent reduces abnormally elevated intracranial pressure (ICP). Using intravenous fluids to support blood pressure, especially if they are hypoosmolar, would exacerbate cerebral edema and raise ICP still further. Similarly, high airway pressures are transmitted by way of the thoracic venous system and cerebrospinal fluid to the intracranial cavity and thus may worsen ICP elevation. The administration of phenytoin or beta blockers would be ineffective.

751. The answer is B. *(Braunwald, ed 11, chap 349.)* Acquired hepatocerebral degeneration is a neurologic syndrome comprised mainly of extrapyramidal signs. A well-known consequence of chronic liver disease, this disorder simulates Wilson's disease in many ways, including the presence of neuropathologic lesions in the cortex, basal ganglia, and other deep nuclei. Many cases become evident after a bout of hepatic encephalopathy, but others occur insidiously in persons who never have had encephalopathy.

752. The answer is B. *(Braunwald, ed 11, chaps 15, 12, 349.)* The combination of autonomic insufficiency and parkinsonian symptoms is known as the Shy-Drager syndrome. The autonomic form of the Landry-Guillain-Barré syndrome causes acute autonomic paralysis but does not cause the parkinsonian symptoms of tremor at rest, bradykinesia, and rigidity. A number of antihypertensive agents cause orthostatic hypotension, but none cause parkinsonism. Micturition syncope is a condition in which syncope occurs because of vagal surge at the time of release of intravesicular pressure.

753. The answer is B. *(Braunwald, ed 11, chap 362.)* Lower brachial plexus injuries predominantly produce C8 and T1 deficits. Typically, ulnar border sensory loss affects the hand, and a Horner's syndrome may develop from damage to sympathetic nerve roots exiting at C8. Wasting of the intrinsic hand muscles leads to a "claw hand" deformity.

754. The answer is B. *(Braunwald, ed 11, chap 350.)* Huntington's chorea, which is inherited as an autosomal dominant trait, is characterized by dementia and choreiform movements. The motor disorder may include grimacing, respiratory spasms, speech irregularity, and a dancing, jangling quality of the gait. Laboratory workup is normal except that atrophy of the caudate may be seen on a careful evaluated CT or MRI scan.

755. The answer is D. *(Braunwald, ed 11, chap 350.)* Several illnesses produce parkinsonian symptoms—rigidity, bradykinesia, and masked facies—but at the same time are not associated with tremor and do not respond to typical antiparkinsonism drugs. The most common of these diseases is progressive supranuclear palsy, which is characterized by vertical ophthalmoplegia, speech difficulty (hypophonia), and anxiety. No form of therapy has been consistently successful in controlling the symptoms of this disorder.

756. The answer is B. *(Braunwald, ed 11, chap 353.)* The most characteristic symptom of syringomyelia is loss of pain sense with preservation of touch. This phenomenon occurs most commonly over the shoulders in a cape-like distribution. Tissue loss in the central gray matter of the spinal cord, where pain fibers cross to join the contralateral spinothalamic tract, is the neuropathologic process involved. Other characteristic features of syringomyelia include thoracic scoliosis and muscle atrophy of the hands. Ataxia does not occur unless the syrinx extends into the brainstem.

757. The answer is A. *(Braunwald, ed 11, chaps 353, 357.)* Neuromyelitis optica (Devic's disease) usually occurs in association with necrotizing myelitis but also is seen in persons who have multiple sclerosis and postinfectious and postvaccinal myelitis. Neuromyelitis optica is characterized by both transverse myelitis and optic neuritis; affected individuals can display such signs and symptoms as progressive sensorimotor deficits, central scotoma, and elevated protein concentration and cell count in cerebrospinal fluid. In the case presented in the question, the presence of optic nerve involvement and the finding of a sensory level on the trunk rules out acute idiopathic polyneuritis, although analysis of cerebrospinal fluid is not inconsistent with polyneuritis in its early stages. A diagnosis of acute spinal epidural abscess is made less likely by the presence of optic neuritis.

758. The answer is E. *(Braunwald, ed 11, chap 352.)* Any lesion impinging on the optic chiasm produces a bitemporal hemianopsia by interfering with images projected onto the nasal retina. The most common cause of bilateral hemianopsia is suprasellar extension of pituitary tumors. Suprasellar aneurysms of the carotid artery are common enough that many neurosurgeons perform angiography before removing apparent pituitary tumors. The best initial diagnostic technique is CT scan with contrast infusion. Other causes of bitemporal hemianopsia include craniopharyngioma, meningioma, and metastatic disease.

759. The answer is A. *(Braunwald, ed 11, chap 354.)* Despite the belief that the finding of CSF pleocytosis rather than albuminocytologic dissociation (high protein without cells) excludes a diagnosis of idiopathic polyneuritis, at least 10 percent of affected persons have cells in their CSF. Signs of meningitis, however, are absent even in these persons. Neuropathies that are more than slightly asymmetrical generally do not evolve into idiopathic polyneuritis. Anesthesia of the legs suggests a spinal cord lesion.

760. The answer is D. *(Braunwald, ed 11, chap 354.)* Entrapment of the lateral femoral cutaneous nerve, which can occur where it enters the thigh beneath the inguinal ligament near the anterior superior iliac spine, causes a sensory neuropathy known as "meralgia paresthetica." Symptoms of this disorder, which typically occurs in obese individuals, include pain and decreased tactile sensation over the lateral aspect of the thigh. Treatment is infiltration with a local anesthetic or, if this procedure proves ineffective, surgical sectioning of the nerve.

761. The answer is E. *(Braunwald, ed 11, chap 354.)* The inflammatory response in Guillain-Barré syndrome strips myelin between the nodes of Ranvier in peripheral nerves. This phenomenon explains both the slowing of nerve conduction and the potential for recovery. Axons are only destroyed in extensively involved areas as a secondary phenomenon. To date, no convincing evidence has emerged to support the contention that the central nervous system is involved in Guillain-Barré syndrome.

DISORDERS OF THE NERVOUS SYSTEM AND MUSCLES

762. The answer is A. *(Braunwald, ed 11, chap 357.)* Myotonia, muscle wasting, cataracts, testicular atrophy, and frontal baldness characterize the hereditary disorder myotonic dystrophy. Onset usually is in early adulthood. In affected individuals, mental retardation is common, atrial arrhythmia is a frequent complication, and diabetes mellitus is more prevalent than in the general population. Myotonic dystrophy is the type of muscular dystrophy most commonly observed in hospitalized individuals.

763. The answer is B. *(Braunwald, ed 11, chap 357.)* Oculopharyngeal dystrophy is a dominantly inherited disease occurring in families of French-Canadian or middle European ancestry. Because it causes late-onset progressive ptosis and difficulty with swallowing, it may be difficult to distinguish from myasthenia gravis, which is not a dystrophic muscle disease. Proximal weakness and ophthalmoplegia suggest the presence of a progressive external ophthalmoplegia.

764. The answer is C. *(Braunwald, ed 11, chap 357.)* Myotonia is the phenomenon in which brief, persistent contractions of a muscle occur after voluntary contraction or, sometimes percussion. Myokymia is continuous, small-muscle movement that is frequently difficult to distinguish from fasciculations. Fibrillation is the electromyographically detected spontaneous firing of muscle fibers and is not visible except in the tongue. Myoedema is a poorly defined sign similar to myotonia in which a ridge of percussed muscle remains contracted for 5 to 8 seconds. It was once thought to be related to hypoalbuminemia, but this relationship probably does not exist.

765. The answer is B. *(Braunwald, ed 11, chap 7, 15.)* Malignancy in the pelvis not infrequently causes compression or infiltration of nerves exiting the spinal cord en route to the leg. This results in stepwise progression of sensory and motor deficits in areas supplied by the involved nerve roots or trunks. Continuous pain in the distribution of a specific nerve or root is also common. In this patient the neurologic deficits began in an S1 distribution but then progressed to L5 and, finally, L4 roots, suggesting an expanding paravertebral mass. Isolated, spontaneous activity of muscle fibers called fibrillations is characteristic of denervation. Nerve conduction will be normal in the leg if the lesion is proximal to the measuring electrodes, i.e., in the pelvis. An expanding cortical mass might also cause progressive numbness in the foot and leg and might be missed on a CT scan that does not take cuts all the way up to the vertex. Back pain and neuropathic pain would not occur with a cortical lesion, and the reflexes under such circumstances should be hyperactive.

766. The answer is D. *(Braunwald, ed 11, chap 358.)* More than three-quarters of patients with myasthenia have circulating antibodies against components of the postsynaptic membrane, including acetylcholine receptors. Antibody action leads to an unfolding, or "simplification," of the membrane and, consequently, a reduced number of acetylcholine receptors. As a result, existing acetylcholine in the synapse is less effective in producing muscle contraction.

767. The answer is E. *(Braunwald, ed 11, chap 359.)* In most persons who have familial periodic paralysis, serum potassium concentration is either slightly high or low (rarely below 2.9 meq/L) during attacks of weakness. The weakness, which develops over minutes to hours is associated with hypotonia and is refractory to electrical stimulation. Between attacks, examination typically is normal, although some persons have myotonia. Cardiac muscle is normal.

768. The answer is B. *(Braunwald, ed 11, chap 6.)* The patient had cluster headache. Cluster headache occurs over the orbit, usually within 2 hours of falling asleep. The key to diagnosis is a history of associated lacrimation, nasal stuffiness, and swelling and erythema over the cheek. The headaches may occur every night for weeks and are quite severe. Ergotamine taken at bedtime is often the first preparation to prevent the headache. Lithium is frequently effective, but its use warrants monitoring of the patient's serum electrolytes and renal function. Alcohol frequently precipitates headache in these patients. Note that the dose of ergotamine in Option D is dangerously excessive. Ergotamine should be limited to a maximum of about 12 mg per week.

769. The answer is E. *(Braunwald, ed 11, chaps 15, 354.)* Fasciculations may occur in a variety of metabolic and toxic disorders, including amyotrophic lateral sclerosis, progressive bulbar palsy, ruptured intervertebral disk, and peripheral neuropathy. However, they should not be viewed with alarm in the absence of weakness, muscle atrophy, or loss of tendon reflexes. The best treatment a physician could offer a person who is asymptomatic except for fascicular twitches is reassurance, and, if appropriate, advice to reduce coffee intake.

770. The answer is C. *(Braunwald, ed 11, chap 362.)* Although porphyric neuropathy may occur without central nervous system involvement, with acute paralysis there is frequently a history of confusion or coma. Predominantly a motor neuropathy, porphyric neuropathy can cause significant sensory loss in some individuals. In this respect it may simulate inflammatory polyneuropathy, though inflammation does not occur. Curiously, cerebrospinal fluid protein concentration is usually normal in affected persons.

771. The answer is C. *(Braunwald, ed 11, chap 3.)* One of the most distressing sequela of thalamic damage is a chronic pain syndrome that occurs months to a few years after the initial lesion. The finding of total hemianesthesia, and the loss of all sensory modalities in the face, arm, and leg is characteristic of thalamic infarction. Lesions of the spinothalamic tract may also cause neuropathic pain syndromes, but hemianesthesia of the face does not occur with spinal cord lesions. Parietal lobe lesions usually affect the cortical senses, i.e., two-point discrimination, graphesthesia, or stereognosia, rather than cause a total hemianesthesia. Depression is not commonly associated with burning pain. Tic douloureux is not associated with sensory loss.

772. The answer is A-Y, B-N, C-Y, D-Y, E-N. *(Braunwald, ed 11, chap 15.)* Polymyalgia rheumatica is characterized by aching pain, but unlike polymyositis weakness is minimal or absent. Subacute combined degeneration due to vitamin-B_{12} deficiency is predominantly a sensory syndrome associated with spasticity; weakness is absent until the disease is far advanced. Botulism is fundamentally a paralytic disorder due to presynaptic neuromuscular blockade. Like botulism, polyneuritis causes paralysis, although a pure sensory neuropathy is not associated with weakness.

773. The answer is A-Y, B-Y, C-N, D-N, E-Y. *(Braunwald, ed 11, chap 16.)* Normal-pressure hydrocephalus and cervical spondylosis typically present with gait difficulty: short steps (sometimes mistaken for parkinsonism), and leg stiffness and slowness of step, respectively. Subacute combined degeneration may produce spasticity of gait as part of its lateral column (corticospinal) damage. Subdural hematoma generally does not cause isolated gait difficulty, and carotid stenosis causes either transient ischemic attacks or strokes but not a progressive syndrome of any sort.

774. The answer is A-N, B-Y, C-Y, D-N, E-N. *(Braunwald, ed 11, chap 20.)* Several sleep disorders are associated with the rapid-eye-movement (REM) phase of sleep. For example, nocturnal attacks of cluster headache typically produce intense, nonthrobbing pain during REM sleep. The night sleep pattern of persons with narcolepsy may begin with REM sleep, skipping the 70 minutes or so usually spent in non-REM (NREM) sleep (stages III and IV). Somnambulism (sleep walking) cannot occur during the REM phase of sleep, because the limb muscles are devoid of tone. Nocturnal epilepsy occurs during or just after the onset of sleep, and night terrors are associated with stage IV NREM sleep.

775. The answer is A-Y, B-N, C-N, D-N, E-Y. *(Braunwald, ed 11, chap 21.)* For most comatose persons seen in a general hospital setting CT scanning is not helpful, because nonsructural causes—i.e., metabolic or exogenous toxins—are at fault. A lesion appears on CT scan only when there is a difference in density compared to adjacent areas of the brain. An area of infarction generally takes at least a day to become lower in density than normal brain; thus, a CT scan performed acutely would be expected to be normal. Acute unilateral middle cerebral artery infarction does not cause coma. Brain death is a clinical, not a radiologic, diagnosis.

DISORDERS OF THE NERVOUS SYSTEM AND MUSCLES

776. The answer is A-N, B-N, C-Y, D-Y, E-Y. *(Braunwald, ed 11, chaps 24, 342.)* So-called simple partial seizures are due to epileptic discharges in a focal brain region. Most often these are in the temporal lobe, where they cause psychologic phenomena, such as déjà vu, or brief emotional symptoms, such as fear, if they impinge on the limbic system. Discharges on the lateral surface of the temporal lobe may cause auditory hallucinations, vertigo, or language disturbances (if on the left side). Well-defined limb or facial sensations or movements are not part of temporal lobe epilepsy.

777. The answer is A-Y, B-Y, C-N, D-N, E-N. *(Braunwald, ed 11, chap 358.)* Conventional electromyography (EMG) and nerve conduction studies as well as muscle biopsy procedures are not useful in an evaluation of myasthenia gravis, because it is not a disease of muscle or nerve. (Electron microscopy of muscle can show unfolding of the postsynaptic muscle membrane, but this procedure is not commonly done.) Curare testing to precipitate myasthenic weakness is dangerous, undependable, and mainly of historical interest. Single-fiber EMG measures the timing of firing of two fibers in the same motor unit. The timing between pairs is inconsistent in myasthenia, giving rise to "jitter" in the oscilloscope tracing; this finding is virtually diagnostic of myasthenia. Repetitive stimulation of motor nerves to observe a decremental response also is a useful procedure in testing for myasthenia gravis.

778. The answer is A-Y, B-Y, C-N, D-Y, E-N. *(Braunwald, ed 11, chap 7.)* Low back pain without ruptured disk or other nerve damage is common. It requires bed rest, administration of muscle relaxants, and time for recovery. It is often precipitated by lifting while the spine is flexed or laterally rotated. X-rays may show the nonspecific signs of paravertebral muscle spasm, i.e., straightening of the normal lumbar lordosis or scoliosis. Because of pain and spasm the patient cannot flex the spine normally. Signs of nervous system damage distinguish the patient with a more serious disorder. Bowel and bladder difficulty accompany damage to sacral roots or the spinal cord. Perineal sensation and rectal tone should be tested along with individual muscle strength, stretch reflexes, Babinski reflexes, and dermatomal sensation. Abnormal results on any of these tests suggest that there is nerve injury in addition to muscular strain.

779. The answer is A-N, B-Y, C-Y, D-Y, E-N. *(Braunwald, ed 11, chaps 15, 341.)* Hypotonia or atonia is characteristic of denervated muscle. Muscle atrophy that occurs after destruction of a motor nerve is much more severe than simple disuse muscle atrophy; denervated muscle usually loses 70 to 80 percent of its original bulk within 90 days. Denervation of muscle produces Erb's reaction of degeneration, in which response to short-duration (faradic) stimulation is lost but response to long-duration (galvanic) stimulation is preserved. The isolated activity of individual muscle fibers (fibrillation) is a characteristic of denervated muscle. Fasciculations, on the other hand, occur when a motor neuron in the anterior horn of the spinal cord becomes diseased; because they depend on reinnervation of muscle by normal nerve fibers, fasciculations generally are not produced when a nerve is totally destroyed.

780. The answer is A-Y, B-N, C-Y, D-N, E-Y. *(Braunwald, ed 11, chap 343.)* Polycythemia, idiopathic thrombocytosis, and sickle cell disease are hematologic disorders regularly associated with cerebrovascular occlusion, though rarely as the first sign. Hyperproteinemia, which causes microvascular occlusion that may be visible in the retina, causes coma or delirium rather than stroke. Cirrhosis is occasionally associated with intracerebral hemorrhage related to hypoprothrombinemia; however, subdural or epidural hematomas usually result, not occlusive stroke.

781. The answers are: A-Y, B-N, C-Y, D-Y, E-Y. *(Braunwald, ed 11, chap 13.)* Papillitis is the disc swelling associated with optic neuritis. It is frequently associated with pain in the eye, loss of visual acuity, and a central scotoma. The appearance of the disc may be indistinguishable from papilledema caused by high intracranial pressure. Papilledema usually spares visual acuity (unless chronic), but it is associated with an enlarged blind spot. Optic neuritis is a frequent presentation in patients later given the diagnosis of multiple sclerosis. The disc becomes chalky white after episodes of optic neuritis, and it is a helpful physical finding in patients with symptoms suggestive of demyelination in the central nervous system.

782. The answer is A-Y, B-Y, C-Y, D-Y, E-N. *(Braunwald, ed 11, chap 349.)* Dialysis "dementia" usually begins as a disorder of articulation, but general mental decline may be evident early as well. Electroencephalography may reveal bursts of slow waves or spikes; cerebrospinal fluid analysis and CT scan typically are normal. The illness is usually progressive to death, although some patients survive for several years. Except for clonazepam treatment of myoclonus and seizures, no effective therapy is known.

783. The answer is A-N, B-Y, C-Y, D-Y, E-Y. *(Braunwald, ed 11, chap 354.)* Acute mononeuropathy involving the oculomotor or peroneal nerves should prompt an investigation for diabetes. A neuropathy that is progressive, distal, and primarily sensory is most characteristic of diabetes but may also occur with an occult neoplasm. The autonomic neuropathy of diabetes usually coexists with the sensory type, but the latter may be mild. Relapsing neuropathy is more typical of idopathic polyneuritis.

784. The answer is A-Y, B-Y, C-Y, D-N, E-N. *(Braunwald, ed 11, chaps 23, 348.)* Several disorders produce chronic, progressive spinal cord disease with sensory and motor involvement. Syndromes of spinocerebellar degeneration may involve the motor and sensory spinal cord systems in addition to causing ataxia. Multiple sclerosis usually causes a relapsing illness but can cause a progressive, usually cervical myelopathy in elderly women. Cervical spondylosis, or bony compression of the cervical cord by osteophytic bars, is another common cause of myelopathy in the elderly. Lumbar disk compression of the cauda equina, which is made up of peripheral nerves, does not cause spinal cord signs. Amyotrophic lateral sclerosis is a disease of spinal cord motor neurons and corticospinal tracts, but has no sensory signs.

785. The answer is A-N, B-Y, C-N, D-N, E-Y. *(Braunwald, ed 11, chaps 349, 352.)* Bilateral lateral-rectus palsies that develop acutely in alcoholic persons should suggest Wernicke's encephalopathy, which requires prompt treatment with thiamine. Bilateral sixth-nerve malfunction may be a falsely localizing sign from increased intracranial pressure, as in subdural hematoma, but does not occur as an isolated disturbance from intrinsic brainstem diseases (e.g., hemorrhage). Orbital fractures usually entrap the fourth nerve, less commonly the sixth; only rarely would the palsy be bilateral. Although neurosyphilis can cause cranial nerve palsies from adhesive meningitis, palsy of oculomotor-related nerves is a rarity.

786. The answer is A-N, B-Y, C-Y, D-Y, E-Y. *(Braunwald, ed 11, chap 353.)* The finding of a clear sensory level above which pinprick is felt but below which sensation is absent is the *sine qua non* of spinal cord disease. The segmental level at which sensory loss begins also gives the corresponding cord level of the lesion. Other typical signs of spinal cord disease, such as hypertonicity and hyperreflexia, may be absent in acute lesions; bladder function, however, is invariably affected if the lesion is severe. Myelopathy due to deficiency of vitamin B_{12} only rarely gives a vague sensory level on the trunk.

787. The answer is A-N, B-Y, C-Y, D-N, E-Y. *(Braunwald, ed 11, chap 343.)* Unilateral occlusion of a vertebral artery typically results in Wallenberg's lateral medullary syndrome. With an infarct on the left, this is likely to include damage to the left ninth and tenth cranial nerves, the left inferior cerebellar peduncle, and the spinothalamic fibers subserving pain and temperature on the right side. Vertigo and nystagmus are common since the lower vestibular complex may be affected. Horner's syndrome is also common with a smaller pupil and ptosis *ipsilateral* to the lesion. Only rarely is the medullary pyramid involved (Babinski-Nageotte syndrome) resulting in a *contralateral* hemiparesis sparing the face; hypoglossal weakness may then be present ipsilateral to the lesion. Lesions of the median longitudinal fasciculus producing internuclear ophthalmoplegia occur in the pons and midbrain in the territory of branches of the basilar artery.

788. The answer is A-Y, B-Y, C-N, D-N, E-Y. *(Braunwald, ed 11, chap 352.)* Cranial nerves III, IV, and VI all pass through the cavernous sinus, so that complete ophthalmoplegia, including ptosis, may result from a disease process there. Since the supraorbital and maxillary divisions of the fifth nerve, but not the mandibular branch, pass through the cavernous sinus, the brow and cheek may be numb, but not the chin. The optic nerve will be involved only if the process extends superiorly.

DISORDERS OF THE NERVOUS SYSTEM AND MUSCLES

789–792. The answers are: 789-D, 790-C, 791-C, 792-A. *(Braunwald, ed 11, chap 7.)* In the assessment of uncomplicated disk protrusion, it is important to keep in mind that many lesions cause sciatica and that a protruding disk generally impinges on the nerve root that exits just below it (e.g., an "L5-S1 disk" most often compresses the S1 root). Walking on the toes requires a powerful gastrocnemius muscle, which is innervated by L5 and S1. When weakness in this maneuver is coupled with a depressed ankle reflex, an S1 compression is likely (protrusion of the L5-S1 disk). Compression of the L5 root by an L4-L5 disk does not affect knee or ankle reflexes but causes anterior tibial weakness (foot drop), extensor hallucis longus weakness, and weakness of foot inversion. The knee reflex is affected by an L3 or L4 radicular lesion (L2-L3 or L3-L4 disks, respectively), but hip flexors are affected by L2 and L3 only. These are the major lower extremity disk syndromes. In complex cases, several nerve roots are involved by protrusion of a single disk.

793–797. The answers are: 793-B, 794-A, 795-C, 796-E, 797-E. *(Braunwald, ed 11, chaps 22, 23.)* Individuals who have large lesions of one or both of the frontal lobes or who have lesions of the central white matter and the anterior region of the corpus callosum may exhibit several clinical syndromes. Some affected individuals develop what is known as the apathetic-akinetic-abulic state, which is characterized by decreased initiative and spontaneity combined with diminished speech and motor activity. Other syndromes include motor abnormalities, impaired intelligence, and personality changes.

Wernicke's aphasia occurs as a result of a lesion in the dominant temporal lobe. Affected individuals are unable to read, write, or comprehend the speech of others. Quadrantic homonymous anopsia also may be associated with Wernicke's aphasia.

A lesion of the dominant parietal lobe can cause Gerstmann's syndrome. This syndrome is considered representative of an agnosia, in that both the formulation and use of symbolic concepts are defective. As a result, affected individuals are unable to write and calculate and to differentiate right from left.

Inability to recognize faces (prosopagnosia) results from a lesion in the visual association areas of the occipital lobe. This disorder can arise from either unilateral or, more frequently, bilateral involvement of the occipitotemporal regions. Visual acuity is intact in affected individuals.

798–801. The answers are: 798-D, 799-C, 800-E, 801-A. *(Braunwald, ed 11, chap 354.)* Several disorders are associated with an acute ascending motor paralysis. Perhaps the best known is acute idiopathic polyneuritis (Landry-Guillain-Barré syndrome), which half the time is associated with a prodrome of mild respiratory or gastrointestinal infection. Muscle weakness involves both proximal and distal muscles and develops rapidly. Careful management can reduce the mortality rate to under 5 percent, although as many as 25 percent of affected individuals may have mild to severe residual deficits. A significant outbreak of acute idiopathic polyneuritis accompanied the swine flu inoculation campaign of 1976.

Individuals who have infectious mononucleosis can develop aseptic meningitis, meningoencephalitis, or a syndrome resembling acute idiopathic polyneuritis during the midphase of the infection. Cerebrospinal fluid can contain as many as several hundred mononuclear cells, and the protein level is elevated. In diphtheritic neuropathy, the early pharyngeal and laryngeal paralysis may be associated with blurring of vision due to loss of accommodation. Polyneuropathy involving all four limbs, usually simultaneously, develops four to eight weeks later. Porphyric polyneuropathy is severe and rapidly progressive. Convulsions and a psychosis associated with delirium and confusion may occur.

802–806. The answers are: 802-A, 803-C, 804-B, 805-D, 806-E. *(Braunwald, ed 11, chap 18.)* Sensory levels on physical examination can be used to pinpoint the spinal cord level affected in a variety of diseases. Each dermatomal level is associated with a major anatomic landmark. Sensory cervical spinal roots are associated with the following landmarks: posterior scalp (C2), neck (C3), clavicle (C4), shoulder (C5), thumb and forefinger (C6), middle finger (C7), and ring finger (C8). Key thoracic dermatomal landmarks include the axilla (T2 and T3), nipple (T4), and umbilicus (T10). Lumbar sensory levels include anterior thigh (L3), knee (L4), and lateral calf and great toe (L5), while sacral levels, which are harder to demarcate, include the posterior calf (S1) and posterior thigh (S2).

807–812. The answers are: 807-B, 808-B, 809-C, 810-B, 811-B, 812-D. *(Braunwald, ed 11, chap 342.)* Rash and idiosyncratic bone marrow suppression are at times seen with phenobarbital, phenytoin, and carbamazepine; leukopenia and thrombocytopenia are most common with carbamazepine (Tegretol). Hepatotoxicity is a rare but feared effect of carbamazepine and acutely with valproic acid (Depakane). In addition to the side effects listed, phenytoin causes the appearance of a slightly prognathic jaw and coarsened facies.

813–816. The answers are: 813-C, 814-D, 815-A, 816-B. *(Braunwald, ed 11, chap 3).* The direct spinothalamic tract projects to the VPL in the thalamus; other spinothalamic fibers end in medial thalamic nuclei. Afferent pain fibers have their cell bodies in the dorsal root ganglia and project centrally to the spinal cord where they release substance P. Destruction of substance P fibers causes analgesia. Descending pathways also mediate the appreciation of pain. Opiate receptors are concentrated in limbic structures along with the periaqueductal gray matter, raphe nucleus and the medial thalamus. The raphe and locus coeruleus neurons project down to the dorsal horn of the spinal cord and modulate pain via release of serotonin and norepinephrine, respectively. The action of these descending pathways may be affected by tricyclic antidepressants accounting for their effectiveness in treating pain syndromes.

817–821. The answers are: 817-E, 818-A, 819-B, 820-D, 821-C. *(Braunwald, ed 11, chap 13.)* Eye movement abnormalities occur as a result of a number of nervous system abnormalities. The pontine gaze center controls ipsilateral horizontal gaze. The medial longitudinal fasciculus (MLF) connects the gaze centers and the oculomotor nuclei. A lesion of the MLF results in an internuclear ophthalmoplegia as described in option C. Lesions of the frontal lobe gaze center cause a gaze preference to the side of the lesion, but the eyes can usually be made to cross the midline. The rostral interstitial nucleus of the MLF controls vertical gaze. Labyrinthine disorders cause vertigo and nystagmus, though nystagmus is also caused by a number of brainstem and cerebellar lesions.

822–826. The answers are: 822-B, 823-C, 824-D, 825-C, 826-A. *(Braunwald, ed 11, chap 350.)* In the elderly, confusion may be caused by almost all the drugs used to treat Parkinson's disease. Amantadine especially causes confusion as well as pedal edema and livedo reticularis, which is purplish mottling of the skin. Anticholinergic agents—such as benztropine mesylate (Cogentin), trihexyphenidyl (Artane), procyclidine (Kemadrin), or biperiden (Akineton)—are limited in their usefulness by dry mouth, urinary retention, and, in some patients, confusion and psychosis. Excessive intake of L-dopa can cause dyskinesias, orthostatic hypotension, and confusion. Propranolol is known to cause bronchospasm in atopic individuals. The drug, however, is useful when a parkinsonian patient has a rapid (8- to 10-Hz) tremor.

827–831. The answers are: 827-C, 828-A, 829-B, 830-A, 831-D. *(Braunwald, ed 11, chap 350.)* Frequent unexplained falls and loss of saccadic eye movements (downward first, then upward, and finally horizontal, with preservation of vestibulo-ocular reflexes) are typical of progressive supranuclear palsy. Tremor is more common in Parkinson's disease than in progressive supranuclear palsy. Patients with either illness may have masked facies and hypophonic speech. Significant dementia occurs only late in patients with these diseases.

832–835. The answers are: 832-B, 833-A, 834-D, 835-C. *(Braunwald, ed 11, chap 350.)* In Alzheimer's disease, loss of neurons in the nucleus basalis of Meynert, which supplies cholinergic innervation to the cerebral cortex, is associated with decreased levels of choline-acetyl transferase in the cortex. In Huntington's disease, loss of spiny neurons is associated with decreased levels of their transmitter, GABA, and its synthetic enzyme, glutamic acid decarboxylase. In Parkinson's disease, loss of pigmented neurons from the substantia nigra is associated with a reduction in the amount of dopamine in the striatum. In some forms of olivo-pontocerebellar atrophy, loss of cerebellar Purkinje cells is associated with decreased levels of glutamic acid dehydrogenase, as assayed in blood leukocytes. This enzyme inactivates glutamate, the excitatory neurotransmitter used in the granule cell to the Purkinje cell synapse. It has been hypothesized that excessive stimulation with glutamate may be toxic to neurons, e.g., Purkinje cells.

BIBLIOGRAPHY

Alper CA, Bloch KJ, Rosen FS: Increased susceptibility to infection in a patient with type II essential hypercatabolism of C3. *N Engl Med* 288:601–606, 1973.

Anderson RJ, Linas SL, Berns AS, et al: Nonoliguric acute renal failure. *N Engl J Med* 296:1134–1138, 1977.

Arieff AI, Carroll HJ: Nonketotic hyperosmolar coma with hyperglycemia: Clinical features, pathophysiology, renal function, acid-base balance, plasma-cerebrospinal fluid equilibria and the effects of therapy in 37 cases. *Medicine* 51:73–94, 1972.

Ashikari R, Park K, Huvos AG, et al: Paget's disease of the breast. *Cancer* 26:680–685, 1970.

Baker JP, Detsky AS, Wesson DE, et al: Nutritional assessment: A comparison of clinical judgment and objective measurements. *N Engl J Med* 306:969–972, 1982.

Bauman WA, Yalow RS: Hyperinsulinemic hypoglycemia: Differential diagnosis by determination of the species of circulating insulin. *JAMA* 252:2730–2734, 1984.

Bentley DP: Anaemia and chronic disease. *Clin Haematol* 11:465–479, 1982.

Bergofsky EH: Respiratory failure in disorders of the thoracic cage. *Am Rev Respir Dis* 119:643–669, 1979.

Beutler E: Abnormalities of the hexose monophosphate shunt. *Semin Hematol* 8:311–347, 1971.

Bloom ME, Mintz DH, Field JB: Insulin-induced posthypoglycemic hyperglycemia as a cause of "brittle" diabetes. *Am J Med* 47:891–903, 1969.

Braunwald E, Isselbacher KJ, Petersdorf RG, et al: *Harrison's Principles of Internal Medicine,* 11th ed. New York, McGraw-Hill, 1987.

Bray GA: Current status of intestinal bypass surgery in the treatment of obesity. *Diabetes* 26:1072–1079, 1977.

Brewer HB, Zech LA, Gregg RE, et al: Type III hyperlipoproteinemia: Diagnosis, molecular defects, pathology, and treatment. *Ann Intern Med* 98:623–640, 1983.

Brownlee M, Cahill G: Diabetic control and vascular complications. *Atherosclerosis Reviews* 4:29–70, 1979.

Brownlee M, Vlassara H, Cerami A: Nonenzymatic glycosylation and the pathogenesis of diabetic complications. *Ann Intern Med* 101:527–537, 1984.

Burgdorfer W, Barbour AG, Hayes SF, et al: Lyme disease—a tick-borne spirochetosis? *Science* 216:1317–1319, 1982.

Carmichael KA, Fallon MD, Dalinka M, et al: Osteomalacia and osteitis fibrosa in a man ingesting aluminum hydroxide antacid. *Am J Med* 76:1137–1143, 1984.

Carroll P, Matz R: Uncontrolled diabetes mellitus in adults: Experience in treating diabetic ketoacidosis and hyperosmolar treatment regimen. *Diabetes Care* 6:579–585, 1983.

Coleman RW, Robboy SJ, Minna JD: Disseminated intravascular coagulation: A reappraisal. *Annu Rev Med* 30:359–374, 1979.

Cook JD: Clinical evaluation of iron deficiency. *Semin Hematol* 19:6–18, 1982.

Cryer PE, Gerich JE: Glucose counterregulation, hypoglycemia, and intensive insulin therapy in diabetes mellitus. *N Eng J Med* 313:232–240, 1985.

Crystal RG, Fulmer JD, Roberts WC, et al: Idiopathic pulmonary fibrosis. *Ann Intern Med* 85:769–788, 1976.

Diabetic Retinopathy Study Research Group: Photocoagulation treatment of proliferative diabetic retinopathy: clinical application of Diabetic Retinopathy Study (DRS) Findings, DRS Report Number 8. *Ophthalmology* 88:583–600, 1981.

Dienstag JL: Halothane hepatitis: allergy or idiosyncrasy? *N Engl J Med* 303:102–104, 1980.

Dienstag JL, Rhodes AR, Bhan AK, et al: Urticaria associated with acute viral hepatitis type B. Studies of pathogenesis. *Ann Intern Med* 89:34–40, 1978.

Dunn FL, Pietri A, Raskin P: Plasma lipid and lipoprotein levels with continuous subcutaneous insulin infusion in type I diabetes mellitus. *Ann Intern Med* 95:426–431, 1981.

Fairbanks VF (ed): *Current Hematology*. New York, Wiley, 1981.

Feig PU, McCurdy DK: The hypertonic state. *N Engl J Med* 297:1444–1454, 1977.

Felig P, Baxter JD, Broadus AE, et al (eds): *Endocrinology and Metabolism*, 2d ed, New York, McGraw-Hill, 1987.

Finch CA, Deubelbeiss K, Cook JD, et al: Ferrokinetics in man. *Medicine* 49:17–53, 1970.

Fine LG, Barnett EV, Danovitch GM, et al: Systemic lupus erythematosus in pregnancy. *Ann Intern Med* 94:667–677, 1981.

Fitzpatrick TB, Eisen AZ, Wolff K, et al: *Dermatology in General Medicine*, 3d ed. New York, McGraw-Hill, 1986.

Flier JS, Scully RE: Case Records of the Massachusetts General Hospital (case 25-1982): amenorrhea, virilization, and hyperpigmentation in a 15-year-old girl. *N Engl J Med* 306:1537–1544, 1982.

Freedberg I, Galdabini J: Case Records of the Massachusetts General Hospital (case 20-1975): dermatitis, weight loss, and hepatomegaly in a 40-year-old man. *N Engl J Med* 292:1117–1123, 1975.

Friedman EA: Diabetic nephropathy: strategies in prevention and management. *Kidney Int* 21:780–791, 1982.

Freinkel N, Dooley SL, Metzger BE: Care of the pregnant woman with insulin-dependent diabetes mellitus. *N Engl J Med* 313:96–101, 1985.

Gabbe SG: Diabetes mellitus in pregnancy: Have all the problems been solved? *Am J Med* 70:613–618, 1981.

Gordon EE, Kabadi UM: The hyperglycemic hyperosmolar syndrome. *Am J Med Sci* 271:252–268, 1976.

Guilleminault C, Tilkian A, Dement WC: The sleep apnea syndromes. *Annu Rev Med* 27:465–484, 1976.

Hartman RC, Arnold AB: Paroxysmal nocturnal hemoglobinuria (PNH) as a clonal disorder. *Annu Rev Med* 28:187–194, 1977.

Heymsfield SB, Bethel RA, Ansley JD, et al: Enteral hyperalimentation: An alternative to central venous hyperalimentation. *Ann Intern Med* 90:63–71, 1979.

Isselbacher KJ, Adams RD, Braunwald E, et al (eds): *Harrison's Principles of Internal Medicine: Update I*. New York, McGraw-Hill, 1981.

Jacobs RL, Freedman PM, Boswell RN, et al.: Nonallergic rhinitis with eosinophilia (NARES syndrome). *J Allergy Clin Immunol* 67:253–262, 1981.

Jordan RM, Kammer H, Riddle MR: Sulfonylurea-induced factitious hypoglycemia: A growing problem. *Arch Intern Med* 137:390–393, 1977.

Jovanovic L, Druzin M, Peterson CM: Effect of euglycemia on the outcome of pregnancy in insulin-dependent diabetic women as compared with normal control subjects. *Am J Med* 71:921–927, 1981.

Jovanovic L, Peterson CM: The clinical utility of glycosylated hemoglobin. *Am J Med* 70:331–338, 1981.

Judd HL, Meldrum DR, Deftos LJ, et al: Estrogen replacement therapy: Indications and complications. *Ann Intern Med* 98:195–205, 1983.

Kaplan SA, Lippe BM, Brinkman CR III, et al: Diabetes mellitus. *Ann Intern Med* 96:635–649, 1982.

BIBLIOGRAPHY

Kelley WN, Harris ED, Ruddy S, et al (eds): *Textbook of Rheumatology*. Philadelphia, Saunders, 1981, pp 1211–1230.

Koffler A, Friedler RM, Massry SG: Acute renal failure due to nontraumatic rhabdomyolysis. *Ann Intern Med* 85:23–28, 1976.

Kushner JP, Cartwright GE: Sideroblastic anemia. *Adv Intern Med* 22:229–249, 1977.

Laszlo J: Myeloproliferative disorders (MPD): Myelofibrosis, myelosclerosis, extramedullary hematopoiesis, undifferentiated MPD, and hemorrhagic thrombocythemia. *Semin Hematol* 12:409–432, 1975.

Lichtenstein LM, Valentine MD, Sobotka AK: Insect allergy: the state of the art. *J Allergy Clin Immunol* 64:5–12, 1979.

Linman JW, Bagby GC Jr.: The preleukemic syndrome. *Blood Cells* 2:11–31, 1976.

Linton AL, Clark WF, Driedger AA, et al: Acute interstitial nephritis due to drugs. *Ann Intern Med* 93:735–741, 1980.

Mason EE: Gastric bypass for obesity after ten years experience. *Int J Obes* 2:197–206, 1978.

Mathes BM, Douglass MC: Seborrheic dermatitis in patients with acquired immunodeficiency syndrome. *J Am Acad Dermatol* 13:947–951, 1985

Mauer SM, Barbosa J, Vernier RL, et al: Development of diabetic vascular lesions in normal kidneys transplanted into patients with diabetes mellitus. *N Engl J Med* 295:916–920, 1976.

Mazur MH, Dolin R: Herpes zoster at the NIH: A 20-year experience. *Am J Med* 65:738–744, 1978.

McGarry JD, Foster DW: Regulation of hepatic fatty acid oxidation and ketone body production. *Annu Rev Biochem* 49:395–420, 1980.

Miller E, Hare JW, Cloherty JP, et al: Elevated maternal hemoglobin A_{1c} in early pregnancy and major congenital anomalies in infants of diabetic mothers. *N Engl J Med* 304:1331–1334, 1981.

Miller GJ: High density lipoproteins and atherosclerosis. *Annu Rev Med* 31:97–108, 1980.

Miller M, Hall JG: Possible maternal effect on severity of neurofibromatosis. *Lancet* 2:1071–1072, 1978.

Miller RD, Hyatt RE: Evaluation of obstructing lesions of the trachea and larynx by flow volume-loops. *Am Rev Respir Dis* 108:475–481, 1973.

Mittman C, Bruderman I: Lung cancer: To operate or not? *Am Rev Respir Dis* 116:477–496, 1977.

Motulsky AG: Current concepts in genetics. The genetic hyperlipidemias. *N Engl J Med* 294:823–827, 1976.

Moylan JA, Evenson MA: Diagnosis and treatment of fat embolism. *Annu Rev Med* 28:85–90, 1977.

Olefsky JM, Kolterman OG: Mechanisms of insulin resistance in obesity and noninsulin-dependent (type II) diabetes. *Am J Med* 70:151–168, 1981.

Olefsky JM, Kolterman OG, Scarlett JA: Insulin action and resistance in obesity and noninsulin-dependent type II diabetes mellitus. *Am J Physiol* 243:E15–E30, 1982.

Penneys NS, Hicks B: Unusual cutaneous lesions associated with acquired immunodeficiency syndrome. *J Am Acad Dermatol* 13:845–852, 1985.

Petersen BH, Lee TJ, Synderman R, et al: *Neisseria meningitidis* and *Neisseria gonorrhoeae* bacteremia associated with C6, C7, or C8 deficiency. *Ann Intern Med* 90:917–920, 1979.

Powell JR, Vozeh S, Hopewell P, et al: Theophylline disposition in acutely ill hospitalized patients. The effect of smoking, heart failure, severe airway obstruction and pneumonia. *Am Rev Respir Dis* 118:229–238, 1978.

Press OW, Press NO, Kaufman SD: Evaluation and management of chylous ascites. *Ann Intern Med* 96:358, 1982.

Rizza RA, Gerich JE, Haymond MW, et al: Control of blood sugar in insulin-dependent diabetes: Comparison of an artificial endocrine pancreas, continuous subcutaneous insulin infusion, and intensified conventional insulin therapy. *N Engl J Med* 303:1313–1318, 1980.

Roberts RC, Moore VL: Immunopathogenesis of hypersensitivity pneumonitis. *Am Rev Respir Dis* 116:1075–1090, 1977.

Ryan EA, Reiss E: Oncogenous osteomalacia. Review of the world literature of 42 cases and report of two new cases. *Am J Med* 77:501–512, 1984.

Saudek CD, Felig P: The metabolic events of starvation. *Am J Med* 60:117–126, 1976.

Scarlett JA, Mako ME, Rubenstein AH, et al: Factitious hypoglycemia. Diagnosis by measurement of serum C-peptide immunoreactivity and insulin-binding antibodies. *N Engl J Med* 297:1029–1032, 1977.

Schaefer EJ: Clinical, biochemical, and genetic features in familial disorders of high density lipoprotein deficiency. *Atherosclerosis* 4:303–322, 1984.

Schaefer EJ, Levy RI: Pathogenesis and management of lipoprotein disorders. *N Engl J Med* 312:1300–1310, 1985.

Snyder PJ: Gonadotroph cell adenomas of the pituitary. *Endocr Rev* 6:552–563, 1985.

Somogyi M: Exacerbation of diabetes by excess insulin action. *Am J Med* 26:169–191, 1959.

Spivak JL: Felty's syndrome: An analytical review. *Johns Hopkins Med J* 141:156–162, 1977.

Stamm WE, Wagner KF, Amsel R, et al: Causes of the acute urethral syndrome in women. *N Engl J Med* 303:409–415, 1980.

Stanbury JB, Wyngaarden JB, Fredrickson DS, et al (eds): *The Metabolic Basis of Inherited Disease*, 5th ed. New York, McGraw-Hill, 1983.

Staub NC: Pathogenesis of pulmonary edema. *Am Rev Respir Dis* 109:358–372, 1974.

Steno Study Group: Effect of 6 months of strict metabolic control on eye and kidney function in insulin-dependent diabetics with background retinopathy. *Lancet* 1:121–123, 1982.

Stunkard AJ, Sorensen TIA, Hanis C, et al: An adoption study of human obesity. *N Engl J Med* 314:193–198, 1986.

Summers RW, Switz DM, Sessions JT Jr, et al: National Cooperative Crohn's Disease Study: Results of drug treatment. *Gastroenterology* 77:847–869, 1979.

Tattersall R, Gale E: Patient self-monitoring of blood glucose and refinements of conventional insulin treatment. *Am J Med* 70:177–182, 1981.

Tofte RW, Williams DN: Clinical and laboratory manifestations of toxic shock syndrome. *Ann Intern Med* 96:843–847, 1982.

Ursing B, Alm T, Bárány F, et al: A comparative study of metronidazole and sulfasalazine for active Crohn's disease: The Cooperative Crohn's Disease Study in Sweden. II. Result. *Gastroenterology* 83:550–562, 1982.

Ware AJ, Cuthbert JA, Shorey J, et al: A prospective trial of steroid therapy in severe viral hepatitis. The prognostic significance of bridging necrosis. *Gastroenterology* 80:219–224, 1981.

Wilson DA: Excessive insulin therapy: Biochemical effects and clinical repercussion. Current concepts of counterregulation in Type I diabetes. *Ann Intern Med* 98:219–227, 1983.

Wilson JD, Foster DW (eds): *Williams Textbook of Endocrinology*, 7th ed. Philadelphia, WB Saunders, 1985.

Yoon JW, Austin M, Onodera T, et al: Isolation of a virus from the pancreas of a child with diabetic ketoacidosis. *N Eng J Med* 300:1173–1179, 1979.

Young GAR, Vincent PC: Drug-induced agranulocytosis. *Clin Haematol* 9:483–504, 1980.

APPENDIX LABORATORY VALUES OF CLINICAL IMPORTANCE

INTRODUCTORY COMMENTS

Since *Principles of Internal Medicine* is a textbook used internationally, in preparing the Appendix the editors have taken into account the fact that the system of international units (SI, système international d'unités) has been adopted by many laboratories. To this end, where possible and appropriate, common laboratory values are expressed in terms of both traditional units and SI units. *Values in SI units appear in brackets* after values in traditional units. The use of SI units in medicine was endorsed by the Thirtieth World Health Assembly (May 1977) with the purpose of implementing an international language of measurement.[1] The SI *base* units, SI *derived* units, other units of measurement referred to in this Appendix, and SI prefixes are listed in Tables A-1 to A-3. These and other tables of laboratory values are to be found at the end of the Appendix.

ASCITIC FLUID

See Table 39-1, page 190.

BODY FLUIDS AND OTHER MASS DATA

Body fluid, total volume: 50 percent (in obese) to 70 percent (lean) of body weight
  Intracellular: 30 to 40 percent of body weight
  Extracellular: 20 to 30 percent of body weight
Blood:
  Total volume:
    Males: 69 mL per kilogram of body weight
    Females: 65 mL per kilogram of body weight
  Plasma volume:
    Males: 39 mL per kilogram of body weight
    Females: 40 mL per kilogram of body weight
  Red blood cell volume:
    Males: 30 mL per kilogram of body weight (1.15 to 1.21 liters per square meter of body surface area)
    Females: 25 mL per kilogram of body weight (0.95 to 1.00 liters per square meter of body surface area)

$$\text{meq/liter} = \frac{\text{mg/dL} \times 10 \times \text{valence}}{\text{atomic weight}}$$

$$\text{mg/dL} = \frac{\text{meq/liter} \times \text{atomic weight}}{10 \times \text{valence}}$$

CEREBROSPINAL FLUID[2]

Osmolarity	292–297 mosmol per liter
Electrolytes:	
Sodium	137–145 meq per liter
Potassium	2.7–3.9 meq per liter
Calcium	2.1–3.0 meq per liter
Magnesium	2.0–2.5 meq per liter
Phosphorus	1.2–2.0 mg/dL
Chloride	116–122 meq per liter
Bicarbonate	20–24 meq per liter
P_{CO_2}	45–49 mmHg
pH	7.31–7.34
Glucose	40–70 mg/dL
Lactate	10–20 mg/dL
Pyruvate	0.078–0.081 meq per liter
Lactate/pyruvate ratio	26.0
Total protein:	20–45 mg/dL
Prealbumin	2–6%
Albumin	56–75%
Alpha$_1$ globulin	2–7%
Alpha$_2$ globulin	4–12%
Beta globulin	8–16%
Gamma globulin	3–12%
IgG	1.0–1.4 mg/dL
IgA	0.1–0.3 mg/dL
IgM	0.01–0.12 mg/dL
IgG synthesis rate	(−) 9.9 to (+) 3.3 mg per day
Ammonia	25–80 µg/dL
Urea	4.4–4.8 mmol per liter
Creatinine	0.5–1.9 mg/dL
Uric acid	0.23–0.27 mg/dL
Putrescine	130–230 pmol/mL
Spermidine	110–190 pmol/mL
Cyclic AMP	3–30 nmol per liter
HVA (homovanillic acid)	35–85 µg/mL
5-HIAA (5-OH indoleacetic acid)	0.03–0.05 µg/mL
MHPG (3-methoxy-4-hydroxy-phenylethyleneglycol)	13.0–17.0 mg/dL
Myelin basic protein	<4 ng/mL
CSF pressure	50–180 mmH$_2$O
CSF volume (adult)	100–160 mL
Leukocytes:	
Total	<4 per cubic millimeter
Differential:	
Lymphocytes	60–70%
Monocytes	30–50%
Neutrophils	1–3%

CHEMICAL CONSTITUENTS OF BLOOD

See also "Function Tests," especially "Metabolic and Endocrine."

Acetoacetate, plasma: <1.0 mg/dL [<0.1 mmol per liter]
Albumin, serum: 3.5 to 5.5 g/dL [35 to 55 g per liter]
Aldolase: 0 to 8 units per liter [0 to 130 nmol/s per liter]
Alpha$_1$ antitrypsin, serum: 85–213 mg/dL [0.85–2.13 g per liter]

---

[1] *The SI for the Health Professions,* Geneva, World Health Organization, 1977.
[2] Since cerebrospinal fluid concentrations are equilibrium values, measurement of blood plasma obtained at the same time is recommended.

α-Amino nitrogen, plasma: 3.0 to 5.5 mg/dL [2.1 to 3.9 mmol per liter]
Alpha fetoprotein (adult), serum: <30 mg/mL
Aminotransferases, serum:
  Aspartate (AST, SGOT): 10 to 40 Karmen units per milliliter; 6 to 18 units per liter [100 to 300 μmol/s per liter]
  Alanine (ALT, SGPT): 10 to 40 Karmen units per milliliter; 3 to 26 units per liter [50 to 430 μmol/s per liter]
Ammonia, whole blood, venous: 80 to 110 μg/dL [47 to 65 μmol per liter]
Amylase, serum: 60 to 180 Somogyi units per deciliters; 0.8 to 3.2 units per liter [13 to 53 nmol/s per liter]
Arterial blood gases:
  [HCO_3^-]: 21 to 28 meq per liter [21 to 28 mmol per liter]
  P_{CO_2}: 35 to 45 mmHg [4.7 to 6.0 kPa]
  pH: 7.38 to 7.44
  P_{O_2}: 80 to 100 mmHg [11 to 13 kPa]
Ascorbic acid (vitamin C), serum: 0.4 to 1.0 mg/dL [23 to 57 μmol per liter]
  Leukocytes: 25 to 40 mg/dL [1420 to 2270 μmol per liter]
Barbiturates, serum: nondetectable
  Phenobarbital, "potentially fatal" level (Schreiner): approximately 9 mg/dL [390 μmol per liter]
  Most short-acting barbiturates: 3.5 mg/dL [150 μmol per liter]
Base, total, serum: 145 to 155 meq per liter [145 to 155 mmol per liter]
β-Hydroxybutyrate, plasma: <3mg/dL [<0.3 mmol per liter]
Bilirubin, total, serum (Malloy-Evelyn): 0.3 to 1.0 mg/dL [5.1 to 17 μmol per liter]
  Direct, serum: 0.1 to 0.3 mg/dL [1.7 to 5.1 μmol per liter]
  Indirect, serum: 0.2 to 0.7 mg/dL [3.4 to 12 μmol per liter]
Bromides, serum: nondetectable
  Toxic levels: >17 meq per liter; 150 mg/dL [17 mmol per liter]
Bromsulphalein, BSP (5 mg per kilogram of body weight, intravenously): 5 percent or less retention after 45 min
C-reactive protein, serum: 7–820 μg/dL
Calciferols (vitamin D), plasma:
  1,25-dihydroxyvitamin D [1,25(OH)₂D]. 20 to 60 pg/mL [48 to 144 nmol per liter]
  25-hydroxyvitamin D [25(OH)D]. 8 to 42 ng/mL [20 to 100 μmol per liter]
Calcium, ionized: 2.3 to 2.8 meq per liter; 4.5 to 5.6 mg/dL [1.1 to 1.4 mmol per liter]
Calcium, plasma: 4.5 to 5.5 meq per liter; 9 to 10.5 mg/dL [2.2 to 2.6 mmol per liter]
Carbon dioxide-combining power, serum (sea level): 21 to 28 meq per liter; 50 to 65 volume percent [21 to 28 mmol per liter]
Carbon dioxide content, plasma (sea level): 21 to 30 meq per liter; 50 to 70 volume percent [21 to 30 mmol per liter]
Carbon dioxide tension, arterial blood (sea level): 35 to 45 mmHg [4.7 to 6.0 kPa]
Carbon monoxide content, blood: nondetectable symptoms with over 20 percent saturation of hemoglobin
Carcinoembryonic antigen (CEA): 0 to 2.5 ng/mL (in healthy nonsmokers) [0 to 2.5 μg per liter]
Carotenoids, serum: 50 to 300 μg/dL [0.9 to 5.6 μmol per liter]
Ceruloplasmin, serum: 27 to 37 mg/dL [1.8 to 2.5 μmol per liter]
Chlorides, serum (as Cl^-): 98 to 106 meq per liter [98 to 106 mmol per liter]
Cholesterol: see Table A-4
Complement, serum:
  Total hemolytic (CH_{50}): 150 to 250 units per milliliter
  C3: 55 to 120 mg/dL [0.55 to 1.20 g per liter]
  C4: 20 to 50 mg/dL [0.20 to 0.50 g per liter]
Copper, serum (mean ± 1 SD): 114 ± 14 μg/dL [17.9 μmol per liter]
Creatine phosphokinase, serum (total):
  Females: 10 to 70 units per millimeter [0.17 to 1.18 mmol/s per liter]
  Males: 25 to 90 units per milliliter [0.42 to 1.51 mmol/s per liter]
  Isoenzymes, serum: fraction 2 (MB) <5 percent of total
Creatinine, serum: <1.5 mg/dL [<133 μmol per liter]
Digoxin serum:
  Therapeutic level: 1.2 ± 4 ng/mL [1.54 ± 0.5 nmol per liter]
  Toxic level: >2.4 ng/mL [>3.2 nmol per liter]
Ethanol, blood:
  Mild to moderate intoxication: 80 to 200 mg/dL [17 to 43 mmol per liter]
  Marked intoxication: 250 to 400 mg/dL [54 to 87 mmol per liter]
  Severe intoxication: >400 mg/dL [>87 mmol per liter]
Fatty acids, free (nonesterified), plasma: <18 mg/dL [<0.7 mmol per liter]
Ferritin, serum: 15 to 200 ng/mL [15 to 200 μg per liter]
Fibrinogen, plasma: see "Platelets and Coagulation"
Fibrinogen split products: see "Platelets and Coagulation"
Folic acid, serum: 6 to 15 ng/mL [14 to 34 nmol per liter]
  Folic acid, red cell: 150 to 450 ng per milliliter of cells [340 to 1020 nmol per liter cells]
γ-Glutamyl transferase (transpeptidase), serum: 4 to 60 units per liter [0.07 to 1.00 μmol/s per liter]
Gastrin, serum: 40 to 200 pg/mL [40 to 200 ng per liter]
Globulins, serum: 2.0 to 3.0 g/dL [20 to 30 g per liter]
Glucose (fasting), plasma:
  Normal: 75 to 115 mg/dL [4.2 to 6.4 mmol per liter]
  Diabetes mellitus: >140 mg/dL (on more than one occasion) [>7.8 mmol per liter]
Glucose, 2 h postprandial, plasma:
  Normal: <140 mg/dL [<7.8 mmol per liter]
  Impaired glucose tolerance: 140 to 200 mg/dL [7.8 to 11.1 mmol per liter]
  Diabetes mellitus: >200 mg/dL [>11.1 mmol per liter] (on more than one occasion)
Hemoglobin, blood (sea level):
  Males: 14 to 18 g/dL [8.7 to 11.2 mmol per liter]
  Females: 12 to 16 g/dL [7.4 to 9.9 mmol per liter]
  Hemoglobin A_{1c}: up to 6 perrcent of total hemoglobin
Immunoglobulins, serum:
  IgA: 90 to 325 mg/dL [0.9 to 3.2 g per liter]
  IgD: 0 to 8 mg/dL [0 to 0.08 g per liter]
  IgE: <0.025 mg/dL [<0.00025 g per liter]
  IgG: 800 to 1500 mg/dL [8.0 to 15.0 g per liter]
  IgM: 45 to 150 mg/dL [0.45 to 1.5 g per liter]
Iron, serum:
  Males and females (mean ± 1 SD): 105 ± 35 μg/dL [19 ± 6 μmol per liter]
Iron-binding capacity, serum (mean ± 1 SD): 305 ± 32 μg/dL [55 ± 6 μmol per liter]
  Saturation: 20 to 45 percent
Ketones, total: 0.5 to 1.5 mg/dL [5.0 to 15.0 mg per liter]
Lactate dehydrogenase, serum:
  200 to 450 units per milliliter (Wrobleski)
  60 to 100 units per milliliter (Wacker)
  25 to 100 units per liter [0.4 to 1.7 μmol/s per liter]
Lactic dehydrogenase isoenzymes, serum (agarose):
  Fraction 1 (% of total): 14–26
  Fraction 2: 29–39
  Fraction 3: 20–26
  Fraction 4: 8–16
  Fraction 5: 6–16
Lactate, venous plasma: 5 to 15 mg/dL [0.6 to 1.7 mmol per liter]
Lead, serum: <20 μg/dL [<1.0 μmol per liter]
Lipase, serum: 1.5 units (Cherry-Crandall)
Lipids: see Table A-4
Lipids, triglyceride, serum: see Table A-4
Lipoprotein: see Table A-4
Lithium, serum:
  Therapeutic concentration: 0.6 to 1.2 mmol per liter
  Toxic concentration: >2 mmol per liter [>2 mmol per liter]

Magnesium, serum: 1.3 to 2.1 meq per liter; 2 to 3 mg/dL [0.8 to 1.3 mmol per liter]

Nitrogen, nonprotein, serum: 15 to 35 mg/dL [0.15 to 0.35 g per liter]

5'-Nucleotidase, serum: 0.3 to 2.6 Bodansky units per deciliter [27 to 233 nmol/s per liter]

Osmolality, plasma: 285 to 295 mosmol per kilogram of serum water

Oxygen content:
   Arterial blood (sea level): 17 to 21 volume percent
   Venous blood, arm (sea level): 10 to 16 volume percent

Oxygen percent saturation (sea level):
   Arterial blood: 97 percent [0.97 mol/mol]
   Venous blood, arm: 60 to 85 percent [0.60 to 0.85 mol/mol]

Oxygen tension, blood: 80 to 100 mmHg ob11 to 13 kPa]

pH, blood: 7.38 to 7.44

Phenytoin, plasma:
   Therapeutic level: 10 to 20 µg/mL [40 to 79 µmol per liter]
   Toxic level: >30 µg/mL [>119 µmol per liter]

Phosphatase, acid, serum:
   Bessey-Lowry method: 0.10 to 0.63 units [28 to 175 nmol/s per liter]
   Bodansky method: 0.5 to 2.0 units
   Fishmann-Lerner (tartrate sensitive): <0.6 units per deciliter (up to 0.15 units per deciliter)
   Gutman method: 0.5 to 2.0 units
   International units: 0.2 to 1.8 [3 to 30 nmol/s per liter]
   King-Armstrong method: 1.0 to 5.0 units

Phosphatase, alkaline, serum:
   Bessey-Lowry method: 0.8 to 2.3 units (3.4 to 9 units[3])
   Bodansky method: 2.0 to 4.5 units (3.0 to 13.0 units[3]) [0.18 to 0.40 nmol/s per liter]
   Gutman method: 2.0 to 4.5 units (3.0 to 13.0 units[3])
   International units: 21 to 91 per liter at 37°C [0.4 to 1.5 µmol/s per liter]
   King-Armstrong method: 4.0 to 13.0 units (10.0 to 20.0 units[3])

Phospholipids, serum: 150 to 250 mg/dL (as lecithin) [48 to 81 mmol per liter]

Phosphorus, inorganic, serum: 1 to 1.5 meq per liter; 3 to 4.5 mg/dL [1.0 to 1.4 mmol per liter]

Potassium, serum: 3.5 to 5.0 meq per liter [3.5 to 5.0 mmol per liter]

Proteins, total, serum: 5.5 to 8.0 g/dL [55 to 80 g per liter]

Protein fractions, serum:
   Albumin: 3.5 to 5.5 g/dL (50 to 60 percent) [35 to 55 g per liter]
   Globulin: 2.0 to 3.5 g/dL (40 to 50 percent) [20 to 35 g per liter]
   Alpha$_1$: 0.2 to 0.4 g/dL (4.2 to 7.2 percent) [2 to 4 g per liter]
   Alpha$_2$: 0.5 to 0.9 g/dL (6.8 to 12 percent) [5 to 9 g per liter]
   Beta: 0.6 to 1.1 g/dL (9.3 to 15 percent) [6 to 11 g per liter]
   Gamma: 0.7 to 1.7 g/dL (13 to 23 percent) [7 to 17 g per liter]

Pyruvate, venous, plasma: 0.5 to 1.5 mg/dL [0.06 to 0.17 mmol per liter]

Quinidine, serum:
   Therapeutic range: 1.5 to 3 µg/mL [4.6 to 9.2 µmol per liter]
   Toxic range: 5 to 6 µg/mL [15.4 to 18.5 µmol per liter]

Salicylate, plasma: 0 mmol per liter
   Therapeutic range: 20 to 25 mg/dL [1.4 to 1.8 mmol per liter]
   Toxic range: >30 mg/dL [2.2 mmol per liter]

Sodium, serum: 136 to 145 meq per liter [136 to 145 mmol per liter]

Steroids: see "Metabolic and Endocrine" under "Function Tests"

Transaminase, serum glutamic oxaloacetic (SGOT, AST): 10 to 40 Karmen units per milliliter; 6 to 18 units per liter [100 to 300 µmol/s per liter]

Transaminase, serum glutamic pyruvic (SGPT, ALT): see Amino-transferases, serum

Transferase, γ-glutamyl, serum: 4 to 60 units per liter [0.07 to 1.00 µmol/s per liter]

Triglycerides: see Table A-4

Urea nitrogen, serum: 10 to 20 mg/dL [3.6 to 7.1 mmol per liter]

Uric acid, serum:
   Men: 2.5 to 8.0 mg/dL [0.15 to 0.48 mmol per liter]
   Women: 1.5 to 6.0 mg/dL [0.09 to 0.36 mmol per liter]

Vitamin A, serum: 20 to 100 µg/dL [0.7 to 3.5 µmol per liter]

Vitamin B$_{12}$, serum: 200 to 600 pg/mL [148 to 443 pmol per liter]

Zinc, serum (mean ± 1 SD): 120 ± 20 µg/dL [18 ± 3 µmol per liter]

FUNCTION TESTS

Circulation

Arteriovenous oxygen difference: 30 to 50 mL per liter

Cardiac output (Fick): 2.5 to 3.6 liters per square meter of body surface area per minute

Contractility indexes:
   Maximum left ventricular dp/dt: 1650 ± 300 mmHg/s
   Maximum $(dp/dt)/p$: 44 ± 8.4 s^{-1}
   (dp/dt)/DP at DP = 40 mmHg: 37.6 ± 12.2 s^{-1} (DP = diastolic press.)
   Mean normalized systolic ejection rate (angiography): 3.32 ± 0.84 end-diastolic volumes per second
   Mean velocity of circumferential fiber shortening (angiography) 1.66 ± 0.42 circumferences per second

Ejection fraction, stroke volume/end-diastolic volume (SV/EDV):
   Normal range: 0.55 to 0.78; average: 0.67

End-diastolic volume: 75 ± 15 mL/m^2

End-systolic volume: 25 ± 8 mL/m^2

Left ventricular work:
   Stroke work index: 30 to 110 (g·m)/m^2
   Left ventricular minute work index: 1.8 to 6.6 [(kg·m)/m^2]/min
   Oxygen consumption index: 110 to 150 mL per liter

Pressures, intracardiac and intraarterial: see Table A-5

Pulmonary vascular resistance: 20 to 120 (dyn·s)/cm^5 [2 to 12 kPa·s per liter]

Systemic vascular resistance: 770 to 1500 (dyn·s)/cm^5 [77 to 150 kPa·s per liter]

Systolic time intervals: see Table A-6

Gastrointestinal   See also "Stool."

Absorption tests:
   D-Xylose absorption test: After an overnight fast, 25 g xylose is given in aqueous solution by mouth. Urine collected for the following 5 h should contain 5 to 8 g [33 to 53 mmol] (or >20 percent of ingested dose). Serum xylose should be 25 to 40 mg per 100 mL 1 h after the oral dose [1.7 to 2.7 mmol per liter].
   Vitamin A absorption test: A fasting blood specimen is obtained and 200,000 units of vitamin A in oil is given by mouth. Serum vitamin A levels should rise to twice fasting level in 3 to 5 h.

Bentiromide test (pancreatic function): 500 mg bentiromide (chymex) orally; p-aminobenzoic acid (PABA) measured in plasma and/or urine
   Plasma: >3.6 (±1.1) µg/mL at 90 min
   Urine: >50 percent recovered as PABA in 6 h

Gastric juice:
   Volume:
      24 h: 2 to 3 liters
      Nocturnal: 600 to 700 mL
      Basal, fasting: 30 to 70 mL/h
   Reaction:
      As pH: 1.6 to 1.8
      Titratable acidity of fasting juice: 15 to 35 meq/h [4 to 10 µmol/s]
   Acid output:
      Basal:
         Females (mean ± 1 SD): 2.0 ± 1.8 meq/h [0.6 ± 0.5 µmol/s]
         Males (mean ± 1 SD): 3.0 ± 2.0 meq/h [0.8 ± 0.6 µmol/s]

---
[3] Values in parentheses are those found in children.

Maximal [after subcutaneous histamine acid phosphate 0.004 mg/kg and preceded by 50 mg promethazine (Phenergan); or after betazole (Histalog) 1.7 mg/kg or pentagastrin 6μg/mg]:
    Females (mean ± 1 SD): 16 ± 5 meq/h [4.4 ± 1.4 μmol/s]
    Males (mean ± 1 SD): 23 ± 5 meq/h [6.4 ± 1.4 μmol/s]
Basal acid output/maximal acid output ratio: 0.6 or less
Gastrin, serum: 40 to 200 pg/mL [40 to 200 ng per liter]
Secretin test (pancreatic exocrine function): 1 unit per kilogram of body weight, intravenously
  Volume (pancreatic juice): >2.0 mL/kg in 80 min
  Bicarbonate concentration: >80 meq per liter [>80 mmol per liter]
  Bicarbonate output: >10 meq in 30 min [>10 mmol in 30 min]

Metabolic and endocrine

ACTH, plasma, 8 A.M.: <80 pg/mL [<80 ng per liter]
Adrenal cortex function tests: see Chap. 325
Adrenal medulla function tests: see Chap. 326
Adrenal steroids, plasma:
  Aldosterone, 8 A.M.: <8.5 ng/dL [<0.24 nmol per liter] (patient supine, 100 meq Na and 60 to 100 meq K intake)
  Cortisol:
    8 A.M.: 5 to 25 μg/dL [138 to 691 nmol per liter]
    4 P.M.: 3 to 12 μg/dL [82 to 331 nmol per liter]
  Dehydroepiandrosterone (DHEA): 0.2 to 0.9 μg/dL [7 to 31 nmol per liter]
  Dehydroepiandrosterone sulfate (DHEA sulfate): 50 to 250 μg/dL [1.3 to 6.5 μmol per liter]
  11-Deoxycortisol (compound S): <1 μg/dL [<30 nmol per liter]
  17-Hydroxyprogesterone:
    Women: follicular phase, 20 to 100 ng/dL [0.6 to 3 nmol per liter]; luteal phase, 50 to 350 ng/dL [1.5 to 10.6 nmol per liter]
    Men: 6 to 300 ng/dL [1.8 to 9.0 nmol per liter]
Adrenal steroids, secretion rates:
  Aldosterone: 50 to 250 μg per day [138 to 690 nmol per day]
  Cortisol: 8 to 24 mg per day [22 to 69 μmol per day]
Adrenal steroids, urinary excretion:
  Aldosterone: 5 to 19 μg per day [14 to 53 nmol per day]
  Cortisol, free: 20 to 100 μg per day [54 to 276 nmol per day]
  17-Hydroxycorticosteroids: 2 to 10 mg per day [5.4 to 28 μmol per day]
  17-Ketosteroids:
    Men: 7 to 25 mg per day [24 to 88 μmol per day]
    Women: 4 to 15 mg per day [14 to 52 μmol per day]
Angiotensin II, plasma, 8 A.M.: 10 to 30 pg/mL [10 to 30 nmol per liter]
Arginine vasopressin (AVP), plasma:
  Random fluid intake: 1 to 3 pg/mL [1 to 3 ng per liter]
  Fluid deprivation, 18 to 24 h: 6 to 12 pg/mL [6 to 12 ng per liter]
Calcitonin, plasma: <50 pg/mL [<50 ng per liter]
Catecholamines, urinary excretion:
  Free catecholamines: <100 μg per day [<590 nmol per day]
  Epinephrine: <50 μg per day [295 nmol per day]
  Metanephrines: <1.3 mg per day [<6.2 μmol per day]
  Vanillylmandelic acid (VMA): <8 mg per day [<40 μmol per day]
Gastrin, plasma: <120 pg/mL [<120 ng per liter]
Glucagon, plasma: 50 to 100 pg/mL [14 to 29 pmol per liter]
Gonadal function tests: see Chaps. 330 and 331
Gonadal steroids, plasma:
  Androstenedione:
    Women: 110 to 190 ng/dL [3.9 to 6.6 nmol per liter]
    Men: 80 to 130 ng/dL [2.9 to 4.6 mmol per liter]
  Estradiol:
    Women: 20 to 60 pg/mL [0.07 to 0.22 nmol per liter], higher at ovulation
    Men: <50 pg/mL [<0.18 nmol per liter]
  Progesterone:
    Men, prepubertal girls, preovulatory women, and postmenopausal women: <2 ng/mL [<6 nmol per liter]
    Women, luteal, peak: >5 ng/mL [>16 nmol per liter]
  Testosterone:
    Women: <100 ng/dL [<3.5 nmol per liter]
    Men: 300 to 1000 ng/dL [10 to 35 nmol per liter]
    Prepubertal boys and girls: 5 to 20 ng/dL [0.17 to 0.7 nmol per liter]
Gonadotropins, plasma:
  Women, mature, premenopausal, except at ovulation:
    FSH: 5 to 20 mU/mL [5 to 20 U per liter]
    LH: 5 to 25 mU/mL [5 to 25 U per liter]
  Ovulatory surge:
    FSH: 12 to 30 mU/mL [12 to 30 U per liter]
    LH: 25 to 100 mU/mL [25 to 100 U per liter]
  Postmenopausal women:
    FSH: >50 mU/mL [>50 U per liter]
    LH: >50 mU/mL [>50 U per liter]
  Men, mature:
    FSH: 5 to 20 mU/mL [5 to 20 U per liter]
    LH: 5 to 20 mU/mL [5 to 20 U per liter]
  Children of both sexes, prepubertal:
    FSH: <5 mU/mL [<5 U per liter]
    LH: <5 mU/mL [<5 U per liter]
Growth hormone, after 100 g glucose by mouth: <5 ng/dL [<50 ng per liter]
Human chorionic gonadotropin, β subunit (β-hCG), plasma:
  Men and nonpregnant women: <3 mIU/mL [<3 IU per liter]
Insulin, serum or plasma, fasting: 6 to 26 μU/mL [43 to 186 pmol per liter]
Insulin-like growth factor I (somatomedin C, IGF-1/SM C): see Chap. 322
Oxytocin, plasma:
  Men and preovulatory women: 0.5 to 2 μU/mL [2 to 4 mU per liter]
  Lactating women: 5 to 10 μU/mL [5 to 10 mU per liter]
Pancreatic islet function tests: Chap. 327
Parathyroid function tests: see Chap. 336
Pituitary function tests: see Chaps. 321 to 323
Pregnancy tests: see Chap. 331
Prolactin, serum: 2 to 15 ng/mL [2 to 15 μg per liter]
Renin-angiotensin function tests: see Chap. 325
Semen analysis: see Chap. 330
Thyroid function tests:
  Dynamic tests of thyroid function: see Chap. 324
  Radioactive iodine uptake, 24 h: 5 to 30 percent (range varies in different areas due to variations in iodine intake)
  Resin T_3 uptake: 25 to 35 percent (varies among laboratories; for calculation of indexes of resin T_3 uptake, see Chap. 324)
  Reverse triiodothyronine (rT_3), plasma: 10 to 40 ng/dL [0.15 to 0.61 nmol per liter]
  Thyroid-stimulating hormone (TSH): <5 μU/mL [<5 mU per liter]
  Thyroxine (T_4), serum radioimmunoassay: 5 to 12 μg/dL [64 to 154 nmol per liter]
  Triiodothyronine (T_3), plasma: 70 to 190 ng/dL [1.1 to 2.9 nmol per liter]

Pulmonary See Tables A-9 and A-10.

Arterial blood gas measurements in normal subjects (sea level):
  P_{CO_2}, seated (mean ± 1 SD): 38.0 ± 2.9 mmHg (no change with age) [5.0 kPa]
  P_{O_2}:
    Seated (mean ± 1 SD): (104.2 ± 0.27 mmHg) × age in years [13.8 kPa]
    Supine (mean ± 1 SD): (103.5 ± 0.42 mmHg) × age in years [13.8 kPa]

Renal

Clearances (corrected to 1.72 m² body surface area):
  Measures of glomerular filtration rate:
    Inulin clearance (C1):
      Males (mean ± 1 SD): 124 ± 25.8 mL/min [2.1 ± 0.4 mL/s]
      Females (mean ± 1 SD): 119 ± 12.8 mL/min [2.0 ± 0.2 mL/s]
    Endogenous creatinine clearance: 91 to 130 mL/min [1.5 to 2.2 mL/s]
    Urea: 60 to 100 mL/min [1.0 to 1.7 mL/s]
  Measures of effective renal plasma flow and tubular function:
    p-Aminohippuric acid clearance (Cl_{PAH}):
      Males (mean ± 1 SD): 654 ± 163 mL/min [10.9 ± 2.7 mL/s]
      Females (mean ± 1 SD): 594 ± 102 mL/min [9.9 ± 1.7 mL/s]
Concentration and dilution test:
  Specific gravity of urine:
    After 12-h fluid restriction: 1.025 or more
    After 12-h deliberate water intake: 1.003 or less
Phenosulfonphthalein:
  After intravenous injection:
    Excretion in urine in 15 min: 25 percent or more
    Excretion in urine in 2 h: 55 to 75 percent
Protein excretion, urine: <150 mg in 24 h [<0.15 g per day]
  Males: 0 to 60 mg in 24 h [0 to 0.06 g per day]
  Females: 0 to 90 mg in 24 h [0 to 0.09 g per day]
Specific gravity, maximal range: 1.002 to 1.028
Tubular reabsorption, phosphorus: 79 to 94 percent of filtered load

HEMATOLOGIC EXAMINATIONS

See also "Chemical Constituents of Blood."

Bone marrow See Table A-11.

Erythrocytes and hemoglobin See also Table A-12.

Carboxyhemoglobin:
  Nonsmoker: 0 to 2.3 percent
  Smoker: 2.1 to 4.2 percent
Erythrocyte "life span":
  Normal survival: 120 days
  Chromium-labeled, half-life ($t_{\frac{1}{2}}$): 28 days
Glucose 6-phosphate dehydrogenase: 12.1 ± 2 IU/gHb (WHO)
Ham's test (acid serum): negative
Haptoglobin, serum (mean ± 2 SD): 128 ± 15 mg/dL [1.3 ± 0.2 g per liter]
Heinz body stain: negative
Hemoglobin, plasma: 1 to 5 mg/dL [0.03 to 0.05 g per liter]
Hemoglobin A_2 (HbA_2): 1.5 to 3.5 percent
Hemoglobin, fetal (HbF): <2 percent
Hemoglobin H prep: negative
Methemoglobin: <1.7 percent
Nitroblue tetrazolium (chronic granulomatous disease): normal
Osmotic fragility:
  Slight hemolysis: 0.45 to 0.39 percent
  Complete hemolysis: 0.33 to 0.30 percent
Plasma iron turnover: 20 to 42 mg per 24 h [0.47 mg/kg]
Protoporphyrin, free erythrocyte (FEP): 16 to 36 μg per deciliter of red blood cells [0.28 to 0.64 μmol per liter]
Red cell distribution width (Coulter): 13 ± 1.5 percent
Sedimentation rate:
  Westergren, <50 years of age:
    Males: 0 to 15 mm/h
    Females: 0 to 20 mm/h
  Westergren, >50 years of age:
    Males: 0 to 20 mm/h
    Females: 0 to 30 mm/h
  Wintrobe:
    Males: 0 to 9 mm/h
    Females: 0 to 20 mm/h
Sucrose hemolysis: negative

Leukocytes See Table A-13.

Platelets and coagulation

Alpha₂ antiplasmin: 70 to 130 percent
Antithrombin III: 80 to 120 percent
Bleeding time:
  Ivy method, 5-mm wound: <9 min
  Duke method: <4 min
  Simplate: <7 min
Clot retraction, qualitative: apparent in 60 min, complete <24 h, usually <6 h
Euglobulin lysis time: >2 h
Factor II: 60 to 100 percent
Factor V: 60 to 100 percent
Factor VII: 60 to 100 percent
Factor IX: 60 to 100 percent
Factor X: 60 to 100 percent
Factor XI: 60 to 100 percent
Factor XII: 60 to 100 percent
Factor XIII: clot stable in urea
Fibrinogen: 200 to 400 mg/dL
Fibrin split products: <10 μg/mL
Plasminogen: 2.4 to 4.4 CTA U/mL
Protein C (antigenic assay): 58 to 148 percent
Protein S (antigenic assay): 58 to 148 percent
Partial thromboplastin time (activated PTT): comparable to control
Prothrombin time (quick one-stage): control ± 1 s
Protamine paracoagulation (3P) test: negative
Platelets: 130,000 to 400,000 per cubic millimeter
Thrombin time: control ± 3 s
von Willebrand's antigen: 60 to 150 percent

Miscellaneous

Leukocyte alkaline phosphatase (LAP): 13 to 100
Lysozyme (muramidase), serum: 5 to 25 μg/dL
Lysozyme, urine: <2 μg/mL
Schilling test: excretion in urine of orally administered radioactive vitamin B_{12}: 7 to 40 percent
Viscosity, plasma: 1.7 to 2.1
Viscosity, serum: 1.4 to 1.8

STOOL

Bulk:
  Wet weight: <197.5 (115 ± 41) g per day
  Dry weight: <66.4 (34 ± 16) g per day
Alpha₁ antitrypsin: 0.98 (±0.17) mg per gram of dry weight stool
Coproporphyrin: 400 to 1000 μg in 24 h [610 to 1500 nmol per day]
Fat (on diet containing at least 50 g fat): <6.0 (4.0 ± 1.5) g per day when measured on a 3-day (or longer) collection
  Percent of dry weight: <30.4 (13.3 ± 8.07)
  Coefficient of fat absorption: >95 percent
Fatty acid:
  Free: 1 to 10 percent of dry matter
  Combined as soap: 0.5 to 12 percent of dry matter
Nitrogen: <1.7 (1.4 ± 0.2) g per day
Protein content: minimal
Urobilinogen: 40 to 280 mg in 24 h [67 to 470 μmol per day]
Water: approximately 65 percent

URINE

See also "Metabolic and Endocrine" under "Function Tests."

Acidity, titratable: 20 to 40 meq in 24 h [20 to 40 mmol per day]
α-Amino nitrogen: 0.4 to 1.0 g in 24 h [28 to 71 mmol per day]
Ammonia: 30 to 50 meq in 24 h [30 to 50 mmol per day]
Amylase: 35 to 260 Somogyi units per hour
Amylase/creatinine clearance ratio [(Cl_{am}/Cl_{cr}) × 100]: 1 to 5
Bentiromide (pancreatic function): 50 percent excreted in 6 h as p-amino benzoic acid (PABA) after 500 mg oral bentiromide
Calcium (10 meq or 200-mg calcium diet): <7.5 meq in 24 h; <150 mg in 24 h [<3.8 mmol per day]
Catecholamines: <100 µg in 24 h
Copper: 0 to 25 µg in 24 h [0 to 0.4 µmol per day]
Coproporphyrins (types I and III): 100 to 300 µg in 24 h [150 to 460 nmol per day]
Creatine, as creatinine:
    Adult males: <50 mg in 24 h [<0.38 mmol per day]
    Adult females: <100 mg in 24 h [<0.76 mmol per day]
Creatinine: 1.0 to 1.6 g in 24 h [8.8 to 14 mmol per day]
Glucose, true (oxidase method): 50 to 300 mg in 24 h [0.3 to 1.7 mmol per day]
5-Hydroxyindoleacetic acid (5-HIAA): 2 to 9 mg in 24 h [10 to 47 µmol per day]
Ketones, total (mean ± 1 SD): 50.5 ± 30.7 mg in 24 h
Lactic dehydrogenase: 560 to 2050 units in 8-h urine
Lead: <0.08 µg/mL; <120 µg in 24 h [0.39 µmol per liter]
Protein: <150 mg in 24 h [<0.05 g per day]
Porphobilinogen: none
Potassium: 25 to 100 meq in 24 h (varies with intake) [25 to 100 mmol per day]
Sodium: 100 to 260 meq in 24 h (varies with intake) [100 to 260 mmol per day]
Urobilinogen: 1 to 3.5 mg in 24 h [1.7 to 5.9 µmol per day]
Vanillylmandelic acid (VMA): <8 mg per day [<40 µmol per day]
D-Xylose excretion: 5 to 8 g within 5 h after oral dose of 25 g [33 to 53 mmol in 5 h]

TABLE A-1 SI and other units

Quantity	Name of unit	Symbol for unit	Derivation of units
SI BASE UNITS			
Length	meter	m	
Mass	kilogram	kg	
Time	second	s	
Thermodynamic temperature	Kelvin	K	
Amount of substance	mole	mol	
SI DERIVED UNITS			
Force	newton	N	$(m \cdot kg)/s^2$
Pressure	pascal	Pa	$N \cdot m^2$
Work, energy	joule	J	$N \cdot m$
Celsius temperature	degree Celsius	°C	K
OTHER UNITS RETAINED FOR USE			
Time	minute	min	
	hour	h	
	day	d	
Volume	liter	L	

TABLE A-2 Radiation derived units

Quantity	Old unit	SI unit	Name for SI unit (and abbreviation)	Conversion
Activity	curie (Ci)	Disintegrations per second (dps)	becquerel (Bq)	1 Ci = 3.7 × 10^{10} Bq; 1 mCi = 37 mBq; 1 µCi = 0.037 MBq or 37 GBq; 1 Bq = 2.703 × 10^{-11} Ci
Absorbed dose	rad	joule per kilogram (J/kg)	gray (Gy)	1 Gy = 100 rad; 1 rad = 0.01 Gy; 1 mrad = 10^{-3} cGy
Exposure	roentgen (R)	coulomb per kilogram (C/kg)	—	1 C/kg = 3876 R; 1 R = 2.58 × 10^{-4} C/kg; 1 mR = 258 pC/kg
Dose equivalent	rem	joule per kilogam (J/kg)	sievert (Sv)	1 Sv = 100 rem; 1 rem = 0.01 Sv; 1 mrem = 10 µSv

TABLE A-3 SI prefixes and their symbols

Factor	Prefix	Symbol for prefix
10^9	giga	G
10^6	mega	M
10^3	kilo	k
10^2	hecto	h
10^1	deka	da
10^{-1}	deci	d
10^{-2}	centi	c
10^{-3}	milli	m
10^{-6}	micro	µ
10^{-9}	nano	n
10^{-12}	pico	p
10^{-15}	femto	f
10^{-18}	alto	a

TABLE A-4 Plasma lipid concentration in normal subjects*

	Total plasma cholesterol, mg/dL		Plasma LDL-cholesterol, mg/dL		Plasma HDL-cholesterol, mg/dL		Plasma triglyceride, mg/dL	
Age	Men	Women	Men	Women	Men	Women	Men	Women
19	113–197	120–203	62–130	59–137	30–63	35–74	37–148	39–132
29	133–244	130–229	70–165	71–164	31–63	37–83	46–249	40–172
39	146–270	141–245	81–189	75–172	29–62	34–82	54–321	41–194
49	158–276	152–268	98–202	79–186	30–64	34–87	58–327	47–228
59	156–276	169–294	88–203	89–210	28–71	37–91	58–286	56–257
69	158–274	171–297	98–210	92–221	30–78	35–98	57–267	60–241
70+	151–270	167–288	80–186	96–206	31–75	33–92	58–258	60–235

* 5th and 95th percentiles not ideal ranges for white men and women; data are too fragmentary to ascertain whether these values apply to other groups.
SOURCE: *The Lipid Research Clinics Population Studies Data Book*, vol 1, The Prevalence Study, NIH Publication No 80-1529, Bethesda, National Institutes of Health, July 1980.

TABLE A-5 Hemodynamic values

Pressures (mmHg):	
Systemic arterial:	
Peak systolic/end-diastolic	100–140/60–90
Mean	70–105
Left ventricle:	
Peak systolic/end-diastolic	100–140/3–12
Left atrium (or pulmonary capillary wedge):	
Mean	2–12
a wave	3–10
v wave	3–15
Pulmonary artery:	
Peak systolic/end-diastolic	15–30/4–14
Mean	9–17
Right ventricle:	
Peak systolic/end-diastolic	15–30/2–7
Right atrium:	
Mean	2–6
a wave	2–8
v wave	2–7
Resistances [(dyn·s)/cm^5]:	
Systemic vascular resistance	700–1600
Total pulmonary resistance	100–300
Pulmonary vascular resistance	20–130
Flows:	
Cardiac index (liters per minute per square meter)	2.4–3.8
Stroke index (milliliters per beat per square meter)	30–65
Oxygen consumption (liters per minute per square meter)	110–150
Arteriovenous oxygen difference (milliliters per liter)	30–50

TABLE A-7 Normal values of echocardiographic measurements in adults*

	Range, cm	Mean, cm	Number of subjects
Age (years)	13 to 54	26	134
Body surface area (m^2)	1.45 to 2.22	1.8	130
RVD—flat	0.7 to 2.3	1.5	84
RVD—left lateral	0.9 to 2.6	1.7	83
LVID—flat	3.7 to 5.6	4.7	82
LVID—left lateral	3.5 to 5.7	4.7	81
Posterior LV wall thickness	0.6 to 1.1	0.9	137
Posterior LV wall amplitude	0.9 to 1.4	1.2	48
IVS wall thickness	0.6 to 1.1	0.9	137
Mid IVS amplitude	0.3 to 0.8	0.5	10
Apical IVS amplitude	0.5 to 1.2	0.7	38
Left atrial dimension	1.9 to 4.0	2.9	133
Aortic root dimension	2.0 to 3.7	2.7	121
Aortic cusps' separation	1.5 to 2.6	1.9	93
Percentage of fractional shortening†	34 to 44%	36%	20
Mean rate of circumferential shortening (Vcf)‡, or mean normalized shortening velocity	1.02 to 1.94 circ/s	1.3 circ/s	38

* RVD = right ventricular dimension; LVID = left ventricular internal dimension; d = end diastole; s = end systole; LV = left ventricle; IVS = interventricular septum.

† $\dfrac{\text{LVIDd} - \text{LVIDs}}{\text{LVIDd}}$

‡ $\dfrac{\text{LVIDd} - \text{LVIDs}}{\text{LVIDd} \times \text{ejection time}}$

SOURCE: From H Feigenbaum, *Echocardiography*, in *Heart Disease—A Textbook of Cardiovascular Medicine*, E Braunwald (ed), Philadelphia, Saunders, 1980.

TABLE A-6 Systolic time intervals in normal individuals (in milliseconds)

Regression equation	SD of index
QS$_2$ (M) = −2.1 HR + 546	14
QS$_2$ (F) = −2.0 HR + 549	14
PEP (M) = −0.4 HR + 131	13
PEP (F) = −0.4 HR + 133	11
LVET (M) = −1.7 HR + 413	10
LVET (F) = −1.6 HR + 418	10

NOTE: QS$_2$ = total electromechanical systole, PEP = preejection phase, LVET = left ventricular ejection time, HR = heart rate, M = male, F = female, SD = standard deviation of the systolic time interval index. Systolic ejection period = 220–320 ms per beat; diastolic filling period = 380–500 ms per beat.
SOURCE: AM Weissler, CL Garrard, *Mod Concepts Cardiovasc Dis* 40:1, 1971.

TABLE A-8 Amplitude of Q, R, S, and T waves in scalar electrocardiogram of 100 normal adults*

	I	II	III	aV$_R$	aV$_L$	aV$_F$	V$_1$	V$_5$	V$_6$
Patients with Q wave	38%	41%	50%	—	38%	40%	0%	60%	75%
Q amplitude:									
Mean	0.4	0.6	0.9	—	0.4	0.7	0	0.3	0.3
Range	0 to 0.10	0 to 1.6	0 to 2.3	—	0 to 1.1	0 to 1.7	0	0 to 1.8	0 to 1.8
R amplitude:									
Mean	5.6	8.9	4.5	1.3	3.4	6.0	1.9	12.6	10.2
Range	1.0 to 10.0	2.0 to 16.9	1.0 to 12.1	0 to 2.9	0 to 8.2	0 to 13.8	1.0 to 6.0	7.0 to 21.0	5.0 to 18.0
S amplitude:									
Mean	2.0	2.1	2.4	7.0	2.6	—	8.0	2.5	1.3
Range	0 to 5.0	0 to 3.7	0 to 6.4	2.2 to 11.8	0 to 5.8	—	3.0 to 13.0	0 to 5.0	0 to 2.0
T amplitude:									
Mean	1.9	2.3	1.0	—	0.3	1.7	1.0	3.3	1.0
Range	1.0 to 3.0	1.0 to 4.0	−2.0 to 2.0	—	−1.0 to 2.0	0 to 4.0	−2.0 to 2.0	2.0 to 7.0	1.0 to 4.0

* Values of Q, R, S, and T amplitudes are in millimeters (1 mm = 0.1 mv).
SOURCE: From J D Cooksey et al, *Clinical Vectorcardiography and Electrocardiography*, 2d ed, Chicago, Year Book Medical Publishers, 1977. Used by permission.

TABLE A-9 Summary of values useful in pulmonary physiology

	Symbol	Typical values Men	Women
PULMONARY MECHANICS			
Spirometry—volume-time curves:			
Forced vital capacity	FVC	≥4.0 liters	≥3.0 liters
Forced expiratory volume in 1 s	FEV_1	>3.0 liters	>2.0 liters
FEV_1/FVC	FEV_1%	>60%	>70%
Maximal midexpiratory flow	MMF (FEF 25–27)	>2.0 liters per second	>1.6 liters per second
Maximal expiratory flow rate	MEFR (FEF 200–1200)	>3.5 liters per second	>3.0 liters per second
Spirometry—flow-volume curves:			
Maximal expiratory flow at 50% of expired vital capacity	$\dot{V}_{max}$ 50 (FEF 50%)	>2.5 liters per second	>2.0 liters per second
Maximal expiratory flow at 75% of expired vital capacity	$\dot{V}_{max}$ 75 (FEF 75%)	>1.5 liters per second	>1.0 liters per second
Resistance to airflow:			
Pulmonary resistance	RL (R_L)	<3.0 cmH_2O/s per liter	
Airway resistance	Raw	<2.5 cmH_2O/s per liter	
Specific conductance	SGaw	>0.13 cmH_2O/s	
Pulmonary compliance:			
Static recoil pressure at total lung capacity	Pst TLC	25 ± 5 cmH_2O	
Compliance of lungs (static)	CL	0.2 L/cmH_2O	
Compliance of lungs and thorax	C(L + T)	0.1 L/cmH_2O	
Dynamic compliance of 20 breaths per minute	C dyn 20	0.25 ± 0.05 liters per cmH_2O	
Maximal static respiratory pressures:			
Maximal inspiratory pressure	MIP	> 90 cmH_2O	> 50 cmH_2O
Maximal expiratory pressure	MEP	>150 cmH_2O	>120 cmH_2O
LUNG VOLUMES			
Total lung capacity	TLC	6–7 liters	5–6 liters
Functional residual capacity	FRC	2–3 liters	2–3 liters
Residual volume	RV	1–2 liters	1–2 liters
Inspiratory capacity	IC	2–4 liters	2–4 liters
Expiratory reserve volume	ERV	1–2 liters	1–2 liters
Vital capacity	VC	4–5 liters	3–4 liters
GAS EXCHANGE (SEA LEVEL)			
Arterial O_2 tension	Pa_{O_2}	95 ± 5 mmHg	
Arterial CO_2 tension	Pa_{CO_2}	40 ± 2 mmHg	
Arterial O_2 saturation	Sa_{O_2}	97 ± 2%	
Arterial blood pH	pH	7.40 ± 0.02	
Arterial bicarbonate	HCO_3^-	24 + 2 meq per liter	
Base excess	BE	0 ± 2 meq per liter	
Diffusing capacity for carbon monoxide (single breath)	DL_{CO}	25 mL CO/min/mmHg	
Dead space volume	V_D	50 ± 25 mL	
Physiologic dead space: dead space-tidal volume			
ratio (rest)	V_D/V_T	≤35% V_T	
(exercise)		≤20% V_T	
Alveolar-arterial difference for O_2	A-a D_{O_2}	≤20 mmHg	

TABLE A-10 Prediction equations for spirometric tests, lung volumes, and gas exchange in adults

Variable	Sex	Age (A)	Height (H)	Weight (W)	Constant (C)	Standard deviation (SD)
PULMONARY MECHANICS						
Spirometry—volume-time curves* (H in inches):						
FVC	M	−0.025	+0.148	—	−4.241	0.74
	F	−0.024	+0.115	—	−2.852	0.52
FEV_1	M	−0.032	+0.092	—	−1.260	0.55
	F	−0.025	+0.089	—	−1.932	0.47
MEFR	M	−0.047	+0.109	—	+2.010	1.66
(FEF 200–1200)	F	−0.036	+0.145	—	−2.532	1.19
MMF	M	−0.045	+0.047	—	+2.513	1.12
(FEF 25–75)	F	−0.030	+0.060	—	+0.551	0.80
Spirometry—flow-volume curves† (H in centimeters):						
$\dot{V}_{max}$ 50	M	−0.015	+0.069	—	−5.400	1.422
(FEF 50%)	F	−0.013	+0.035	—	−0.444	1.22
$\dot{V}_{max}$ 75	M	−0.012	+0.044	—	−4.143	1.026
(FEF 75%)	F	−0.014	—	—	+3.042	0.936
Lung volumes‡ (H in meters; W in kilograms):						
TLC	M	—	+6.92	−0.017	−4.30	0.67
	F	−0.015	+6.71	—	−5.77	0.48
FRC	M	+0.015	+5.30	−0.037	−3.89	0.56
	F	—	+5.13	−0.028	−4.50	0.41
RV	M	+0.022	+1.98	−0.015	−1.54	0.38
	F	+0.007	+2.68	—	−3.42	0.32
VC	M	−0.020	+4.81	—	−2.81	0.50
	F	−0.022	+4.04	—	−2.35	0.40
Gas exchange§ (H in meters; W in kilograms):						
DL_{CO}	M	−0.20	+32.5	—	−17.6	5.1
	F	−0.16	+21.2	—	−2.66	3.6

NOTE: Answer = (A × age) + (H × height) + (W × weight) + C ± 2 SD. Example: The normal value and lower limit for the FEV_1 are sought in a man, age 40 years, height 183 cm, and weight 91 kg. The following equation gives the normal value:
FEV_1 = (−0.032 × 40) + (0.092 × 72) + (−1.260) = 4.08 liters
The lower limit of normal:
4.08 − (2 × SD) = 4.08 − (2 × 0.55) = 2.98 liters
Only 2.5% of a normal population will fall below this value (2 SD below the mean).
For other abbreviations, see Table A-9.
* Morris et al, *Am Rev Respir Dis* 103:57, 1971.
† Knudson et al, *Am Rev Respir Dis* 113:587, 1976.
‡ Grimby G, Söderholm B, *Acta Med Scand* 173:199, 1963.
§ Coates, JE, *Lung Function and Application in Medicine*, Davis, 1965.

TABLE A-11 Differential nucleated cell counts of bone marrow

	Normal, mean%*	Range, %†
Myeloid:	56.7	
Neutrophilic series:	53.6	
Myeloblast	0.9	0.2–1.5
Promyelocyte	3.3	2.1–4.1
Myelocyte	12.7	8.2–15.7
Metamyelocyte	15.9	9.6–24.6
Band	12.4	9.5–15.3
Segmented		
Eosinophilic series	3.1	1.2–5.3
Basophilic series	<0.1	0–0.2
Erythroid:	25.6	
Pronormoblasts	0.6	0.2–1.3
Basophilic normoblasts	1.4	0.5–2.4
Polychromatophilic normoblasts	21.6	17.9–29.2
Orthochromatic normoblasts	2.0	0.4–4.6
Megakaryocytes	<0.1	
Lymphoreticular:	17.8	
Lymphocytes	16.2	11.1–23.2
Plasma cells	2.3	0.4–3.9
Reticulum cells	0.3	0–0.9

* Frm MM Wintrobe et al. Clinical Hematology, 8th ed. Philadelphia, Lea & Febiger, 1981.
† Range observed in 12 healthy men.

TABLE A-12 Erythrocytes and hemoglobin: Normal values at various ages

Age	Red blood cell count,* millions/mm³	Hemoglobin,* g/dL	Vol. packed RBCs,* mL/dL	MCV, fl	MCH, pg	MCHC, g/dL	MCD, μm
Days 1–13	5.1 ± 1.0	19.5 ± 5.0	54.0 ± 10.0	106–98	38–33	36–34	8.6
Days 14–60	4.7 ± 0.9	14.0 ± 3.3	42.0 ± 7.0	90	30	33	8.1
3 months to 10 years	4.5 ± 0.7	12.2 ± 2.3	36.0 ± 5.0	80	27	34	7.7
11–15 years	4.8	13.4	39.0	82	28	34	
Adults:							
Females	4.8 ± 0.6	14.0 ± 2.0	42.0 ± 5.0	90 ± 7	29 ± 2	34 ± 2	7.5 ± 0.3
Males	5.4 ± 0.9	16.0 ± 2.0	47.0 ± 5.0	90 ± 7	29 ± 2	34 ± 2	7.5 ± 0.3

* The range of values represents almost the extremes of observed variations (93 percent or more) at sea level. The blood values of healthy persons should fall well within these mean ± SD figures.
NOTE: MCV = mean corpuscular volume, MCH = mean corpuscular hemoglobin, MCHC = mean corpuscular hemoglobin concentration, MCD = mean corpuscular diameter.
SOURCE: MM Wintrobe et al, Clinical Hematology, 8th ed, Philadelphia, Lea & Febiger, 1981.

TABLE A-13 Normal leukocyte count, differential count, and hemoglobin concentration at various ages

Age	Leukocytes, total	Neutrophils Total	Band	Segmented	Eosinophils	Basophils	Lymphocytes	Monocytes	Hemoglobin, g/dL blood
12 mo	11.4(6.0–17.5)	3.5(1.5–8.5)	0.35	3.2	0.3(0.05–0.7)	0.05(0–0.20)	7.0(4.0–10.5)	0.55(0.05–1.1)	11.6(9.0–14.6)
		<u>31</u>	<u>3.1</u>	<u>28</u>	<u>0.4</u>	<u>0.4</u>	<u>61</u>	<u>4.8</u>	
4 yr	9.1(5.5–15.5)	3.8(1.5–8.5)	0.27(0–1.0)	3.5(1.5–7.5)	0.25(0.02–0.65)	0.05(0–0.20)	4.5(2.0–8.0)	0.45(0–0.8)	12.6(9.6–15.5)
		<u>42</u>	<u>3.0</u>	<u>39</u>	<u>2.8</u>	<u>0.6</u>	<u>50</u>	<u>5.0</u>	
6 yr	4.3(1.5–8.0)	0.25(0–1.0)	4.0(1.5–7.0)	4.0(1.5–7.0)	0.23(0–0.65)	0.05(0–0.20)	3.5(1.5–7.0)	0.40(0–0.8)	12.7(10.0–15.5)
		<u>51</u>	<u>3.0</u>	<u>48</u>	<u>2.7</u>	<u>0.6</u>	<u>42</u>	<u>4.7</u>	
10 yr	8.1(4.5–13.5)	4.4(1.8–8.0)	0.24(0–1.0)	4.2(1.8–7.0)	0.20(0–0.60)	0.04(0–0.20)	3.1(1.5–6.5)	0.35(0–0.8)	13.0(10.7–15.5)
		<u>54</u>	<u>3.0</u>	<u>51</u>	<u>2.4</u>	<u>0.5</u>	<u>38</u>	<u>4.3</u>	
21 yr	7.4(4.5–11.0)	4.4(1.8–7.7)	0.22(0–0.7)	4.2(1.8–7.0)	0.20(0–0.45)	0.04(0–0.20)	2.5(1.0–4.8)	0.30(0–0.8)	♂15.8 (14.0–18.0)
		<u>59</u>	<u>3.0</u>	<u>56</u>	<u>2.7</u>	<u>0.5</u>	<u>34</u>	<u>4.0</u>	♀13.9 (11.5–16.0)

NOTE: Values are expressed as "cells × 10³/μL." The numbers underlined are percentages.
SOURCE: WJ Williams et al (eds), Hematology, 3d ed, New York, McGraw-Hill, New York, 1983. By permission.

Color Plates

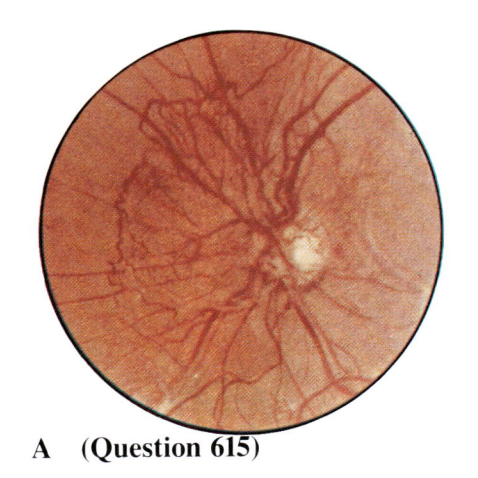

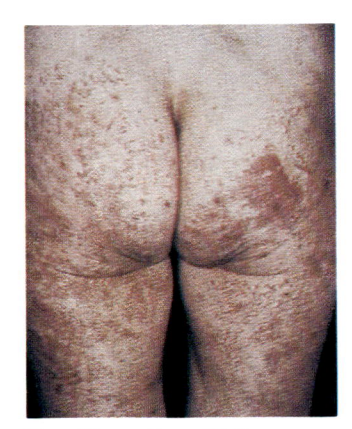

A (Question 615)

B (Question 621)

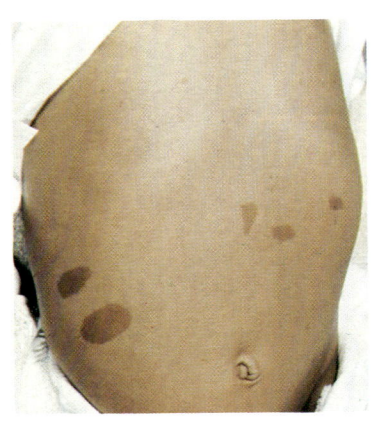

C (Question 699)

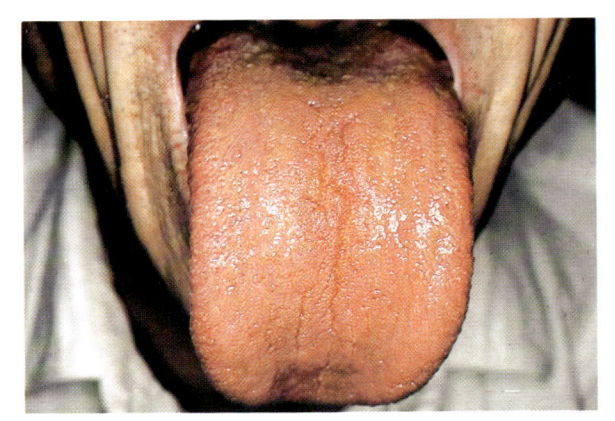

D (Question 700)

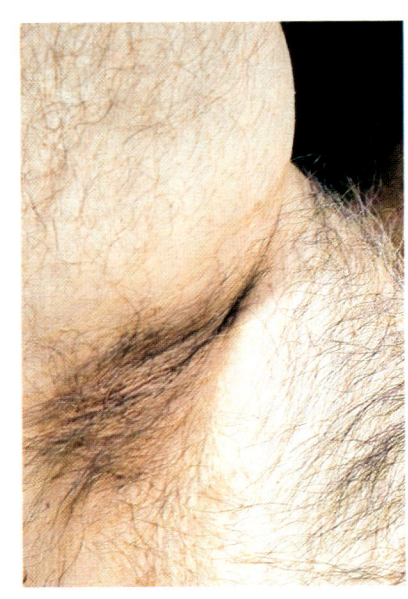

E (Question 701)

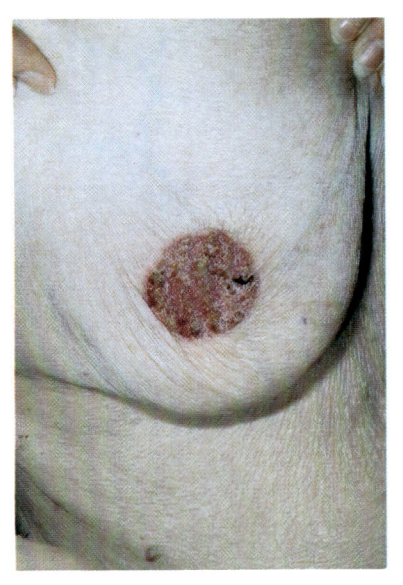

F (Question 702)

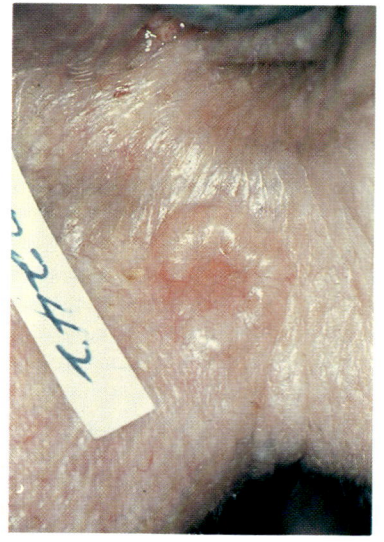

G (Question 703)

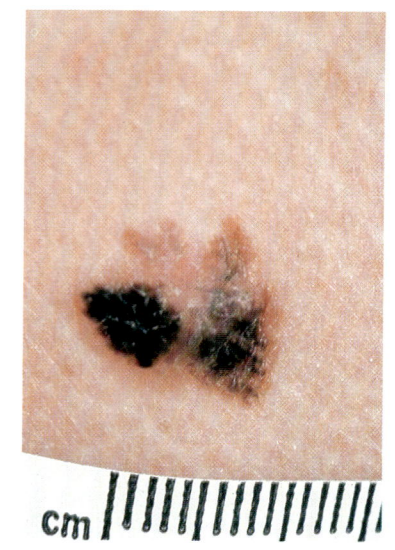

H (Question 704)

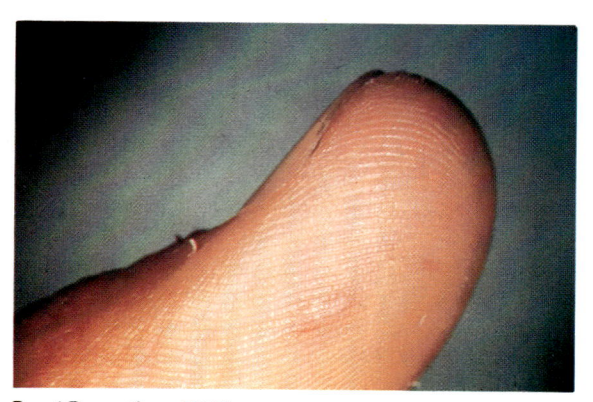

I (Question 705)

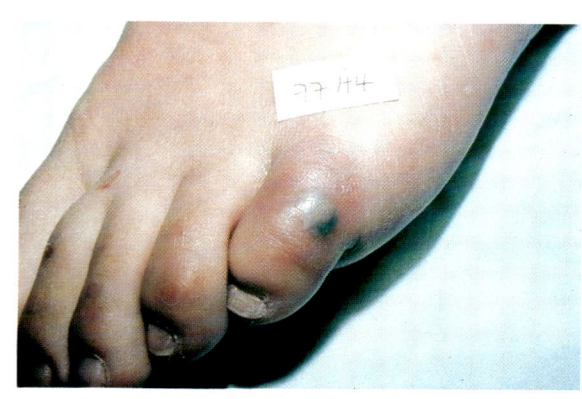

J (Question 706)

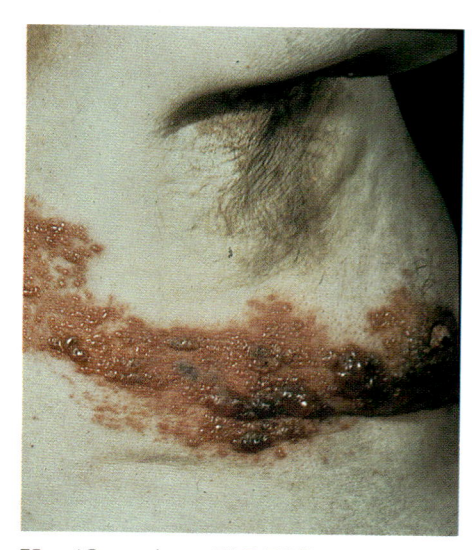

K (Questions 707-708)

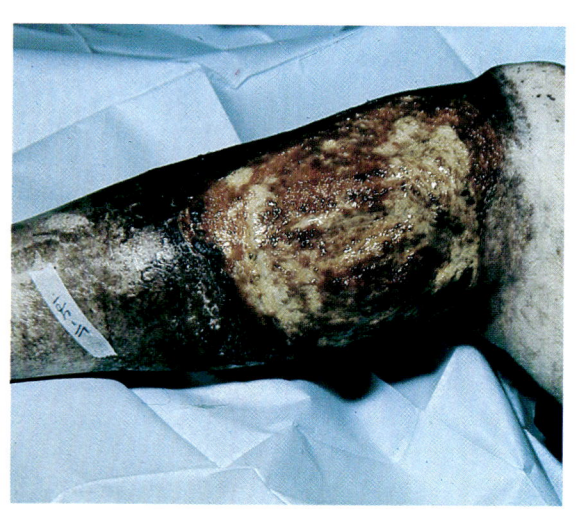

L (Question 709)

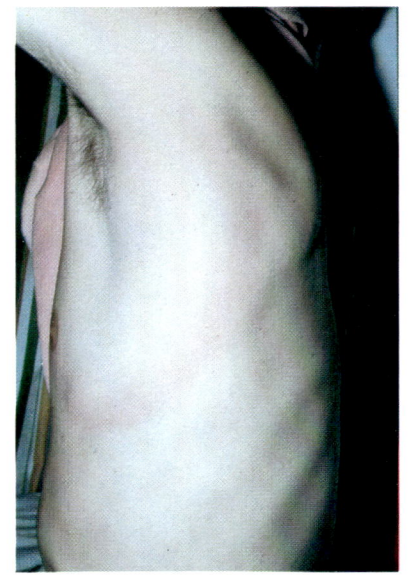

M (Questions 710-711)

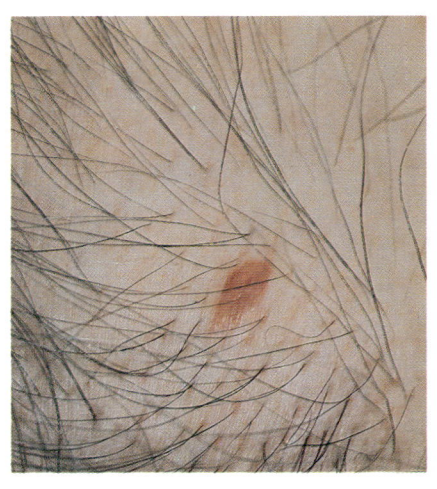

N (Question 712)

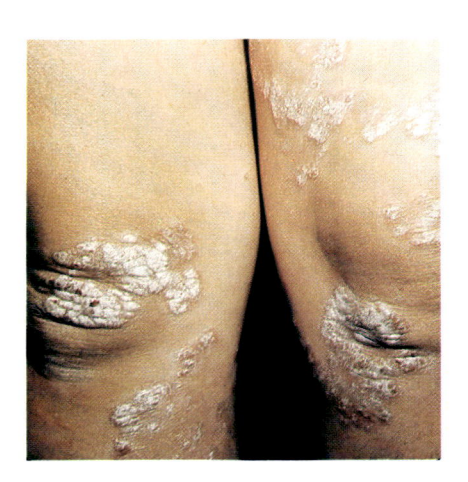

O (Question 713)

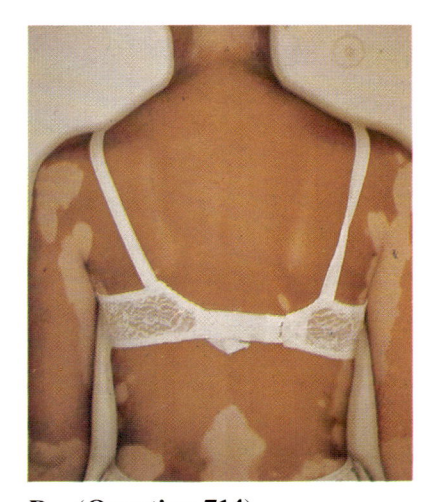

P (Question 714)

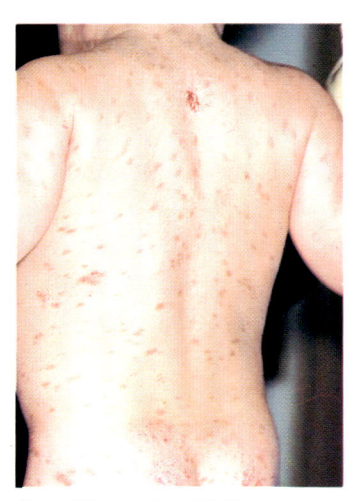

Q (Question 715)

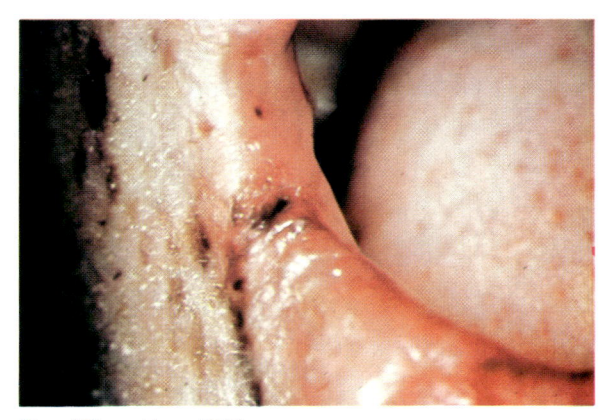

R (Question 717)

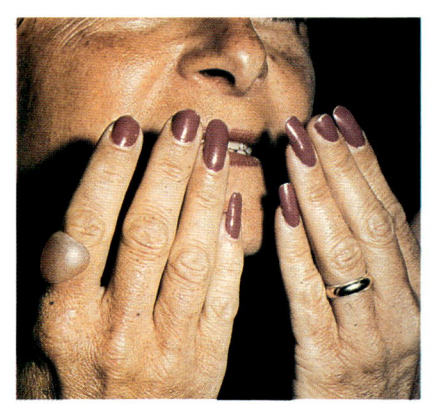

S (Questions 718-719)

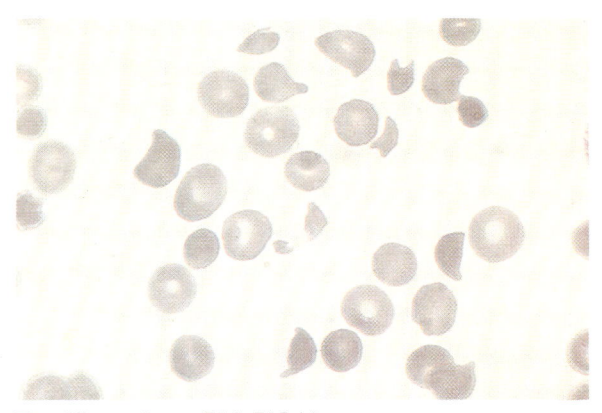

T (Questions 514-518A)

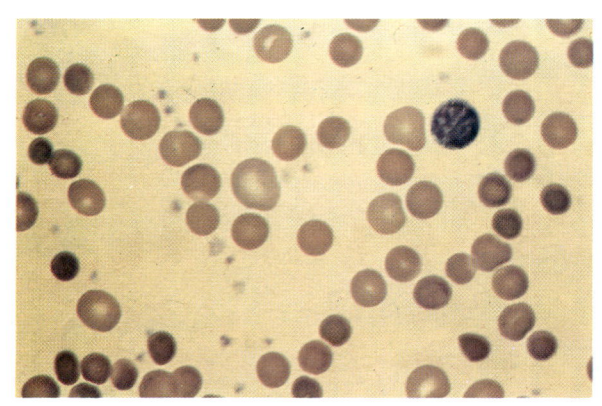

U (Questions 514-518B)

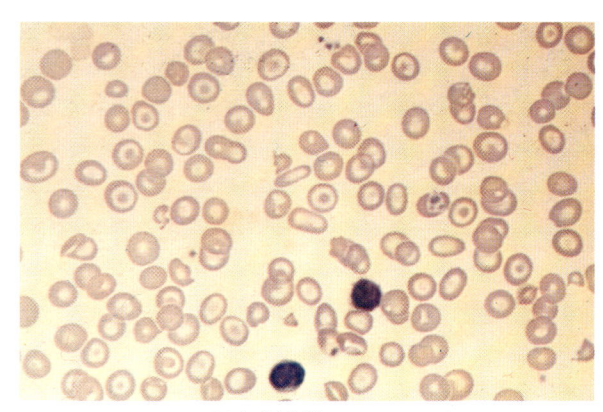

V (Questions 514-518C)

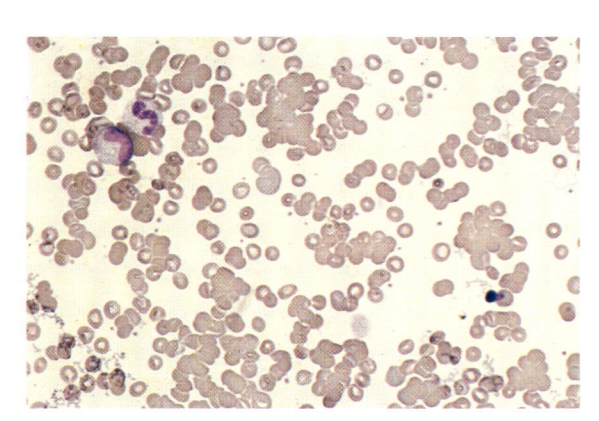

W (Questions 514-518D)

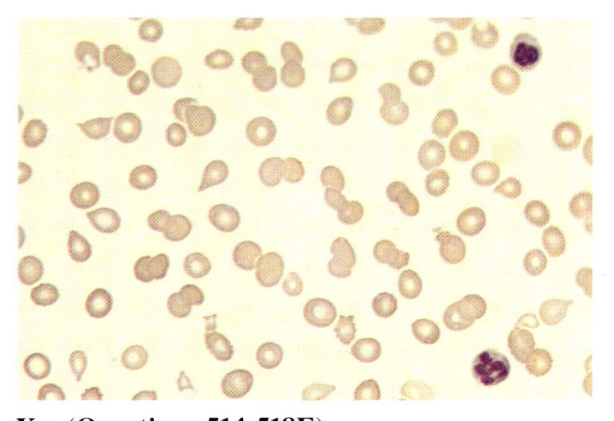

X (Questions 514-518E)